Handbook of

Sports Medicine

and Science

Swimming

David L. Costill PhD
Director, Human Performance Laboratory,
Ball State University, Muncie, Indiana

Ernest W. Maglischo PhD
Men's Swimming Coach,
Arizona State University,
Tempe, Arizona

Allen B. Richardson MD
1380 Lusitana Street, Suite 608,
Honolulu, Hawaii

b

**Blackwell
Science**

© 1992 by
Blackwell Science Ltd
Editorial Offices:
Osney Mead, Oxford OX2 0EL
25 John Street, London WC1N 2BL
23 Ainslie Place, Edinburgh EH3 6AJ
238 Main Street, Cambridge
    Massachusetts 02142, USA
54 University Street, Carlton
    Victoria 3053, Australia

Other Editorial Offices:
Arnette Blackwell SA
    1, rue de Lille
    75007 Paris
    France

Blackwell Wissenschafts-Verlag GmbH
    Kurfürstendamm 57
    10707 Berlin
    Germany

    Feldgasse 13
    A-1238 Wien
    Austria

First published 1992
Reprinted 1993, 1995

Set by Setrite Typesetters Ltd, Hong Kong
Printed and bound in Great Britain by
Butler & Tanner Ltd, Frome and London

DISTRIBUTORS

Marston Book Services Ltd
PO Box 87
Oxford OX2 0DT
(*Orders:* Tel: 01865 791155
            Fax: 01865 791927
            Telex: 837515)

USA
Human Kinetics Books
Human Kinetics Publishers, Inc.
Box 5076, Champaign
Illinois 61825—5076
(*Orders:* Tel: 1 800—747—4457)

Canada
Human Kinetics Publishers, Inc.
Box 2503, Windsor
Ontario N8Y 4S2
(*Orders:* Tel: 1 800—465—7301)

Australia
Blackwell Science Pty Ltd
54 University Street
Carlton, Victoria 3053
(*Orders:* Tel: 03 347—0300
            Fax: 03 349—3016)

British Library
Cataloguing in Publication Data

Costill, David L.
    Handbook of sports medicine and science.
    1. Swimming
    I. Title   II. Maglischo, Ernest W.
    III. Richardson, Allen B.
    612.044

    ISBN 0-632-03027-5

Library of Congress
Cataloging-in-Publication Data

Costill, David L.
    Swimming/David L. Costill,
    Ernest W. Maglischo, Allen B. Richardson.
            p.   cm.
    (Handbook of sports medicine and science)
    Includes index.
    ISBN 0-632-03027-5
    1. Swimming—Physiological aspects.
    2. Swimming—Training.
    I. Maglischo, Ernest W.
    II. Richardson, Allen B.   III. Title.
    IV. Series.
    RC 1220.S8C67   1992
    612'.044—dc20

Contents

Foreword by the IOC Publications Advisory Committee

The success of the publication of *The Olympic Book of Sports Medicine* as the initial volume of the *Encyclopaedia of Sports Medicine* resulted in the formation by the Medical Commission of the International Olympic Committee of a Publications Advisory Committee. The responsibilities assigned to this committee involved the planning and organization of succeeding volumes in the encyclopaedia series.

At the present, individual volumes of the series are in preparation on the topics of endurance in sport, strength and power in sport, and the prevention of injuries in sport. Each volume in the encyclopaedia is to represent the leading edge of knowledge in the particular topic area with regard to both biological and clinical considerations.

When the Publications Advisory Committee was established, it was also recognized that there was a great need for reference books on the practical application of sports medicine and sports science as related to specific sports activities for the use of professional personnel working directly with competitive athletes. It was, therefore, decided that the Committee would concurrently initiate a second series of publications under the title of *Handbook of Sports Medicine and Science*.

Each volume of this series will address a specific sports activity and provide practical information about medical issues, biological factors in the per-

formance of the sport, and physical conditioning. The target groups of the handbook series are team coaches who have academic preparation in the basic sciences, medical doctors in family practice but with no special training in sports medicine or sports biology, athletic trainers, physical therapists and other health-related professionals working with athletes and sports teams, and knowledgeable athletes.

The Publications Advisory Committee designated swimming as the sport for the initial handbook and, with the collaboration of the Medical Committee of the Fédération Internationale de Natation Amateur (FINA), designated an editor and contributing authors to produce the volume, *Handbook of Sports Medicine and Science: Swimming*. It was our great pleasure to have been able to recruit to this editorial team three outstanding individuals who complemented each other so well in covering the basic biology and biomechanics of swimming, the physiology of training and conditioning, performance testing and the medical aspects of swimming. The group brought to the task outstanding credentials in terms of personal experience as competitive swimmmers, research productivity, coaching success, and medical care of high-performance swimmers and swimming teams.

It is with great pleasure that the IOC Publications Advisory Committee presents the first volume of the handbook series. We wish success to competitive swimmers, swimming coaches, and medical care personnel in the application of the information and knowledge contained in this book for the improvement of performance as well as the health and safety of swimmers all over the world.

Howard G. Knuttgen (Chairman)
Francesco Conconi
Per Renström
Richard H. Strauss
Kurt Tittel
IOC Publications Advisory Committee

Foreword by FINA

The pursuit of excellence has always been one of the hallmarks of FINA (Fédération Internationale de Natation Amateur), be it in the field of sports competition, pool safety and sanitation, or communication. In 1968, when FINA established a Sports Medicine Committee, it was partly with 'communication' in mind that it did so, in order to provide its sport disciplines (swimming, diving, water-polo, synchronized swimming, long-distance swimming and masters) with the medical and sports science expertise they needed. There then followed a series of FINA World Sports Medicine Congresses: London, UK (1969), Dublin, Ireland (1971), Barcelona, Spain (1974), Stockholm, Sweden (1977), Amsterdam, The Netherlands (1982), Dunedin, New Zealand (1985), Orlando, USA (1987), London, UK (1989), Rio de Janeiro, Brazil (1991), and Kyoto, Japan to come in 1993.

These Congresses have made a major contribution to improving communication, but in spite of them there has remained a gap between the somewhat "ivory tower" language of the Congresses and that understood by the workers on the pool deck. It was only natural, therefore, that FINA would welcome an opportunity to collaborate with the International Olympic Committee in the production of this handbook, specifically designed to bridge that communication gap.

Jose A. Merino (Chairman)
Mohamed Kouidri
Bert De Pape
K.M.S. Aziz
Jose Blanco
J.M. Cameron
Ioan Dragan
Daniel Garcia Mazzeroli
David F. Gerrard
Lothar Kipke
Willem L. Mosterd
Allen B. Richardson
Olu Asekun
FINA Medical Committee

Section 1

Biology of

Swimming

Chapter 1

Characteristics of muscle

Upper body strength has been demonstrated to be one of the major determinants of success in sprint swimming. Swimming power, as determined during tethered swimming, has been shown to account for 86% of one's performance in a 25-m front crawl sprint and there is a strong positive relationship between a swimmer's strength and the ability to develop power. However, as the competitive distance increases, the contribution of strength appears to diminish. At 100, 200, and 400 m, the contribution of muscular strength drops to 74, 72, and 58%, respectively. Nevertheless, it comes as no surprise that the most successful competitive swimmers are most often the strongest.

The ability to generate maximal muscular force during swimming is complex, depending on the coordinated interactions of many physiological factors. An understanding of these factors is necessary in order to optimize the swimmer's potential and to plan a training program to improve strength. The intent of the following discussion will be to describe the applied aspects of muscle physiology and to present a basis for training. A more detailed explanation of the mechanisms of muscle contraction is available in the text by Wilmore and Costill (1988).

Muscles: structure and function

Skeletal muscles, also referred to as voluntary muscles, are those muscles of which we are consciously aware and are able to control, which attach to and cause movement of the skeleton. The *muscle fibers* or cells do not function alone nor act independently of the other muscles in the body. Rather, the fibers' actions are coordinated by a master network of nerve cells, both inside and outside the brain.

A single muscle is composed of thousands of individual muscle fibers. The number of muscle fibers per whole muscle varies considerably, depending on the size and function of the muscle. Each fiber has a protective covering or membrane which surrounds it, the *sarcolemma*, while the interior of these muscle cells contains the sarcoplasm, a gelatin-like substance that contains the protein filaments and energy-producing mechanisms that are essential for movement. The electron micrograph shown in Fig. 1.1 provides a view of the interior of a muscle fiber showing the contractile proteins (*actin* and *myosin*), the energy-generating units (*mitochondria*), and the

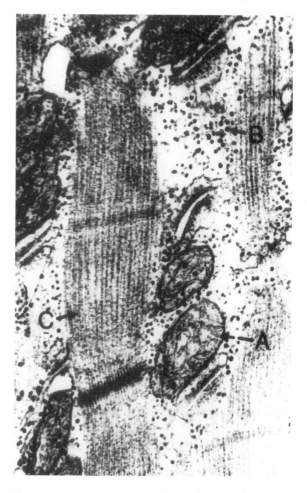

Fig. 1.1 An electron micrograph of the interior of a muscle fiber. A = mitochondria, B = glycogen, and C = protein strands of actin and myosin ($\times$ 187 500).

primary fuel (*glycogen*) used to produce energy during swimming.

Though the precise mechanism responsible for shortening the fiber's length during contraction is not fully understood, there is sufficient evidence to indicate that, when stimulated, the actin and myosin filaments slide past one another. This motion is accomplished by the pulling action of crossbridges that reach out from the myosin filaments and attach themselves to the actin filament. After binding, the crossbridges suddenly shorten, thereby drawing the two protein threads past one another. This action takes place simultaneously in thousands of muscle fibers, resulting in a forceful pull on the tendons.

Since the swimmer's endurance and speed depend on the muscles' ability to produce force and energy, individual differences in performance can, in some ways, be related to these characteristics in arm and leg muscles. Thanks to technological advances over the past 20 years, it is now possible to obtain samples of muscle tissue from swimmers before and after exercise using a needle biopsy procedure, illustrated in Fig. 1.2.

Microscopic and chemical techniques have enabled us to study the makeup of muscle cells and gauge the effects of acute exercise and training on their performance. One characteristic of muscle that has gained considerable attention from the "world of sport" is the muscle's composition of *fast* and *slow twitch fibers*. The microscopic photograph of human muscle in Fig. 1.3 illustrates these different fiber types. Those fibers that stain black in this photo are the slow twitch (ST) type fibers. There are two types of fast twitch fibers: a (FT_a; unstained in Fig. 1.3) and b (FT_b; gray in Fig. 1.3). In an average group of people, roughly 50% of the fibers in the arm and leg muscle are slow twitch, whereas FT_a fibers constitute about 25% of the muscle. The remaining 25% are mostly FT_b. The nerve cells that control these fibers determine whether they will be ST or FT. The muscle fiber and its connecting nerve system are referred to as a *motor unit*. An ST motor unit may include one relatively small nerve cell connected to a cluster of 10–180 muscle fibers, while FT motor units are arranged with a larger nerve cell which controls from 300 to 800 fibers per nerve cell.

In general, the ST motor units are characterized as having good aerobic endurance and appear to be recruited most often during low-intensity endurance events. The FT_a motor units develop considerably more force than an ST motor unit, though they fatigue rather easily. Thus, these FT_a fibers are used during shorter, faster races. Although the significance of the FT_b fibers is not fully understood, it appears that these

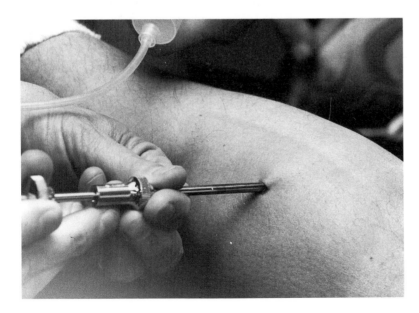

Fig. 1.2 Obtaining a muscle specimen from the shoulder of a swimmer.

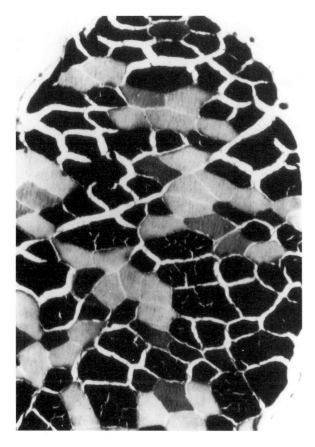

Fig. 1.3 A cross-sectional view of muscle fibers from the thigh of an untrained man. The black-stained fibers are the slow twitch (ST), while the fast twitch type a (FT$_a$) fibers are unstained. The gray fibers are the fast twitch b (FT$_b$) type. In general, slow twitch fibers demonstrate higher aerobic and lower anaerobic capacity than do the fast twitch fibers.

fibers are not easily turned on by the nervous system and are, therefore, used rather infrequently in normal, low-intensity activity.

It is not the speed of contraction, however, that determines the pattern of muscle fiber recruitment. Rather, it is the level of force that is demanded of the muscle that causes the motor nerve cells selectively to activate the ST and FT fibers. Figure 1.4 illustrates the relationship between force development by a muscle and the recruitment of ST, FT$_a$, and FT$_b$ fibers. During slow, low-intensity swimming, most of the muscle force is generated by the ST fibers. As the muscle tension requirements increase at heavier loads, the FT$_a$ fibers are added to the work force. Finally, in sprint events (i.e., 50–200 m) where maximal strength is needed, the FT$_b$ fibers are also turned on.

Such information is of practical importance to our understanding of the specific requirements of training and competition. It suggests that all training done at a slow pace or with light force will emphasize the use of the ST fibers, thereby inducing little training effect in the FT$_a$ or FT$_b$ fibers. Thus, long slow training bouts do not prepare the muscle for the demands of competition where maximal forces are required from both the ST and FT fibers.

Such knowledge relative to the composition and use of muscle fibers suggests that athletes who have a high percentage of ST fibers might have an advantage in long, endurance events, whereas those with a predominance of FT fibers could be better suited for short explosive activities. Table 1.1 presents the muscle fiber makeup of successful athletes from a

Fig. 1.4 The ramp-like recruitment of muscle fibers with varied levels of muscular effort. Whereas light force requirements only use the slow twitch fibers, heavy loads on the muscle will result in the recruitment of all three types of muscle fibers.

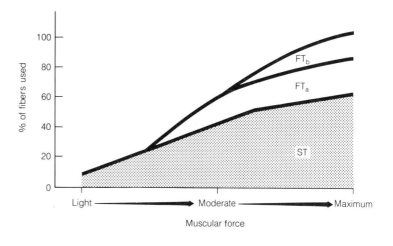

Table 1.1 The average percentage of slow twitch (%ST) and fast twitch (%FT) fibers in selected muscles of male (M) and female (F) athletes. Also shown are the average cross-sectional areas of the muscle fibers

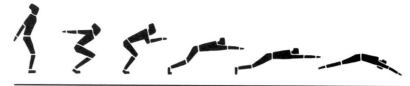

Athletes	Sex	Muscle	%ST	%FT	Fiber size (μ²)	
					ST	FT
Swimmers	M	Deltoidius	67	33	6345	5455
	F	Deltoidius	69	31	4332	3857
Sprint (runners)	M	Gastrocnemius	24	76	5878	6034
	F	Gastrocnemius	27	73	3752	3930
Distance (runners)	M	Gastrocnemius	79	21	8342	6485
	F	Gastrocnemius	69	31	4441	4128
Cyclists	M	Vastus lateralis	57	43	6333	6116
	F	Vastus lateralis	51	49	5487	5216
Weight lifters	M	Gastrocnemius	44	56	5060	8910
	M	Deltoidius	53	47	5010	8450
Triathletes	M	Deltoidius	60	40	—	—
	M	Vastus lateralis	63	37	—	—
	M	Gastrocnemius	59	41	—	—
Canoeists	M	Deltoidius	71	29	4920	7040
Shot-putters	M	Gastrocnemius	38	62	6367	6441
Non-Athletes	M	Vastus lateralis	47	53	4722	4709

variety of athletic events. As anticipated, leg muscles of élite sprint runners are composed principally of FT fibers, whereas distance runners have a predominance of ST fibers. Though there are tendencies for swimmers to have a higher percentage of ST fibers in their shoulder muscles (i.e., deltoidius) than nonathletes, *muscle fiber composition does not appear to be a prerequisite for success in competitive swimming.* Unlike sprint runners, who have a predominance of FT fibers in their leg muscles, the percentage of ST and FT fibers varies widely among successful sprint and distance swimmers.

Whereas previous studies have shown that training may increase the endurance capacity of muscle, there is little evidence to suggest that the percentage of ST and FT fibers changes following a few months of training. There is some debate concerning the likelihood of converting ST and FT fibers as a result of long-term training. Any changes that may occur in the percentage of ST and FT fibers with training, however, are probably small. That is to say, it would be highly unlikely for training to change one's fiber composition by more than a few percentage points. Most studies have reported that the composition of muscle appears fixed and unaffected by training, suggesting that at least this quality of the champion may be inherited. Studies with identical twins (from the same egg) have shown that they have identical fiber compositions, whereas fraternal twins (those from separate eggs) differ in their fiber profiles as well as in other physical characteristics. These findings support the contention that one's fiber composition is determined by genetics, with the percentage of ST and FT fibers being established soon after birth and remaining relatively unchanged throughout life.

One exception to this rule is that the subtypes of FT fibers (FT_a and FT_b) may show some modification with training. The FT_a fibers are generally described as being more aerobic — able to use oxygen for energy production — than the FT_b fibers. With endurance training the FT_b fibers begin to take on the characteristics of the FT_a fibers. This suggests that these fibers are used more heavily during training and gain greater endurance ability. Though the full significance of this change of FT_b to FT_a fibers is not known, it may explain why we find very few, if any, FT_b fibers in the muscles of highly trained swimmers.

The size (diameter) of the muscle fibers varies markedly among élite swimmers, but on the average, ST fibers are some 14% larger than FT fibers in élite male and female swimmers' shoulder muscles (Table 1.1). Physiologists have proposed that training for endurance or strength may result in selective enlargement (hypertrophy) of the ST and FT fibers, respectively. It should also be noted that there is a gender difference in muscle fiber diameter. Muscle fibers from male runners, cyclists, and swimmers are 40–50% larger than those observed in female athletes from the same sports. Thus, the differences in muscle mass between men and women may be more a *function of individual fiber size* than a difference in the number of fibers.

Is the percentage of ST and FT fibers the same in all the muscles of the body? Generally, the muscles of the arms and legs have similar fiber compositions, though swimmers tend to have a somewhat higher percentage of ST fibers in their deltoidius muscles than do athletes who train only their leg muscles (e.g., cyclists and runners). This finding and studies with other athletes (e.g., canoeists) who train only their arm muscles suggests that such training may increase the percentage of ST fibers in those muscles. The soleus, a muscle near the bone in the lower leg, is composed almost completely of ST fibers (>90%) in all people. It has also been observed that untrained men having a predominance of ST fibers in their leg muscles will likely have a high percentage of ST fibers in their arms as well.

How are muscles used?

The more than 215 pairs of muscles in the body vary widely in size, shape, and use. It is important to realize that every coordinated movement requires the application of force by muscles that serve as the prime movers, *agonistic* muscles, and the relaxation of muscles that might resist that motion, the *antagonistic* muscles. The smooth flexion of the elbow requires shortening of the biceps muscle (agonist) and the relaxation of the triceps (antagonist).

The principal function of muscle is shortening, referred to as a *concentric* action. There are, however, frequent periods when muscles may act without reducing their length. Such static force development is termed an *isometric action*, and occurs, for example, when we attempt to lift an object that is heavier than the force generated by the muscle, or when we hold an object steady with the elbow flexed. On the other hand, when the muscle lengthens while being stimulated to act, as the biceps do when the elbow is extended when lowering a heavy weight, the action is referred to as *eccentric*. In many activities, such as running and jumping, all three types of action may occur. Swimming, in contrast, is performed almost exclusively with concentric contractions.

The development of muscle force depends on its initial length and the speed of shortening. If a muscle was not attached to bone, it would assume a relaxed, *equilibrium length*. When attached to the skeleton, a muscle at resting length is normally under slight tension, since it is moderately stretched. Measurements of isometric force are maximal when the length of the muscle at the time of activation is approximately 20% greater than the equilibrium length. Increasing or decreasing the muscle length causes a reduction in maximal force development. When the muscle is elongated to twice its equilibrium length, the force produced by the muscle is nearly zero. This failure to yield force when overstretched is due to a decrease in the overlap between the actin and myosin filaments. The more they are stretched apart, the fewer crossbridges are available to bind the filaments and create force.

Muscles and their connective tissues (i.e., fascia and tendons) have the property of *elasticity*. When stretched, this elastic characteristic results in stored energy that creates additional force during a subsequent contraction. In the intact body, muscle length is restricted by the anatomical arrangement and attachment of muscle to bone. When stretched, this anatomical arrangement allows the muscle length to increase 1.2 times the muscle's equilibrium length, the optimal length for maximal force development.

Since the muscles exert their force using skeletal levers, the physical arrangement of these muscle–bone levers are critical to our understanding of movement. The tendon attachment for the biceps is only one-10th the distance from the fulcrum (elbow) to the weighted resistance held in the hand. Thus, in order to hold a 5-kg weight, the muscle must exert 10 times (50 kg) as much force as the weight. The best joint angle for the application of this force is approximately 100°, since greater or lesser flexion of the elbow will reduce the angle of the force applied to the lever arm.

The ability to develop force also depends on the speed of muscle lengthening or shortening. Figure 1.5 illustrates this relationship, showing that the highest muscle forces occur during fast eccentric contraction. Maximal force development during concentric contractions, on the other hand, becomes progressively less at higher speeds. Such measurements are possible only with specialized testing equipment that can control the rate of muscle shortening or lengthening.

Summary

There are several important lessons for the coach and swimmer that can be learned from the preceding discussion. First, the strength of the muscles used in swimming is a major determinant of success in events from 50 to 1500 m. Though this may not seem surprising, it must be remembered that strength *per se* does not dictate fast swimming. The forces generated by the muscle must be effectively applied to the water if they are to propel the body. Thus, strength specificity is the key to swimming success.

Second, the selective recruitment of ST and FT muscle fibers is dictated by the intensity of each contraction. Thus, at slow swimming speeds, where force production is low, the muscles rely mostly on the ST fibers, recruiting more and more of the FT fibers at progressively faster speeds. This leads us to conclude that, in order to train both fiber types, the swimmer must perform at least some training at or near racing speeds. It appears that such training is essential in developing the neurological patterns of recruitment needed for maximal force development during sprint swimming. This should not be interpreted to mean that all training should be done at high speeds. As will be explained in the following section, swim training at near race pace also imposes severe energy demands on the muscle fibers that are critical to performance in all competitive events.

Finally, the ST and FT fiber makeup of the swimmer's muscles does not appear to be a deciding factor in successful competition. Though élite sprint and endurance performers in other sports (e.g., running and cycling) can be characterized by the percentage of ST or FT fibers, sprint and distance swimmers do not differ in this regard. Thus, the swimmer's fiber composition appears to have little bearing on success in competition, though the studies of muscle fiber recruitment and energy use provide important information for training and nutrition, which ultimately influence performance.

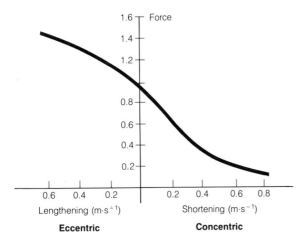

Fig. 1.5 The relationship between the rate of movement and the maximal force development during eccentric and concentric actions.

Recommended reading

Brooke, M.H. & Kaiser, K.K. (1970) Muscle fiber types: how many and what kind? *Arch. Neurol.* **23**:369–379.

Buchthal, F. & Schmalbruch, H. (1970) Contraction times and fiber types in intact muscle. *Acta Physiol. Scand.* **79**:435–452.

Burke, R.E. & Edgerton, V.R. (1975) Motor unit properties and selective involvement in movement. In Wilmore, J. & Keogh, J. (eds), *Exercise and Sports Sciences Reviews.* New York: Academic Press, pp. 31–83.

Costill, DL. (1986) *Inside Running: Basics of Sports Physiology.* Indianapolis: Benchmark Press.

Fox, E.L. (1984) *Sports Physiology*, 2nd edn. New York: CBS College Publications.

Henneman, E. (1980) Skeletal muscle. The servant of the nervous system. In Mountcastle, V.B. (ed.) *Medical Physiology*, 14th edn, vol. 1. St Louis, Missouri: Mosby Publishing, pp. 674−702.

Jones, N.L., McCartney, N. & McComas, A.J. (1986) *Human Muscle Power*. Champaign, Illinois: Human Kinetics.

Porter, R. & Whelan, J. (1981) *Human Muscle Fatigue:*

Physiological Mechanisms (Ciba Foundation Symposium 82). London: Pitman Medical.

Wickiewicz, T.L., Roy, R.R., Powell, P.L., Perrine, J.J. & Edgerton, V.R. (1984) Muscle architecture and force−velocity relationships in humans. *J. Appl. Physiol. Environ. Exercise Physiol.* **57**:435−443.

Wilmore, J.H. & Costill, D.L. (1988) *Training for Sport and Activity*. Dubuque, Iowa: W.C. Brown.

Chapter 2

Energy for swimming

Success or failure in swimming competition depends to a large extent on the muscles' ability to generate the energy needed to propel the body through the water. The energy referred to here is that produced from the foods we eat (carbohydrates, fats, and proteins). When broken down by the body these fuels yield low levels of energy that are inadequate for muscular activity. Instead, the cells convert these low energy sources into a high-energy compound, adenosine triphosphate (ATP) that provides the immediate energy for muscular activity. In turn, the energy stored within the ATP molecule is released when the third phosphate is separated from the structure (Fig. 2.1).

The muscles have four possible sources of ATP:

1 that stored within the muscle;

2 that generated from another phosphate compound (i.e., ATP–phosphocreatine (ATP–PCr) system);
3 ATP produced from the breakdown of muscle sugar (i.e., glycolytic system);
4 the ATP generated with the aid of oxygen (i.e., oxidative system).

The ATP–PCr system

Phosphocreatine (PCr) is present within the muscle fibers, though it serves a somewhat different function than does ATP. Unlike the energy derived from the breakdown of ATP, PCr is not used directly to provide power within the cells. Instead, it is used to rebuild the ATP molecule, thereby maintaining a relatively constant supply of this high-energy source. Thus, when energy is released in the splitting of the ATP molecule, it can be reconstructed with the energy from PCr (Fig. 2.2). Unfortunately, this energy reserve is very limited and can last only a few seconds during maximal sprint swimming. Though ATP is maintained at a relatively normal level, PCr declines rapidly, breaking down in an effort to generate more ATP. However, at exhaustion both ATP and PCr are quite low and unable to provide the energy for further contractions.

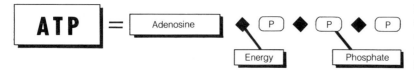

Fig. 2.1 The chemical structure of adenosine triphosphate (ATP). The diamond-shaped symbols connecting the four components indicate energy. (From Maglischo, 1990.)

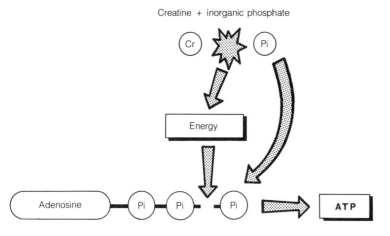

Fig. 2.2 The breakdown of creatine (Cr) and phosphate (Pi) to maintain the supply of adenosine triphosphate (ATP).

The glycolytic system

During the early minutes of exercise and when the intensity of the muscular effort is high, the body is incapable of providing sufficient oxygen to regenerate the needed ATP. To compensate, both the ATP−PCr and glycolytic energy systems generate ATP without the aid of oxygen, a process termed *anaerobic metabolism*. *Glycolysis* is the breakdown of muscle sugar − glycogen − in the absence of oxygen, resulting in the production and accumulation of lactic acid. Thus, glycolysis provides ATP under conditions when there is inadequate oxygen being supplied to the system. Unfortunately, this process is relatively inefficient, providing only a small, but essential, part of the ATP needed during competitive swimming. In the presence of oxygen, aerobic energy production can generate 13 times more ATP than can be generated by glycolysis. Thus, the glycolytic system supplements the ATP−PCr system in providing energy for highly intense muscular effort when the oxygen supply is inadequate.

In events ranging from 50 to 200 m the demands on the glycolytic system are high, causing muscle lactic acid levels to rise from a resting value of about 1 mmol·kg^{-1} of muscle to over 25 mmol·kg^{-1}. The high acid content of the muscle fibers inhibits further breakdown of glycogen and may interfere with the muscle's contractile process. Thus, extended reliance on glycolysis for energy will result in muscular fatigue and exhaustion as the fibers become acidic.

The aerobic energy system

Since muscles use energy during a 50 or 100-m sprint at nearly 200 times that required at rest, it is impossible for the ATP−PCr and glycolytic systems to produce sufficient ATP to meet all the muscles' energy requirements. Without another more efficient energy system, the maximal duration of sprint swimming might be limited to 30 s or less. As we have seen, the anaerobic production of ATP, without oxygen, is quite inefficient and inadequate for events lasting more than a few minutes. Consequently, aerobic metabolism is the primary method of energy production during endurance events, placing heavy demands on the athlete's ability to deliver oxygen to the exercising muscles.

Mitochondria use fuels and oxygen to produce large amounts of ATP. Carbohydrates and fat are the primary fuels used to drive this system of ATP production. These molecules are disassembled within the fluids (sarcoplasm) and mitochondria of the muscle fibers with the aid of oxidative enzymes, which are special proteins produced within the fibers. In this process, hydrogen (H$^+$) atoms, in the presence of the oxygen (O$_2$) we breathe, release energy to produce ATP and water (H$_2$O). If left unattended, the hydrogen component of these fuels would be free to disrupt the function of the cells. Carbon dioxide (CO$_2$), formed from the carbon and oxygen within the fuels, is another byproduct of oxidative metabolism. Fortunately, carbon dioxide diffuses easily out of the cells and is transported by the venous blood back to the lungs, where it can leave the body in the expired air.

Oxygen transport to muscles

Oxygen delivery to the muscle is essential in maintaining a high rate of aerobic energy production. During mild exercise the blood receives oxygen as it passes through the lungs, transports it to the muscles where it is exchanged for carbon dioxide, then returns to the heart and lungs where it can unload the carbon dioxide and refill its oxygen supply. As the intensity of the exercise and energy demands increase, the rate of oxidative ATP production increases. In an effort to satisfy the muscle's need for oxygen, the heart beats faster, pumping more blood and oxygen to the muscles. Since the body stores little oxygen, the amount absorbed by the blood as it passes through the lungs is considered a direct indication of the amount used for aerobic energy production. Consequently, an accurate estimate of aerobic metabolism can be made by determining the amount of oxygen being consumed.

As the body shifts from rest to exercise, there is an increase in the need for energy. This increase in metabolism is in direct proportion to the demand for muscular power (Fig. 2.3). As with the ATP−PCr and glycolytic energy systems, there is a limit to the amount of energy that can be generated via oxidative metabolism. In the face of increasing energy demands the body reaches a limit for oxygen delivery ($\dot{V}\text{O}_{2\,\text{max}}$). At this point, there is a leveling of the $\dot{V}\text{O}_2$, even

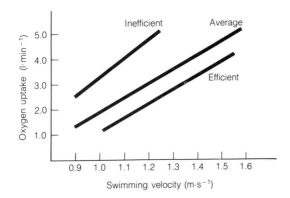

Fig. 2.3 The relationship between front crawl swimming speed and oxygen uptake.

though the energy demand continues to increase. The value at which the $\dot{V}_{O_2}$ plateaus is referred to as the *aerobic capacity* or *maximal oxygen consumption* ($\dot{V}_{O_2\,max}$). $\dot{V}_{O_2\,max}$ is regarded as the best single measurement of cardiorespiratory endurance and aerobic fitness, because it describes the maximal capacity of the cardiovascular and aerobic systems' potential for energy production.

Since the swimmer's need for energy is influenced by his or her body size, age, and level of fitness, $\dot{V}_{O_2\,max}$ is frequently expressed relative to body weight ($ml\cdot kg^{-2}\cdot min^{-1}$), though values for swimmers have also been reported in milliliters of oxygen per unit of height ($ml\cdot m^{-1}$) or per unit of body surface area ($ml\cdot m^{-2}$). These calculations allow a more equitable comparison among individuals of different sizes. Normally active 18–22-year-old college students have been reported to have average $\dot{V}_{O_2\,max}$ values of 38–42 $ml\cdot kg^{-1}\cdot min^{-1}$ (women) and 44–50 $ml\cdot kg^{-1}\cdot min^{-1}$ (men). Highly trained male and female swimmers, on the other hand, have been reported to have $\dot{V}_{O_2\,max}$ values ranging from 45 to 65 and 50 to 75 $ml\cdot kg^{-1}\cdot min^{-1}$, respectively.

Fuels for swimming

Carbohydrates, in the form of blood glucose and muscle glycogen, provide the primary energy to form ATP during swimming competition and training. Foods that contain simple and complex sugars and starches are reduced to glucose during the process of digestion. This glucose is then transported via the blood stream to the liver and other cells of the body. Although some of this glucose is used directly as fuel, a portion of it is stored within the cells as glycogen. When exercise begins muscle glycogen is broken down, providing a reservoir of energy for glycolysis.

Since glycogen is stored within the muscle, it is more readily available for ATP production. The usual quantity of glycogen stored in muscle fibers is sufficient to produce ATP for several minutes or hours depending on the swimmer's speed. Because of its limited supply some muscle fibers may become depleted of glycogen in as little as 5 or 10 min of maximum effort. However, glycogen will remain in the less active fibers within that same muscle, allowing exercise to continue until the number of depleted fibers becomes so great that the muscle can no longer exert the force needed to maintain the desired swimming speed.

Although it has been estimated that an entire muscle could become depleted in just 15–20 min of swimming, the effort needed to produce this rate of depletion is so intense that it could not be maintained for even that short period of time. Biopsies taken from the shoulder muscles of swimmers before and after interval training, however, have shown that the glycogen supplies can be nearly exhausted after completing 3000–6000 m of repeated 100-m swims, with 20 s rest between each swim. Though it is highly unlikely that a swimmer will exhaust his or her muscle stores during a single event, exhaustive training bouts are certain to reduce or empty this fuel supply, posing an important nutritional problem for the swimmer.

The body also contains carbohydrate stored as liver glycogen that can be broken down to glucose and transported to the muscles when needed. In addition to maintaining a relatively constant blood sugar level, liver glycogen supplements the muscles' glycogen supply for use during exercise.

Fat is stored in muscles and beneath the skin as adipose tissue. It provides the body's largest store of potential energy for ATP recycling. The process is entirely aerobic, but far too slow to provide the energy needed during sprint swimming events.

Generally speaking, body fat is a contributor of energy during prolonged training sessions and long-distance swimming events. It appears that in aerobic swimming, where the intensity is below the individual's maximal capacity, 30–50% of the energy may be derived from fats; the longer the duration, the higher the contribution of fat. During intense swimming lasting only a few minutes, as is the case for most events, fat may contribute less than 10% of the energy used.

Although the oxidation of fatty acids can supply a sizeable amount of energy during endurance events, it is released so slowly that swimmers would be unable to sustain a fast pace if this was the only energy source for ATP recycling. Fat metabolism may contribute part of the total energy for a 1500-m race but that contribution is quite small compared to the amount of energy derived from muscle glycogen and blood glucose.

In competitive swimming, the essential role of fat metabolism is to supply energy for ATP replacement during training. It can provide a significant amount during long interval sets that are swum at moderate speeds. By doing so, less muscle glycogen will be used. It has been estimated that fat supplies between 30 and 50% of the total energy used during a typical 2-h training session.

Training can increase the amount of energy supplied by fat, thereby lessening the muscles' demands on muscle glycogen for energy. In this way, athletes can swim long sets of repeats and still have muscle glycogen left for fast anaerobic swims later in a training session. An increase in fat metabolism will also reduce muscle glycogen use from day to day so that swimmers can train twice a day for several days at a time with greater average intensity.

Proteins are composed of amino acids. There are more than 20 known amino acids. Nine of these are considered essential because they cannot be synthesized in the body and therefore, must be supplied through the diet. Amino acids have a limited life span in the human body. They can last from several days up to a few months before they must be replaced by new amino acids through the diet or from other tissues. Muscle tissue, including mitochondria, is formed from them, so swimmers need an adequate supply of the essential amino acids to maintain progress in training. This should *not* be interpreted to mean that swimmers need to eat extra protein. Nutritional research has shown that a well balanced diet will adequately provide the protein needed for building and repair of body tissues, and that

protein supplements do not enhance the adaptations associated with training.

As noted above, proteins are the building blocks of the body and aid in the repair of tissues. They also play a role in controlling the acidity within the muscle fibers by serving as a buffer against the acids produced during highly anaerobic activities. Protein can also donate energy for recycling ATP. However, like fat, the release of energy from protein is a slow process. Protein metabolism is, in fact, the slowest and least economical method for recycling ATP.

The energy cost of swimming

The amount of energy expended for different activities varies relative to the intensity and strokes used in swimming. Measures of energy use during swimming are usually estimated by monitoring the oxygen consumption during submaximal swimming, at speeds well below those used in competition. These values typically ignore the *anaerobic* aspects of exercise, since the energy derived from the ATP–PCr and glycolytic systems is not included in these estimates. This is an important point, since a swimmer's efficiency and the energy used at speeds requiring energy in excess of one's aerobic capacity may be markedly different than that estimated during submaximal swimming.

Table 2.1 provides an estimate of aerobic energy expenditure for each of the competitive strokes at a relatively slow speed (1 m·s^{-1}). Since swimming involves moving against the resistance of the water, these figures may vary considerably with the weight, age, sex and the technical skill (i.e., efficiency) of the swimmer.

The ability to perform any exercise skillfully results in a reduced demand for energy. Energy expended during swimming is used, in part, to pay the cost to maintain the body on the surface of the water and to generate the force required to overcome the water's resistance to motion. Although the energy needed for swimming is dependent on body size and buoyancy, the effective application of force against the water is the major determinant of economy in this activity. Figure 2.4 illustrates the difference in oxygen requirements of trained competitive male and female swimmers and for a group of highly trained triathletes. Although the triathletes trained daily at swimming,

Table 2.1 Oxygen uptake and heart rate for a collegiate male swimmer performing each stroke at a common speed

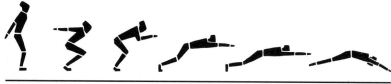

Stroke	Speed (m·s^{-1})	Oxygen uptake (l·min^{-1})	Heart rate (beats·min^{-1})
Front crawl	1.0	1.83	125
Backstroke	1.0	2.42	138
Butterfly	1.0	2.85	150
Breaststroke	1.0	3.42	162

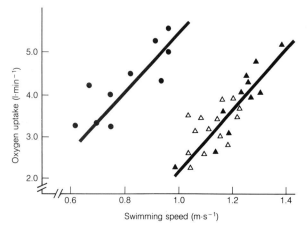

Fig. 2.4 Oxygen uptake of male triathletes (●) and competitive swimmers (male, ▲; female, △).

none had a prior background in competitive swimming. It is also interesting to note that many of these triathletes had aerobic capacities that were markedly higher than the competitive swimmers, but few could perform as well as even the poorest competitive swimmer. Several female swimmers who possessed $\dot{V}_{O_2\,max}$ values of 2.1–2.3 l·min^{-1} were able to swim 400 m as fast as triathletes having values above 5.0 l of O_2·min^{-1}.

Thus, it appears that swimming performance is limited more by the athlete's skill than by his or her $\dot{V}_{O_2\,max}$. Such information makes it clear that the training time and effort spent on the mechanical aspects (techniques) of swimming may be equally as or more important than the time dedicated to improving strength and endurance.

Support systems for energy production

Although energy metabolism takes place in each individual muscle fiber, the circulatory and respiratory systems are responsible for delivering the fuels and oxygen to the muscles and removing waste products.

The blood delivers oxygen, glucose and other substances to capillaries which have direct contact with the body cells. After delivering these fuels to the muscles, the blood leaves the tissues carrying carbon dioxide, lactate and other byproducts of metabolism. After returning to the heart, blood is pumped to the lungs, where carbon dioxide diffuses into the gases of the lung and is then exhaled. Simultaneously, oxygen diffuses into the blood from the lungs, replacing that being used in the muscles and other body tissues.

The ventricles of the heart contract at rates that are somewhat proportional to the energy demands of the muscles. At rest, heart rates may vary from about 50 to 80 beats·min^{-1} for most swimmers, though rates as low as 35 beats·min^{-1} have been reported. Generally, resting heart rates of trained athletes are lower than those of untrained individuals, though such measurements are not a precise indication of one's endurance potential or fitness level.

When immersed in the water, the swimmer's heart rate may drop by 5–8 beats·min^{-1}. Water tends to facilitate the return of blood to the heart, thereby reducing the work of the cardiovascular system. In addition, placing the face in the water will also lower one's heart rate. This effect is the result of a facial reflex that is common to many mammals. Consequently, at a given exercise effort (i.e., oxygen uptake) in the water, one's heart rate may be 10–12 beats·min^{-1} lower than during exercise on land.

The heart has a maximal rate (i.e., maximal heart rate) that it cannot exceed during even the most exhaustive exercise. Though this maximal rate differs from swimmer to swimmer, the average for teenagers and young adults is 200 beats·min^{-1}, with males having lower maximal values ($<$200 beats·min^{-1}) than females ($>$200 beats·min^{-1}).

The amount of blood that is pushed out of the heart with each beat is known as the stroke volume (SV). A normal range of values for SV at rest is between 60 and 100 ml·beat^{-1}. During exercise, the heart may increase its SV by 2−3 times the resting level. As one might expect, the SV for endurance-trained athletes is greater than for nonathletes, which explains why these athletes have lower resting heart rates. They can supply more blood with each beat, thereby reducing the number of beats required to maintain the cardiac output—the amount of blood ejected from the heart per minute. A normal cardiac output at rest is approximately 5 l·min^{-1}. While untrained individuals can increase their cardiac output fourfold during exercise, trained swimmers can increase this value by six or seven times the resting level. Cardiac output can be calculated from the following equation:

$$CO = SV \times HR$$
(cardiac output = stroke volume × heart rate)

The lower heart rates observed during swimming at standard speeds after training provide an excellent indication of the swimmer's improved cardiovascular fitness and capacity for endurance performance. Thus, one of the easiest and least expensive ways of monitoring the cardiovascular adaptation to training is to record the swimmer's heart rate after a 400- or 800-m swim at a standard or set speed. As swimmers get into better physical condition, their postswim heart rates will be lower. This point is illustrated in Fig. 2.5.

Respiration is the process by which carbon dioxide is removed from and oxygen delivered to the body tissues. This process can be differentiated into two separate phases: *external* and *internal* respiration. External respiration is the process of breathing, which includes the exchange of gases between the alveoli of the lungs and the blood. Internal respiration refers to the process of oxygen and carbon dioxide exchange between the blood and the body tissues. Thus, external respiration identifies the process of gas exchange in the lung, whereas internal respiration defines the process of gas exchange at the level of the muscles and other body tissues.

Inspiration is an active process involving the diaphragm, which is the primary muscle of ventilation, and the muscles responsible for enlarging the chest cavity—the secondary muscles of respiration. The ribs and sternum assist with breathing by changing the size of the volume of the chest. The

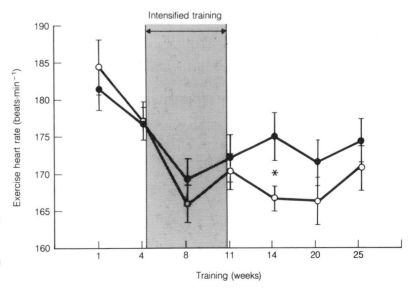

Fig. 2.5 Effects of swimming training on heart rate during a 365.8-m (400-yard) front crawl swim. During the intensified period of training one group of swimmers trained twice per day (10 000−12 000 m·day^{-1}; ●), whereas the other group continued to train once per day (5000−6000 m·day^{-1}; ○).

muscles between the ribs rotate and lift the ribcage, contributing to the expansion of the thoracic cavity. These actions decrease the pressure within the thoracic cavity, causing air to flow into the lungs. *Expiration* is usually a passive process involving the relaxation of the diaphragm and a reduction in the size of the ribcage, which forces air out of the lungs. During swimming, the muscles of ventilation play a major role in inspiration, whereas the abdominal muscles play a major role in forced expiration.

At rest, approximately 5–12 liters of air is breathed each minute. During heavy exercise this volume may be in excess of 100 $l \cdot min^{-1}$ and can exceed 200 $l \cdot m^{-1}$ in very large, well conditioned athletes.

Gas exchange in the lungs involves the removal of carbon dioxide from the venous blood returning from various parts of the body and the replacement of oxygen which has been removed by the muscles. By the time the blood exits from the lungs on its return to the heart, the amount of oxygen will nearly equilibrate with that in the alveoli. Carbon dioxide reacts in a similar manner, though it diffuses at a rate approximately 20 times faster than oxygen. At the tissue level, the same gas laws apply to the unloading of oxygen and the uptake of carbon dioxide.

Oxygen is carried by the red blood cells in combination with *hemoglobin* and in plasma. Hemoglobin in the 4–6 billion red blood cells of the body makes it possible for the blood to transport nearly 70 times more oxygen than can be dissolved in plasma. Each 100 ml of blood contains an average of 14–16 g of hemoglobin in men and approximately 12–14 g in women. Since each gram of hemoglobin can combine with about 1.34 ml of oxygen, the blood's oxygen-carrying capacity is approximately 20 ml per 100 ml of blood when fully saturated with oxygen. As the blood passes through the lungs, it is in contact with the alveolar air for approximately 0.75 s, sufficient time for hemoglobin to pick up nearly all the oxygen it can hold. As a result, blood leaving the lungs is about 98% saturated with oxygen.

Individuals who have a low hemoglobin content, which occurs in *iron-deficiency anemia*, have a reduced capacity to transport oxygen, since the blood's carrying capacity is reduced. At rest, these people may feel little effect of being anemic, since their cardiovascular systems can compensate for the lower oxygen content by increasing the flow of blood.

During activities where oxygen delivery may become a limitation, the reduced oxygen content of the blood limits aerobic energy production and performance.

At rest, the oxygen content of arterialized blood is about 20 ml per 100 ml, which drops to 15–16 ml per 100 ml as it passes through the capillaries into the venous system. This arterial–venous difference in oxygen content (a− $\dot{V}_{O_2 \text{ diff}}$) amounts to about 4–5 ml of oxygen per 100 ml of blood. The amount of oxygen taken up by the tissues is similar to the amount being used for energy production in the tissues. As the rate of oxygen usage increases, the a− $\dot{V}_{O_2 \text{ diff}}$ widens. During intense exercise, the a− $\dot{V}_{O_2 \text{ diff}}$ of contracting muscles may increase to 15 ml per 100 ml of blood. The unloading of oxygen from the blood to the muscles is facilitated by the low partial pressure of oxygen in the tissue, and increases in tissue acidity, temperature or carbon dioxide concentration — factors all known to occur during muscular activity.

The increasing demands for oxygen during exercise can also be met by an increase in the volume of blood flow through the muscle, thereby requiring less removal of oxygen from each 100 ml of blood. Consequently, oxygen delivery and uptake depend on the oxygen content of blood, blood flow, and the local conditions within the muscle. During maximal swimming, several of these factors may contribute to limit oxygen delivery, thereby restricting the muscle's ability to meet the oxidative demands of the effort.

Carbon dioxide exits the cells by diffusion in response to the partial pressure gradient between the tissue and the capillary blood. Whereas a small amount of carbon dioxide is dissolved in plasma, it is mostly transported to the lungs in combination with hemoglobin and water (*carbonic acid*). Carbonic acid provides the largest avenue for carbon dioxide transport. With the aid of the enzyme *carbonic anhydrase* (ca), the carbon dioxide and water molecules combine in the tissue capillaries to form carbonic acid (H_2CO_3). After leaving the capillaries, carbonic acid dissociates a hydrogen ion (H^+), thereby forming a bicarbonate ion (HCO_3^-). The events may be portrayed as:

$$CO_2 + H_2O \rightarrow H_2CO_3 \rightarrow H^+ + HCO_3^-$$

The hydrogen (H^+) is subsequently buffered by hemoglobin, which maintains the acidity (pH) of the blood relatively normal. As a consequence of this reaction, nearly 70% of the carbon dioxide is carried in the form of bicarbonate (HCO_3^-). In the lungs, the partial pressure of carbon dioxide is lowered, resulting in the reformation of carbonic acid. At this stage, carbon dioxide and water are reformed, allowing the carbon dioxide to leave the blood, entering the alveoli to be exhaled during pulmonary ventilation.

Controls of breathing

The involuntary regulation of the rate and depth of breathing is not fully understood, though many of the intricate neural controls have been identified. The maintenance of arterial oxygen and carbon dioxide and pH within very narrow limits depends on a high level of coordination of pulmonary ventilation and circulation. The control center for pulmonary ventilation (the *respiratory center*) is located in the middle of the medulla, though other areas of the brain (e.g., cerebral hemispheres and pons) contribute to fine regulation of breathing. At rest, changes in arterial blood P_{CO_2}, P_{O_2}, pH, and temperature activate neurons within the medulla and the arterial system, thereby relaying signals to the inspiratory and expiratory centers which control the rate and depth of breathing.

A decrease in arterial P_{O_2} activates the chemical receptors (*chemoreceptors*) in the aortic and carotid bodies. These same receptors are also responsible for sensing a rise in carbon dioxide (P_{CO_2}), blood temperature, and blood pressure, and a drop in pH. Under resting conditions, the partial pressure of carbon dioxide is the strongest stimulus for the regulation of breathing. As noted above, small changes in carbonic acid, formed from carbon dioxide and water, result in an increase in hydrogen ion concentrations, the result of a dissociation of carbonic acid to bicarbonate and hydrogen ions. This increase in blood hydrogen ion concentration stimulates breathing, thereby eliminating carbon dioxide, which lowers the hydrogen ion concentration as water is formed. This sequence of reactions regulates the acidity of the blood, while controlling the mechanism for inspiration and expiration.

Being short of breath during exercise is most common among individuals who are in poor physical condition and who attempt to exercise at levels which produce a sudden increase in arterial carbon dioxide and a drop in pH. As noted earlier, both of these stimuli send strong signals to the respiratory center, resulting in an increased demand on ventilation. Although exercise-induced dyspnea is sensed as an inability to breath, the underlying cause is an increase in blood hydrogen and carbon dioxide levels.

Breathing during swimming

It has been suggested that the motor cortex is the principal site for stimulating the respiratory center to the high breathing rates observed during voluntary breathing and exercise. Movement of the arms and legs appears to provide the greatest stimulus to breathing during exercise, although changes in blood acidity (pH) and temperature have a strong influence on ventilation as well. The anticipation of exercise results in a sudden increase in respiration above the body's needs. Such overbreathing is termed *hyperventilation*, and may result in an excessive unloading of carbon dioxide, and a rise in pH above normal levels. Such voluntary deep, rapid breathing can lead to light-headedness and even unconsciousness when performed for only a few seconds, revealing the sensitivity of the respiratory system's regulation of carbon dioxide and acid−base balance. At the end of mild exercise the energy demands of the muscles drop almost immediately to resting levels, whereas breathing returns to normal at a relatively slow rate. If the rate of breathing was perfectly matched to the metabolic demands of the tissues, respiration would drop to the resting level within seconds after exercise. The fact that recovery of breathing takes several minutes to return to the resting level suggests that postexercise breathing is regulated by acid−base balance and blood temperature.

During long, steady-state swims, respiration appears to match the rate of energy metabolism. Ventilation tends to be in proportion to the volume of oxygen consumed and the carbon dioxide produced by the body. As the intensity of exercise is increased toward maximum, there is a disproportionate increase in ventilation with regard to oxygen consumption. Like all aspects of tissue activity, lung ventilation and gas transport within the body require energy. At rest, only about 2% of the total energy used by the body is for breathing. As the rate and depth of ventilation increase, so does its energy cost. More than 15% of the oxygen consumed during high-speed swimming may be used by the muscles of the chest wall, diaphragm, and abdomen to ventilate the lungs. During recovery from exercise, the work of breathing continues to demand a sizeable amount of energy, using 9–12% of the total oxygen being consumed.

Though it is clear that the muscles of respiration are heavily taxed during exercise, there is sufficient breathing reserve to prevent a rise in alveolar carbon dioxide or a decline in alveolar oxygen tension during activities that last for only a few minutes. Heavy breathing for several hours, however, may result in glycogen depletion and fatigue of the respiratory muscles. It should be noted that the respiratory muscles are better designed for long-term activity than are the muscles of the arms and legs. Diaphragm muscle, for example, has 2–3 times the aerobic capacity and blood flow supply of skeletal muscle. Consequently, a larger part of the energy production for respiration can be derived from fat and lactate than in other muscles.

In an attempt to reduce the respiratory distress of exercise, swimmers often hyperventilate before competition, resulting in a decrease in blood carbon dioxide but little change in its oxygen content. As a result of the decreased carbon dioxide content of the blood, the swimmer may feel little desire to breathe during the first 10–20 s of the race. During this period, however, the arterial oxygen content may decline to critically low levels, impairing muscle metabolism and oxygen delivery to the nervous system. Thus, in events lasting more than 20–30 s, the practice of hyperventilation and subsequent breathholding mav impair performance rather than improve it.

Recommended reading

Belcastro, A.N. & Bonen, A. (1975) Lactic acid removal rates during controlled and uncontrolled recovery exercise. *J. Appl. Physiol.* **39**:932–937.

Beltz, J.D., Costill, D.L., Thomas, R., Fink, W.J. & Kirwan, J.P. (1988) Energy demands of interval training for competitive swimming. *J. Swim Res.* **4**:5–9.

Bergstrom, J., Hermansen, L., Hultman, E. & Saltin, B. (1967) Diet, muscle glycogen and physical performance. *Acta Physiol. Scand.* **71**:140–150.

Brooks, G.A. (1987) Amino acid and protein metabolism during exercise, and recovery. *Med. Sci. Sports Exercise* **19** (suppl):S150–156.

Cheetham, M.E., Boobis, L.H., Brooks, S. & Williams, C. (1986) Human muscle metabolism during sprint running. *J. Appl. Physiol.* **6**:54–60.

Clausen, J.P. (1973) Muscle blood flow during exercise and its significance for maximal performance. In Keul, J. (ed.) *Limiting Factors of Physical Performance.* Stuttgart, Germany: Georg Thieme Verlag, pp. 253–265.

Costill, D.L., Fink, W.J., Getchell, L.H., Ivy, J.L. & Witzman, F.A. (1979) Lipid metabolism in skeletal muscle of endurance-trained males and females. *J. Appl. Physiol.* **47**:787–791.

Costill, D.L., Flynn, M.G., Kirwan, J.P. *et al.* (1988) Effects of repeated days of intensified training on muscle glycogen and swimming performance. *Med. Sci. Sports Exercise* **20**:249–254.

Gaesser, G.A. & Poole, D.C. (1988) Blood lactate during exercise: time course of training adaptation in humans. *Int. J. Sports Med.* **9**:284–288.

Maglischo, E. (1990) *Swimming Faster.* Palo Alto, California: Mayfield Publishing.

Pendergast, D.R., diPrampero, P.E., Craig, A.B., Sr. & Rennie, D.W. (1978) The influence of selected biomechanical factors on the energy cost of swimming. In Eriksson, B. & Furberg, B. (eds) *Swimming Medicine IV: International Series on Sport Sciences*, vol. 6. Baltimore, Maryland: University Park Press, pp. 367–378.

Sahlin, K. (1983) Effect of acidosis on energy metabolism and force generation in skeletal muscle. In Vogel, J.A. & Poortmans, J. (eds) *Biochemistry of Exercise*, vol. 13. Champaign, Illinois: Human Kinetics, pp. 151–161.

Salo, D.C. (1988) Specifics of high-intensity training. *Swimming World* **29**:21.

Saltin, B. & Karlsson, J. (1971a) Muscle glycogen utilization during work of different intensities. In Pernow, B. & Saltin, B. (eds) *Muscle Metabolism During Exercise.* New York: Plenum Press, pp. 289–299.

Saltin, B. & Karlsson, J. (1971b) Muscle ATP, CP, and lactate during exercise after physical conditioning. In Pernow, B. & Saltin, B. (eds) *Muscle Metabolism During Exercise.* New York: Plenum Press, pp. 395–399.

Chapter 3

Fatigue: factors limiting

swimming performance

We use the term "fatigue" to describe the general sensations of tiredness, as well as the decline in performance during an all-out effort, though there appear to be multiple definitions and causes for fatigue during exhaustive swimming. Those who have competed in 100-m front crawl or butterfly know that the sensations of fatigue and exhaustion are markedly different from those experienced during events of 1500 m or longer. Although fatigue cannot be eliminated, its effect on performance can be reduced as a consequence of training and proper pacing. The following discussion will attempt to outline the causes of fatigue and the value of different training programs in increasing the swimmer's tolerance to fatigue.

Much of the time spent in training is directed toward improving muscular endurance, that is building resistance to fatigue. Fatigue results in a reduction in swimming speed, though the causes are not the same in all events. Swimmers experience fatigue in events as short as 25 m, causing a drop in velocity over the final 5–10 m. This occurs despite the fact that they do not suffer pain or become exhausted. In longer races, (i.e., 400–1500 m) they experience a different form of fatigue, a loss in muscular power and a general sensation of distress. It appears that each of these all-out efforts is associated with a different form of fatigue which is not the same as the chronic heavy, sluggish feeling that swimmers experience during periods of intense overload training.

Generally, fatigue is a complex series of events that involves several aspects of the energy processes. It is difficult to identify any one factor as the "weak link" that might be responsible for the breakdown and reduction in swimming speed. Although availability of energy may reduce the muscles' capacity to generate tension, the energy systems cannot be held wholly responsible for all forms of fatigue. The most widely accepted theories to explain the causes of fatigue are as follows:

1 depletion of energy necessary for sprint swimming, e.g., adenosine triphosphate (ATP), phosphocreatine (PCr), and glycogen;

2 the accumulation of waste products such as lactic acid;

3 changes in the physiochemical state of the muscle, e.g., minerals;

4 disturbances in the processes of muscular coordination, e.g., central nervous system.

Depletion of energy

As noted earlier, ATP provides the immediate energy used for muscular contraction, and is critical in muscle tension development. In sprint swimming lasting less than 10 s, muscle ATP levels are maintained at the expense of a breakdown of PCr. As shown in Fig. 3.1, PCr declines rapidly during the first minute of an intense exercise bout; then there is a more gradual reduction until the end of exercise. The rate at which PCr declines during exercise is dependent on the intensity of the muscular effort.

The rate of PCr breakdown increases with higher speeds of swimming, resulting in a rapid onset of fatigue and ultimate exhaustion. Studies of human thigh muscle and isolated muscle preparations have shown that exhaustion during repeated maximal contractions coincides with the depletion of PCr. Although ATP is directly responsible for the energy used during short sprints, it declines much less than PCr during muscular effort. At exhaustion, however, both ATP and PCr may be depleted. Thus, to delay the onset of fatigue, the swimmer must control the rate of effort through proper pacing to insure that PCr and ATP are not exhausted prematurely. Selecting a pace that is too rapid at the start of a race will result in a quick decline in the available phosphogens (ATP and PCr), an early onset of fatigue, and the inability to maintain the pace over the final stage of the swim. Training and experience enable the swimmer to judge the optimal exercise pace that will result in an even distribution of ATP and PCr use over the entire event, giving the best possible performance.

In addition to PCr, the levels of muscle ATP are also maintained by the aerobic and anaerobic breakdown

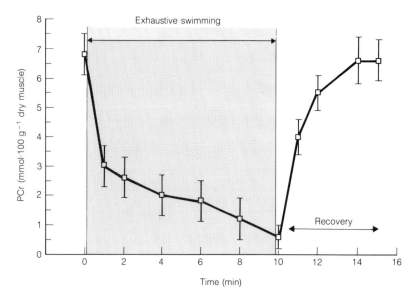

Fig. 3.1 Effects of exhaustive swimming on muscle phosphocreatine (PCr) levels.

of muscle glycogen. In swimming events lasting more than a few seconds, muscle glycogen becomes a primary source of energy for the production of ATP. Although most swimming events are too short to cause a complete emptying of a well nourished muscle's glycogen supply, during periods of extensive training the reserves may become low. Under these conditions the muscle may be able to generate force at near normal levels for only a brief period, relying on the available ATP–PCr system. As with PCr use, the rate of muscle glycogen depletion is controlled by the intensity of the activity.

Increments in the power production result in a rapid decrease in muscle glycogen. It has been estimated that during sprint swimming muscle glycogen may be used 35–40 times faster than during long-distance, low-intensity swimming. During the first few minutes of endurance exercise, muscle glycogen is used at a higher rate than later in the activity. This point is illustrated by Fig. 3.2, which shows the change in muscle glycogen content during 1–1.5 h of interval swimming. Muscle glycogen use from the shoulder muscle (deltoidius) was greatest during the first 75 min of the exercise. Thereafter, the swimmers became progressively fatigued as glycogen levels approached zero. Thus, it appears that the sensation of fatigue in long training sessions or during repeated days of intense training may coincide with the exhaustion of the muscle glycogen reserves.

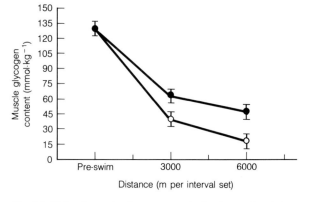

Fig. 3.2 Rate of muscle glycogen use during interval training. ●, 500-m repeats; ○, 100-m repeats.

It should be noted, however, that muscle fibers deplete their energy reserves in selected patterns. That is to say, the muscle fibers that are most frequently recruited during exercise may become individually depleted of glycogen, thereby reducing the number of fibers that are available and capable of producing the force needed for exercise.

When the slow twitch (ST) fibers have relinquished their glycogen stores, the fast twitch (FT) fibers appear unable to generate enough tension or cannot be easily recruited to compensate for the loss in muscle tension. For that reason, it has been theorized that the sensations of muscle fatigue and heaviness that occur during repeated days of heavy training may reflect the inability of some muscle fibers to generate energy at the rates needed for fast swimming.

In addition to selectively depleting glycogen from ST or FT fibers, exercise may place unusually heavy demands on select groups of muscles. During front crawl swimming, for example, considerably more glycogen may be used from the triceps and deltoidius muscles than that used by the biceps. This demonstrates that the extensor muscles of the arm may become selectively depleted, with fatigue isolated to those muscles.

Muscle glycogen alone cannot provide all the carbohydrate needed for exercise lasting several hours. Glucose delivered to the muscles via the blood has been shown to contribute a sizeable amount of energy during intense exercise. The liver breaks down glycogen to provide a constant supply of glucose in the blood. In the early stages of exercise, energy production requires relatively little blood glucose, but in the later stages of an endurance event, blood glucose may make a large contribution to the energy needs of the muscles. The longer the exercise period, the greater must be the output of glucose from the liver to keep pace with the glucose uptake by the muscles.

Since the liver has a limited supply of glycogen and is unable to produce glucose from other fuels, blood glucose levels may begin to decline when the muscle uptake becomes greater than the liver's glucose output. Unable to obtain sufficient glucose from the blood, the muscles must rely more heavily on their glycogen reserves, resulting in an acceleration of muscle glycogen use and the earlier onset of exhaustion.

In light of the muscle's dependence on glycogen and blood glucose, it is not surprising that endurance performances are improved when the supply of muscle glycogen is elevated at the start of the activity. However, it is highly unlikely that extremely large glycogen reserves will enhance the swimmer's performance above that experienced with relatively normal glycogen stores, since glycogen depletion and low blood sugar appear to limit performance and cause fatigue only in events lasting 30 min or longer. Fatigue in shorter events is more likely the result of an accumulation of waste products, such as lactate and hydrogen ion build-up within the muscles.

Accumulation of waste products

The association between fatigue and lactic acid accumulation in the blood has been recognized since the early 1930s. During strenuous exercise, some energy is provided with the formation of lactic acid in the sarcoplasm of the muscle fibers. The continual dissociation of hydrogen away from the lactate molecule causes the muscle to become more acid, thereby lowering its pH. Though most people believe that lactic acid is responsible for fatigue and exhaustion in all types of exercise, it is only during relatively short-term, highly intense muscular effort that lactate accumulates within the muscle fiber, altering its acidity. Runners, for example, may have near resting lactate and pH levels at the end of a marathon race, despite their state of exhaustion. Sprint swimming, on the other hand, results in a large accumulation of lactate, caused by glycolytic energy production. Hydrogen ion dissociation from lactate decreases muscle pH from 7.1 at rest to 6.4 at exhaustion, a value that is incompatible with normal cell function.

Thus, activities that depend on glycolysis for a sizeable portion of their energy become acidotic within the muscles and throughout the body. The cells and body fluids possess buffers, such as bicarbonate (HCO_3^-), which function to minimize the disrupting influence of the hydrogen ion. If the hydrogen ions were added to an unbuffered solution, the free concentration of hydrogen ions would lower pH by about 1.5 u (pH 7.1 to 5.6), effectively killing the muscle. Because of the body's buffering capacity, the free hydrogen ion concentration is kept low, even in the fastest sprint swimming, limiting the drop in pH to 6.6−6.4 at exhaustion.

Nevertheless, such changes in pH have a negative effect on energy and the contractile processes within the muscle. A reduction in intracellular pH to less than 6.9 has been shown to inhibit the rate of glycolysis and ATP production. At pH 6.4 the influence of free hydrogen ions is strong enough to stop any further breakdown of glycogen and to interfere with the muscle's contractile process. It is generally agreed, therefore, that a decrease in pH within the muscle is the major limiting factor and site of fatigue during most swimming events.

As shown in Fig. 3.3, recovery from an exhaustive

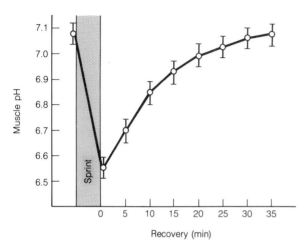

Fig. 3.3 Changes in muscle pH before and during recovery from an exhaustive sprint swim. Note that nearly 30 min of rest was required for muscle pH to return to the pre-exercise level.

sprint exercise bout takes approximately 20–30 min. At that point, muscle pH has returned to the pre-exercise level, although blood and muscle lactate may still be quite elevated. Experience has shown that athletes can continue to exercise at relatively high intensities even when their muscle pH is below 7, with lactate levels above 6 or 7 mmol·l^{-1}, which is 4–5 times the resting value. Currently, swimming coaches and physiologists are attempting to use measurements of blood lactate to gauge the intensity and volume of training needed to produce an optimal training stimulus. Although such measurements provide an index of the training intensity, they may not be related to the anaerobic processes or the state of acidosis within the muscles. As lactate and hydrogen ions are generated within the muscles, they diffuse out of the cells, are diluted in body fluids, are transported to other areas of the body, and are metabolized. Consequently, blood values for lactate are dependent on their rate of production, diffusion, and removal. Since there are a variety of factors that can influence this presence of lactate and hydrogen ions in blood, the validity of their use in evaluating training is questionable.

Neuromuscular and psychological fatigue

Thus far we have considered only factors within

the muscle that might be responsible for fatigue. There is also evidence to suggest that under some circumstances fatigue may be the result of an inability of the nervous system to activate the muscle fibers. Impulses must be transmitted across the junction between the nerve and muscle membrane, the motor end-plate. It has been suggested that fatigue may occur at this junction, making it impossible to activate the fibers. Fatigue at the motor end-plate was first suggested in the early part of this century, though the precise causes for such fatigue have not been clearly demonstrated and remain speculative.

Fatigue may also occur within the central nervous system, that is the brain and spinal cord. Since the activation of muscle depends, in part, on conscious control, the psychological trauma of exhaustive exercise may consciously or subconsciously inhibit the swimmer's willingness to tolerate further pain. Slowing the pace to a tolerable level may, therefore, be the result of limited central nervous control rather than local fatigue in the muscle. It is generally agreed that the perceived discomfort of fatigue precedes the onset of a physiological limitation within the muscles. Unless they are highly motivated, most swimmers will terminate the exercise before their muscles are physiologically exhausted. In order to achieve a peak performance, swimmers must train to develop the buffering capacity within the muscles, learn proper pacing, and develop tolerance for the discomfort of fatigue.

In conclusion, the sites of fatigue are multiple and, at present, only partly known. It is generally agreed, however, that fatigue and exhaustion during swimming are dependent on the availability of energy, the accumulation of metabolic waste products, and limitations within the nervous systems. There is no single factor responsible for fatigue. Rather there are a multitude of conditions and causes underlying the sensation and discomforts associated with exercise fatigue and exhaustion.

Recommended reading

Asmussen, E. (1979) Muscle fatigue. *Med. Sci. Sports* **11**:313–321.

Åstrand, P.-O. & Rodahl, K. (1986) *Textbook of Work Physiology*. New York: McGraw-Hill.

Bergstrom, J. (1967) Local changes of ATP and phosphoryl-creatine in human muscle tissue in connection with exercise. In *Physiology of Muscular Exercise*. Monograph no. 15. New York: American Heart Association, pp. 191–196.

Bigland-Richie, B., Jones, D.A., Hosking, G.P. & Edwards, R.H.T. (1978) Central and peripheral fatigue in sustained maximum voluntary contractions of human quadriceps muscle. *Clin. Sci. Mol. Med.* **541**:609–614.

Costill, D.L., Gollnick, P.D., Jansson, E.D., Saltin, B. & Stein, E.M. (1973) Glycogen depletion pattern in human muscle fibers during distance running. *Acta Physiol. Scand.* **89**:374–383.

Costill, D.L., Jansson, E., Gollnick, P.D. & Saltin, B. (1974) Glycogen utilization in leg muscles of men during level and uphill running. *Acta Physiol. Scand.* **91**:474–481.

Pernow, B. & Saltin B. (1971) *Muscle Metabolism During Exercise*. New York: Plenum Press.

Sahlin, K. (1982) Effect of exercise on intracellular acid–base balance in the skeletal muscle of man. In Komi, P. (ed.) *Basic Metabolism and Exercise*. Champaign, Illinois: Human Kinetics, pp. 3–14.

Chapter 4

Age and gender differences

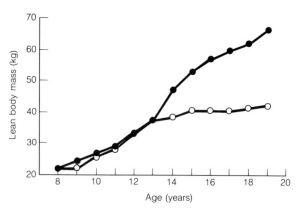

Fig. 4.1 Changes in lean body mass with growth and aging in normally active males (●) and females (○). From Wilmore & Costill (1988).

Introduction

The skill required to be an outstanding swimmer takes years of training and repetition. The foundation and development of future champions depend on the learning of swimming skills at an early age, a fact that may account for the past achievements in this sport. But there are some special considerations and questions that must be addressed in planning a program that meets the capacities of preadolescent boys and girls. Although an attempt has been made throughout this book to present information that can be applied to all age levels of both genders, there are some special concerns that must be noted when working with young swimmers. In addition, the coach and parents must recognize the physiological and developmental differences between boys and girls when planning the swimmer's training and competitive program.

Physical differences

It appears that differences between the genders in height, weight and body fat do not exist until 12–14 years, at the onset of puberty. Prior to this period, there is a striking similarity between boys and girls for all measurements of size and maturity. Lean body mass (LBM), for example, is not different for the genders prior to puberty. As shown in Fig. 4.1, after 12 or 13 years of age, the LBM of females begins to plateau, whereas the males experience a continued increase until at least the age of 18 years.

Despite the similarities in LBM prior to puberty, females typically possess more body fat at all ages, with the greatest differences being observed after age 12. The cause for these differences is related to the regulation of the sex hormones, testosterone and estrogen. Testosterone secretion by the testes, which stops at birth, is activated again at puberty, producing an increased retention of protein by muscle. This ultimately results in the larger muscle and bone mass observed in males, creating a decided difference in potential strength between the genders.

Prior to puberty, the anterior pituitary gland is unable to secrete any gonadotrophic hormones. Thus, in the female, at the time when a sufficient quantity of follicle-stimulating hormone begins to be secreted from the anterior pituitary, the ovaries develop, and estrogen secretion begins. Estrogen has a significant influence on body growth, broadening the pelvis, increasing the size of the breasts, and proliferating the deposition of fat, particularly in the thighs and hips. Additionally, estrogen increases the growth rate of bone, allowing the ultimate bone length to be reached within 2–4 years following the onset of puberty. As a result, the female grows rapidly for the first few years following puberty and then ceases to grow. The male has a much longer growth phase, allowing him to attain greater height. As a result of these hormonal changes at puberty, males at full maturity are nearly 13 cm (5 in) taller, 14–18 kg (30–40 lbs) heavier in total weight, and have 6–9% less body fat than females.

From birth through adolescence there is a steady increase in relative muscle mass of the body. This change appears to be caused by the enlargement of individual muscle fibers rather than an increase in the number of fibers. There is, however, some debate concerning the effect of strength training on the number of muscle fibers, a topic that will be mentioned later. The total muscle mass in males, for example, increases from 25% of body weight at birth to 40% or more in the adult. Though girls do not experience this same rate of change, their muscle mass does continue to increase, but at a slower rate than the boys. When females reach 16−18 years of age, muscle mass is at its peak. Males, on the other hand, experience an increase in muscle growth until the age of 22 years. Both sexes experience a relatively constant muscle mass through the age of 30 or 40 years, at which time it begins to decline. Though muscle mass can be increased through resistance training, the gender differences noted above for normally active males and females also exist among highly trained swimmers.

Studies of body fat content among swimmers have reported average values that vary from 8 to 18% of body weight in postadolescent males, and from 14 to 26% in females. Roughly 80% of the body fat is stored in cells beneath the skin formed in the early development of the fetus. The number of fat cells may become fixed early in life, though they can increase in size at any age. Recent evidence, however, suggests that fat cells may continue to increase in number throughout life, suggesting that it is important to maintain good dietary and exercise habits as one grows older. The coach and parents must also realize that heredity is a major determinant of fat cell number, though the degree of fat accumulation depends on energy intake and expenditure. Unlike many other sports, small increments in body fat will not impair the swimmer's performance. To the contrary, average or slightly above normal body fat levels may provide some benefit for buoyancy, provided added fat does not increase body drag. In light of the sensitivity of most adolescents to their physical appearance, coaches and parents must use caution in making comments and suggestions regarding body fatness.

Swimming performance

As illustrated in Fig. 4.2, swimming performances improve rapidly before and during the period of adolescence, paralleling the swimmer's increase in strength, endurance and motor skills. Since there are wide individual differences in the rate at which

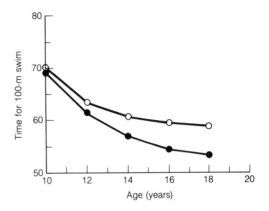

Fig. 4.2 Changes in swimming records (100-m front crawl) for males (●) and females (○) from age 10 to 18 years.

swimmers mature, it is impossible to predict when one's best performances will be attained. In most other sports that require strength and endurance for optimal performance records are set by individuals in their late 20s or early 30s. Swimmers, on the other hand, have traditionally achieved their best times while still below the age of 20 years, but that trend is changing.

Improvements in swimming performance are less pronounced after the age of 17 or 18 years. US National Collegiate (male) qualifiers and nonqualifiers have been observed to improve by about 0.7−0.8% per year in the front crawl events (50−1650 yards). This is in contrast to a 5−6% gain in performance per year from the age of 10−12 years, and a 1.7% per year gain from 14 to 18 years of age. Thus, a swimmer who performed 400 m in 4 min 15 s at the age of 18 years might be expected to improve by only 3−5.1 s by 22 years old. Although some swimmers show greater improvements than this, there are an equal number who show no gains or in some cases swim slower after 4 years of intense training. There is at present no explanation for this relatively small improvement in performance during a period when these men were training intensely, when athletes in other sports are experiencing much larger improvements. These findings lead us to ask the following questions: Do swimmers who show the largest improvements come from the programs with the most intense and greatest volume training? What kind of changes can we expect to see among female swimmers? Are the changes due to improvements in skill? What physical changes taking place during this period can be related to the changes in swimming performance? Perhaps future research will tell us which factors are most important and should be emphasized during the swimmer's development to optimize gains in performance.

The skill required for swimming generally increases with age. Studies with normally active boys and girls have demonstrated that most motor skills are learned rapidly from 6 to 17 years, although girls tend to plateau at the age of puberty for most test items. These improvements are the result of the development of neuromuscular and hormonal systems that occur with growth and development. It may, however, be invalid to compare the learning of swimming skills to the motor skills measured in these normally active children. Nevertheless, we frequently observe that most age-group swimmers (that is swimmers below the age of 16 years) achieve the biomechanical skill required for each of the strokes prior to puberty, with little additional improvement despite additional years of training and competition. There is some thought that swimming skills are best learned prior to puberty, since the swimmer's movement patterns may become difficult to change after this period. This may explain why it is difficult for the coach and swimmer to make small refinements in the swimmer's technique after the age of 12−14 years. Gross changes in technique, however, may be possible even after the age of 20 years.

Previous studies suggest that swimming success is dependent more on the swimmer's skill than on muscular strength and endurance. Physiological and performance studies have shown that many athletes have greater strength and endurance than some champion swimmers, but they lack the skill to use it in the water. Although a great many physiological studies have been conducted with swimmers, more information is needed to help us understand the process of how we learn swimming skills and the changes that can be expected in swimmers after they reach puberty.

Muscular strength appears to be the second most important determinant for success in competitive swimming. This may explain why swimmers often experience their largest improvements in performance during the period of most rapid muscle growth and physical development. In general, the marked increases in strength that males experience during puberty is the result of a large (up to 10-fold) increase in testosterone. Females, on the other hand, experience a more gradual increase in strength, and do not exhibit a sudden change in the rate of strength gain with the onset of puberty, primarily because their bodies do not produce a large amount of testosterone.

It should come as no surprise that muscular strength is proportional to the cross-section of the muscle, which accounts for the greater strength in males. When leg and arm strength are calculated relative to lean body weight, it is interesting to note that females have similar leg strength but are markedly lower in upper body strength (Fig. 4.3). This probably explains why female swimmers obtain relatively less of their propulsion from their armstroke than males. It is no surprise for most coaches to learn that females are at a decided disadvantage when they are required to swim using their arms only (i.e., pulling), but are more competitive with their male counterparts when kicking only. It should be realized that there is little difference in the strength of the muscle fibers from males and females. That is to say, strength is determined by the size of the muscle and is not a result of any gender difference in the strength of individual fibers.

In addition to the strength changes that occur as a result of maturation, a number of changes occur in the cardiovascular system which enhance endurance. As the child ages, heart size and blood volume increase in proportion to their increase in body size. Consequently, the amount of blood that can be delivered to the muscles during exercise is increased. This should not be interpreted to mean that children lack endurance, or that they have less stamina than older swimmers. Since the changes in the cardiovascular system are related to body size, there is no evidence that endurance is less developed in age-group swimmers than in older competitors. Likewise, the ability to sustain exercise without exhibiting a fall-off in performance is similar in males and females. Coaching experience with male and female swimmers might lead one to conclude that females have greater endurance than males, since they seem capable of holding a relatively higher speed than males during training. This may be explained by the fact that female swimmers generally have more body fat and greater buoyancy than their male counterparts. As a result, it costs the female swimmer less energy to stay afloat, enabling her to use more of her energy for propulsion.

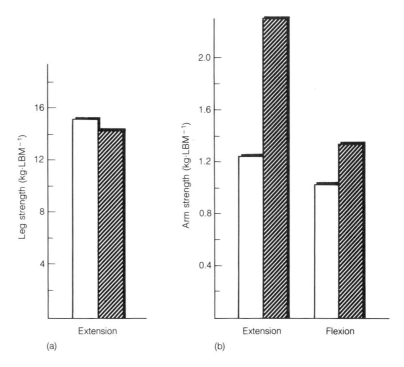

Fig. 4.3 A comparison of (a) leg strength and (b) arm strength for males (▨) and females (□). Note that both genders have similar leg strength, but are decidedly different in upper body strength.

(a)

(b)

Responses to exercise

Prior to puberty children have only limited ability to perform anaerobic types of activities. This fact is demonstrated by the child's inability to achieve the same blood or muscle lactate levels as observed in adults during submaximal and maximal rates of exercise. It has been shown that some of the key enzymes of glycolysis are lower in prepubescent boys than in adults. As a result, the child's muscle fibers are unable to generate large amounts of adenosine triphosphate (ATP) by the anaerobic breakdown of glycogen, resulting in less lactate production and a more rapid depletion of available ATP and phosphocreatine (PCr). This diminished anaerobic capacity seems to be similar in both boys and girls, though it can be improved with training. From a coaching point of view, it should be realized that, although these young swimmers lack anaerobic capacity, their ability to perform aerobically does not appear to be diminished as a consequence of their age.

It is generally agreed that the capacity to consume oxygen during maximal exercise ($\dot{V}_{O_2\,max}$) is the best single laboratory measure of the swimmer's aerobic capacity. In normally active boys and girls $\dot{V}_{O_2\,max}$ increases steadily from about 5 or 6 years of age, in most cases paralleling the child's increase in body size. As shown in Fig. 4.4, when corrected for changes in body weight ($ml \cdot kg^{-1} \cdot min^{-1}$), $\dot{V}_{O_2\,max}$ shows little change in boys and a decline in girls from the age of 6 through 18 years. Of course, endurance training can increase $\dot{V}_{O_2\,max}$ 10–30% above the values observed in these normally active children, with prepubescent boys and girls having about the same values. With the onset of puberty, however, the values for boys continue to rise, whereas the girls show smaller increments in aerobic capacity with training.

How do these changes in aerobic capacity with growth affect the young swimmer's performance? For any swimming activity that requires a fixed rate of energy expenditure, the swimmer with the highest $\dot{V}_{O_2\,max}$ will have an endurance advantage. This does not mean that individuals with the highest $\dot{V}_{O_2\,max}$ will automatically be the best distance swimmers. As with strength, one must have the motor skill necessary for efficient swimming to gain the benefit of this physiological advantage. On the other hand, if two swimmers have similar skill levels, then the one with the highest aerobic capacity will have a decided

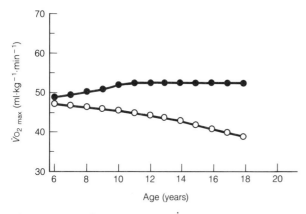

Fig. 4.4 Maximal oxygen uptake ($\dot{V}_{O_2\,max}$) values for normally active boys (●) and girls (○) from 6 to 18 years of age.

advantage during events lasting more than a few minutes. It should not, therefore, be assumed that the best distance swimmer has the highest $\dot{V}_{O_2\,max}$. Surprisingly, the best predictor of aerobic capacity in highly trained swimmers is body weight and not swimming performance (Costill *et al.*, 1985).

Training responses

Is it necessary to give special consideration in training young boys and girls? Do females adapt differently to training than male swimmers? A number of concerns have been expressed regarding the influence of gender and age on the adaptations to training. Unfortunately, there is little more than intuitive information to guide us in determining the volume and intensity of training needed by these groups to attain optimal adaptations.

Generally, prepubescent and postpubescent males and females all show improvement when on programs of strength and endurance training. The amount of adaptation, however, is influenced by the swimmer's gender and age. The amount of improvement to any training program depends to a large extent on the swimmer's genetic potential: that is to say, the rate and amount of adaptation to training are predetermined by heredity. This may explain why a given training program may, in one case, produce a champion, whereas the same program may overtrain another swimmer. Thus, we are faced with the problem of matching the training volume and intensity to the swimmer's potential for adaptation. Since

swimmers all have different inherited characteristics *we cannot expect them to respond similarly to the same training program.*

To date, there is little or no information available to tell the coach how much and how intense the training program should be for age-group swimmers (or, for that matter, mature swimmers). At this point we must base the training programs for these children on past experience, which suggests that significant improvements in strength and endurance can be achieved in a wide variety of training programs. Additional attention will be given on this point in Chapters 13, 16, and 18.

Strength training in prepubescent children is a topic of controversy. It has been suggested that since these boys and girls have relatively low circulating androgen levels, there is no reason to expect them to be able to benefit from strength training at this early age. Recent studies, however, have demonstrated that prepubescent boys can gain substantial strength as a consequence of resistance training. In a 1986 study, prepubescent boys and girls took part in a 9-week progressive resistance–strength training program for 25–30 min per day for 3 days per week. They experienced a mean strength increase of 43% compared to a 10% increase in a nontraining group of children. A number of similar studies have been conducted in recent years, with none showing any evidence of damage to the children's bones, tendons, or muscles.

Although the risk of injury and structural damage from heavy-resistance exercise is extremely low, it has been suggested that a program using low weights and high repetitions should be preferred to one using heavy weights and low repetitions. It has even been suggested that the safest technique for strength training in young children would be to use isokinetic resistance which is matched to the force applied, eliminating the risk of injury associated with the use of free-weights.

Do prepubescent boys and girls benefit from aerobic training? This is also a highly controversial topic, since several early studies indicated that training in these children did not improve $\dot{V}_{O_2\,max}$. Interestingly, even without significant increases in $\dot{V}_{O_2\,max}$, these children had substantial improvements in endurance performance (e.g., reduced time to run a fixed distance). Based on these and other studies it can be concluded that there will be only small increases in aerobic capacity with training in children 10 years of age and younger, even though their performances in aerobic activities are improved. More substantial changes in $\dot{V}_{O_2\,max}$ appear to occur once the child reaches puberty. The underlying causes for this finding is not clearly understood, though it is quite possible that improvements in aerobic capacity depend on growth of the heart, which is more likely during and after puberty.

Psychological aspects

Is formal, organized competition and heavy physical training damaging to the emotional health and psychological development of the swimmer? It is generally agreed that the pressures and stresses of competitive swimming present no major problems for the mature swimmer, but many parents, educators, physicians, and psychologists have expressed concerns over the potential for undesirable emotional experiences in the age-group swimmer. Do children who compete in formal, highly organized training programs develop undesirable behavior patterns or drop out of swimming because of the pressures to win?

Only limited research has been conducted in this area of sports science, and none of the available studies have used young girls. Studies from the 1950s with Little League and Middle League (13–15 years of age) found essentially no difference in emotional stability between these athletes and children who engaged in informal recreational softball. Few athletes had any serious emotional problems that could be related to the stress of competition. The results of this study concluded that formal competition at this age level was not detrimental to the child's emotional growth — rather it facilitated social and emotional growth.

There are, however, experimental studies with young boys that have shown some negative effects of intense competition (Sherif *et al.*, 1961). When groups of boys were separated and placed in competition with each other, the members of the groups developed strong allegiances to their own group and extreme hostility toward the other group. The study was eventually terminated when individual members of

the groups began to develop serious psychological disturbances. It took considerable time to bring the two groups back together in cooperative ventures, removing all forms of competition between the groups.

Obviously, the findings from these studies are not directly applicable to age-groups swimming, but it is generally agreed that competition can have both positive and negative influences on the emotional development of the young athlete. Of major importance is the climate in which the competition takes place. If the climate is such that winning is the only goal and parents are allowed to say and do whatever they please without giving the child sound guidance in coping with the stress of competition and training, the child will be likely to have a negative experience. In short, the nature of the child's experience will depend on the local situation, though we all recognize that individual differences in personality and emotional makeup will also influence the child's reaction to the stresses of swimming competition. It is generally agreed that when competition is organized for the enjoyment of the child and not the adults, the experience should be positive and facilitate sound emotional growth and psychological development.

Recommended reading

Bar-Or, O. (1983) *Pediatric Sports Medicine for the Practitioner.* New York: Springer-Verlag.

Costill, D.L., Kovaleski, J., Porter, D., Kirwan, J., Fielding, R. & King, D. (1985) Energy expenditure during front crawl swimming: predicting success in middle-distance events. *Int. J. Sports Med.* **6**:266–270.

Eriksson, B.O. (1973) Physical training, oxygen supply and muscle metabolism in 11 to 13 year-old boys. *Acta Physiol. Scand.* **87**:27–39.

Eriksson, B.O., Lundin, A. & Saltin, B. (1975) Cardiopulmonary function in former girl swimmers and the effects of physical training. *Scand. J. Clin. Lab. Invest.* **35**:135–140.

Sherif, M., Harvey, O.J., White, B.J., Hood, W.R. & Sherif, C.W. (1961) *Intergroup Conflict and Cooperation: The Robber's Cave Experiment.* Norman, Oklahoma: University of Oklahoma Book Exchange.

Skubic, E. (1955) Emotional responses of boys to Little League and Middle League competitive baseball. *Res. Q* **26**:342–352.

Wilmore, J.H. & Costill, D.L. (1988) *Training for Sport and Activity*, 3rd edn. Dubuque, Iowa: W.C. Brown.

Chapter 5

Nutritional needs of the swimmer

Carbohydrate is the primary fuel used by muscles during competitive swimming. This energy source is provided as blood glucose and muscle glycogen. Although the muscles can use fats as an alternate fuel, energy production from this source cannot adequately meet the demands imposed during high-intensity effort. Consequently, when blood glucose declines or muscle glycogen is depleted, the swimmer will feel fatigued and unable to produce the muscle force needed to sustain a desired swimming pace. Good nutrition, however, entails more than fuels for energy: the swimmer must also consider the vitamins and minerals that are essential for growth and normal cellular function. Thus, in the following discussion attention will be given to the variety of dietary needs that contribute to optimal swimming performance and training.

Despite the wealth of published information dealing with proper nutrition, few efforts have been made to describe the nutritional needs and the optimal dietary regimen of the competitive swimmer. That is not to say that the area of nutrition has not been considered important by nutritionists, coaches, and swimmers. To the contrary, in their quest for success, most swimmers have at one time searched for the "magic food" that would produce a winning performance. Unfortunately, most efforts to manipulate diet have been promoted by suggestions from more successful performers, poorly designed research studies, invalid commercial advertising claims, and the misinterpretation of nutritional research. The net results are confusion and many claims that are not only unsound, but potentially dangerous.

Basic nutritional needs

Simply defined, food includes all the solid and liquid materials taken into the digestive tract that are utilized to maintain and build body tissues, regulate body processes, and supply body heat. Food can be categorized into six classes of nutrients, each with a unique chemical structure and a specific function within the body. The six categories include *water, minerals, vitamins, proteins, fats*, and *carbohydrates*. Each of these will be briefly discussed relative to their importance in general body function.

Water

Since swimmers spend many hours each day in the water and generally do not experience dehydration, we are inclined to consider water as a minor nutritional concern. There are, however, situations where sweating and dryland training may produce a significant body water loss sufficient to impair performance.

While it has no caloric value, and does not provide any of the other nutrients, water is second in importance only to oxygen in maintaining life. Water constitutes about 60% of the total body weight, with two-thirds of the water contained within the body tissues (*intracellular*) and one-third outside the cells (*extracellular*). While we can survive for weeks or even months without food, we cannot tolerate water deprivation for more than a few days. It has been estimated that we can lose up to 40% of our body weight in fats, carbohydrates, and proteins and still survive, while a 15–20% loss in body water can be fatal.

Water is necessary for digestion, absorption, circulation, and excretion. With respect to exercise, body water plays two critical roles. First, it is important in maintaining the mineral balance in the body. Second, it is a transporter of nutrients and byproducts to and from the cells, via the circulatory system. Water intake is controlled largely by one's sensation of thirst. It should be mentioned, however, that the body's thirst mechanisms do not always keep up with its need for water. While a small degree of dehydration will not usually have serious consequences over a single day, when faced with repeated exposure to exercise in the heat—not a common problem in swimmers—dehydration can produce serious consequences. Because of thirst's sluggish drive to replace body water, it is generally recommended that we drink more fluid than our thirst mechanisms dictate in an attempt to avoid dehydration. If too much water is ingested, the body can adapt readily by passing off the excess in urine.

Ingested water is rapidly absorbed by the intestines, but it must first be emptied from the stomach. Considerable research has shown that when materials are dissolved in the solutions we drink, they tend to be delayed as they pass through the stomach, slowing the replacement of body water. Thus, to increase water absorption in the intestines, it is important to ingest either water or solutions having few dissolved particles, such as sugar or minerals. For the swimmer, the easiest way to gauge the state of water balance is to monitor one's early morning body weight and/or observe the color of one's urine. Sudden changes in body weight are normally attributed to alterations in body water content, since measurable changes in body fat and/or muscle take weeks before they become noticeable. Since the kidneys are responsible for regulating the water content of the body, a dark-yellow urine is indicative of the kidneys' attempt to conserve water, whereas a very dilute, clear urine suggests that the body has too much water and that the kidneys are unloading the excess.

Minerals

While there are more than 20 different minerals in the body, approximately 17 have been proven to be essential in the diet. Approximately 4% of one's body weight is in the form of minerals, and most of this is in bone. Minerals such as calcium, potassium, sulfur, sodium, chlorine, phosphorus, and magnesium are needed in relatively large amounts. These *macro-minerals*, by definition, are minerals that are needed by the body in amounts of more than 100 mg per day. *Microminerals*, on the other hand, are trace elements that are needed in amounts of less than 100 mg per day, and include iron, zinc, selenium, manganese, copper, iodine, molybdenum, cobalt, fluorine, and chromium. Calcium is the most abundant mineral in the body, constituting 1.5−2% of the total body weight, and approximately 40% of the total minerals present in the body. Of the total calcium in the body, 99% is found in the bones and teeth. The major function of calcium is to build and maintain bones

and teeth. It is essential for muscle contraction, blood clotting, control of cell membrane permeability, and nervous control of the heart. Milk and other dairy products are the best sources of calcium.

Phosphorus is closely linked to calcium, and constitutes approximately 22% of the total mineral content of the body. About 80% of phosphorus is found in combination with calcium in the form of calcium phosphate, which provides strength and rigidity to the bones and teeth. It is also an essential part of metabolism, cell membrane structure, and the buffering system to maintain the blood at a constant pH. Meat, poultry, fish, eggs, and milk are the major sources of phosphorus.

Iron is present in the body in relatively small amounts — 35−50 mg per kg body weight. Iron plays an extremely critical role in the transportation of oxygen in the blood as a component of hemoglobin. In addition, myoglobin, found in muscle, is an iron-containing protein that is essential in the storage and transport of oxygen within the fibers. Iron deficiency results in a reduction in the oxygen-carrying capacity of the blood, and a feeling of general tiredness and lack of energy. Though these symptoms are not uncommon in swimmers who are in the midst of intense training, few cases of anemia have been reported among healthy male and female swimmers. Nevertheless, this condition does pose a threat to some individuals, principally postadolescent females. The major dietary source of iron is liver. However, oysters, shellfish, lean meat, and other organ meats provide good sources, as do leafy green vegetables and egg yolks.

Sodium, potassium, and chloride are classified as *electrolytes* and are found distributed throughout all body fluids and tissues, with sodium and chloride found predominantly outside the cells and potassium distributed mostly within the cells. These electrolytes function to maintain normal water balance and distribution, and to provide for normal neuro-muscular function. The major sources of sodium chloride are table salt, seafood, milk, and meat. Potassium is found most readily in fruits, milk, meat, cereals, and vegetables.

The importance of these minerals cannot be over-stated, but it should be made clear that swimmers who eat a normal balanced diet will not likely become mineral-deficient. In addition to the kidneys' role in regulating the body water content, they also assist in controlling the body mineral reserves.

Vitamins

Vitamins are defined as a group of unrelated organic compounds that perform specific functions to promote growth and to maintain health. They are needed in relatively small quantities, but are essential for specific metabolic reactions within the cells. Vitamins function primarily as catalysts in chemical reactions within the body. They are essential for the release of energy, for tissue building, and for controlling the body's use of food. Vitamins can be classified into one of two major categories: *fat-soluble* or *water-soluble*. Fat-soluble vitamins A, D, E, and K are stored by the body in lipids. Because they are stored, there is the possibility that they could be taken in doses that would lead to vitamin toxicity. Vitamin C and the B-complex vitamins are water-soluble, and when taken in excess will be excreted, mainly in the urine. Table 5.1 provides a list of each vitamin, its sources and functions, and the recommended daily allowance.

Vitamin A was the first fat-soluble vitamin to be discovered (1913). Natural vitamin A is usually found esterified with a fatty acid. It is essential for night vision. It is also essential for maintaining normal epithelial structure, and is thus important in the prevention of infection. It is important for healthy skin, normal bone development, and tooth formation. The major dietary sources of vitamin A are liver, kidney, butter, egg yolk, whole milk, fruits, and leafy dark green and yellow vegetables. Approximately 90% of the stored vitamin A is found in the liver. Toxicity results in bone fragility and stunted growth, loss of appetite, coarsening and loss of hair, scaly skin eruptions, enlargement of the liver and spleen, irritability, double vision, fatigue, and skin rashes.

Vitamin D is absorbed with fats from the intestine and can also be absorbed directly from the skin into the blood. It is stored in the liver, skin, brain, and bones, being essential for normal growth and development. Rickets results from vitamin D deficiency, and toxicity leads to excessive calcification of bone, kidney stones, headache, nausea, and diarrhea.

Vitamin E functions in metabolism, and helps to enhance the activity of vitamins A and C. Vitamin E deficiency in humans is rare, and few serious toxic effects have been identified. Many claims have been made for vitamin E with respect to enhancement of swimming performance, but the claims for improved endurance lack supporting scientific evidence.

The B-complex vitamins were at one time considered to be a single vitamin important in the prevention of the disease beriberi. At the present time, however, more than a dozen B-complex vitamins have been identified which have very specific functions within the body. B-complex vitamins play an essential role in the metabolism of all living cells, serving as cofactors in the various enzyme systems involved in the oxidation of food and the production of energy. The B-complex vitamins have such a close interrelationship that a deficiency in one may impair the utilization of the others. Since many athletes consume foods containing simple sugars, their diets are often lower than the recommended daily allowance for one or more of the B-complex vitamins. There have, however, been no reported cases of vitamin B deficiencies in athletes. Table 5.1 lists major food sources for each of the B-complex vitamins.

Vitamin C, or ascorbic acid, was isolated in 1928, and is both the prevention and cure for scurvy. Vitamin C functions as either a coenzyme or a cofactor in metabolism. It is required for the production and maintenance of collagen, and has been postulated to assist in wound healing, to combat fever and infection, and to prevent or cure the common cold. Vitamin C deficiency is characterized by general weakness, poor appetite, anemia, swollen and inflamed gums and loosened teeth, shortness of breath, swollen joints, and neurotic disturbances (symptomatic of many swimming coaches during the taper period).

Proteins

Proteins are nitrogen-containing compounds formed by amino acids. They constitute the major structural component of the cell, antibodies, enzymes, and many hormones. Protein is necessary for growth, but it is also necessary for the repair and maintenance of body tissues; the production of hemoglobin (iron plus protein); the production of enzymes, hormones, mucus, milk, and sperm; the maintenance of normal

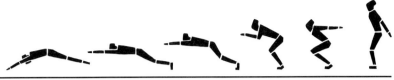

Table 5.1 Vitamins and their primary functions, sources, and recommended daily allowance (RDA)

Vitamin	Primary function	Sources	1980 RDA (units·day^{-1})
Fat-soluble vitamins			
A	Adaptation to dim light, resistance to infection, prevention of eye and skin disorders, promotion of bone and tooth development	Liver, kidney, milk, butter, egg yolk, yellow vegetables, apricots, cantaloupe, and peaches	800 and 1000 µg for females and males, respectively—teens and adults
D	Facilitates absorption of calcium; bone and tooth development	Sunlight, fish, eggs, fortified dairy products, and liver	10 µg for ages 11−18; 5−7.5 µg for adults
E	Prevents oxidation of essential vitamins and fatty acids, and protects red blood cells from hemolysis	Wheatgerm, vegetable oils, green vegetables, milk fat, egg yolk, and nuts	8−10 mg for teens and adults
K	Blood clotting	Liver, soybean oil, vegetable oil, green vegetables, tomatoes, cauliflower, and wheat bran	70−140 µg for teens and adults
Water-soluble vitamins			
B$_1$ (thiamine)	Energy metabolism, growth, appetite, and digestion	Pork, liver, organ meats, legumes, whole-grain and enriched cereals and breads, wheatgerm, and potatoes	1.0−1.5 mg for teens and adults
B$_2$ (riboflavin)	Growth, health of eyes, and energy metabolism	Milk and dairy foods, organ meats, green vegetables, eggs, fish, and enriched cereals and breads	1.2−1.7 mg for teens and adults
Niacin	Energy metabolism and fatty-acid synthesis	Fish, liver, meat, poultry, grains, eggs, peanuts, milk, and legumes	13−19 mg for teens and adults
B$_6$ (pyridoxine)	Protein metabolism and growth	Pork, glandular meats, bran and germ cereals, milk, egg yolk, oatmeal, and legumes	1.8−2.2 mg for teens and adults
Pantothenic acid	Hemoglobin formation, and carbohydrate, protein, and fat metabolism	Whole-grain cereals, organ meats, and eggs	4−7 mg for teens and adults
Biotin	Carbohydrate, fat, and protein metabolism	Liver, peanuts, yeast, milk, meat, egg yolk, cereal, nuts, legumes, bananas, grapefruit, tomatoes, watermelon, and strawberries	100−200 µg for teens and adults
Folic acid (folacin)	Growth, fat metabolism, maturation of red blood cells	Green vegetables, organ meats, lean beef, wheat, eggs, fish, dry beans, lentils, asparagus, broccoli, and yeast	400 µg for teens and adults
B$_{12}$ (cobalamin)	Red blood cell production, nervous system metabolism, and fat metabolism	Liver, kidney, milk and dairy foods, and meat	3.0 µg for teens and adults
C (ascorbic acid)	Growth, tissue repair, tooth and bone formation	Citrus fruits, tomatoes, strawberries, potatoes, melons, peppers, and pineapple	50−60 mg for teens and adults

osmotic balance, and protection from disease through antibodies. Proteins are also potential sources of energy, but they are generally spared when fat and carbohydrate are available in ample supply. Over 20 amino acids have been identified, and of these, eight or nine are considered to be essential as part of the daily food intake. While many of the amino acids can be manufactured or synthesized by the body, these essential or indispensable amino acids either cannot be synthesized by the body or cannot be synthesized at a rate sufficient to meet the body needs, and thus become a necessary part of the diet. If any one of these is absent from the diet, protein cannot be synthesized or body tissue maintained. Protein sources in the diet that contain all of the essential amino acids in the proper ratio and in sufficient quantity are referred to as *complete* proteins. Meat, fish, and poultry are the three primary complete proteins. The proteins in vegetables and grains are referred to as *incomplete* proteins, as they do not supply all of the essential amino acids in appropriate amounts. This concept becomes important for individuals on vegetarian diets.

Approximately 5−15% of the total calories consumed per day in the US are in the form of protein. This is considered by many to be 2−3 times the amount of protein necessary for proper body function. The daily recommended allowance published in 1980 by the National Research Council is 45 and 56 g per day for the teenage and adult male, respectively, and 44−46 g per day for the teenage and adult female. One's need for protein is dependent on the individual's body weight, with an allowance of 1 g per kg body weight considered adequate for adults.

Fats

Swimmers and coaches generally think of fat in negative terms, considering the fat swimmer to be in poor condition or less capable of optimum performance. This may not be the true picture. Fat is an essential component of cell walls and nerve fibers; it is a primary energy source, providing up to 70% of total energy when the body is in the resting state; it adds buoyancy during swimming, reducing the energy needed to maintain the body on the surface of the water; it is a support and cushion for vital organs; it is involved in the absorption and transport of the fat-

soluble vitamins, and it is a subcutaneous insulation layer for the preservation of body heat.

Most nutritionists recommend that approximately 25% of the caloric intake be taken in the form of fat. While many agree that the reduction of fat intake should come from saturated fats, there is presently a great deal of controversy on specific recommendations for the intake of fats, particularly in reference to egg and dairy products.

Carbohydrates

Carbohydrates are composed of sugars and starches. Monosaccharides are the simple sugars (e.g., glucose and fructose) that cannot be broken down to a simpler form. Disaccharides can be hydrolyzed to two molecules of the same or different monosaccharide, such as the sucrose that we commonly use as table-sugar. Oligosaccharides can be hydrolyzed to yield 3−10 monosaccharide units, whereas polysaccharides can provide more than 10 monosaccharide units. The major polysaccharides are starch, dextrin, cellulose, and glycogen; these are composed completely of glucose units.

Glucose serves many functions in the body. First, it is a major source of energy, particularly during high-intensity exercise. Glucose also exerts an influence on both protein and fat metabolism, sparing the use of protein as an energy source, and controlling the utilization of fat. Glucose is the sole source of energy for the nervous system. The major sources of carbohydrates are grains, fruits, vegetables, milk, and concentrated sweets. Refined sugar, syrup, and cornstarch are examples of pure carbohydrates, and many of the concentrated sweets such as candy, honey, jellies, molasses, and soft drinks contain few if any other nutrients.

The swimmer's diet

Since athletes place considerable demands on their body every day during training and competition, it is important that their diet restores essential nutrients. Too often, swimmers spend considerable time and effort in perfecting skills and attaining top physical condition, only to ignore proper nutrition and rest. It is not uncommon to trace the deterioration of an athlete's performance back to poor nutrition.

Unfortunately, we know very little about the eating habits of athletes. To gain a little insight into their nutritional practices, the diets of a group of highly trained collegiate male swimmers were recorded during a period of training. Although the dietary habits of these swimmers varied widely, these findings suggest that the swimmers' performances were not altered as a result of their diets. One interesting finding was how closely swimmers came to meeting the recommended daily allowance—the standard considered necessary for good health.

This sample of swimmers ate diets containing 50% carbohydrates, 36% fats and 14% proteins. In light of the need for a high-carbohydrate diet when training for swimming, we might at first consider their carbohydrate intake to be low. These men, however, ate more than enough carbohydrate to meet the energy needed for training. Since their total calorie intake was nearly 50% higher than would be expected for individuals of similar size, their total carbohydrate intake was well above average.

What is a well balanced diet? In the early 1940s, the Food and Nutrition Board of the National Research Council of the National Academy of Sciences was formed to define the nutrient requirements of the American population. At the conclusion of their deliberations, they published a report that became known as the "Recommended Daily Allowances," or the RDA. The allowances were designed to provide a guideline for planning and evaluating food intake. In 1980, the National Research Council published its most recent of a number of revisions. With respect to energy intake, males 11−50 years of age should consume between 2700 and 2900 kcal (11 350−12 200 kJ), and females of the same age between 2000 and 2200 kcal (8400−9250 kJ). These figures are calculated on the basis of the average height and weight of the population, and for individuals doing light work. Obviously, swimmers in intensive training would have considerably higher energy demands.

Vegetarian diets

Vegetarian diets are chosen for a number of reasons, including health, ecological, and economical reasons. Most vegetarians eat any food from plant sources. However, there are several types of vegetarians. *Vegans* are strict vegetarians and eat only food from plant sources. *Lactovegetarians* eat plant foods plus dairy products. *Ovovegetarians* eat plant foods plus eggs, and *lacto-ovovegetarians* eat plant foods, dairy products, and eggs. *Fruitarians* eat fruits, nuts, olive oil, and honey.

Can swimmers survive on a vegetarian diet? The answer is a qualified yes. If the athlete is a strict vegan, he or she must be very careful in the selection of the plant foods eaten to provide a good balance of the essential amino acids, adequate sources of vitamin A, riboflavin, vitamin B_{12}, vitamin D, calcium, iron, and sufficient calories. More than one professional athlete has noted a significant deterioration in athletic performance after switching over to a strict vegetarian diet. The problem was later traced to an unwise selection of plant foods. Inclusion of milk and eggs is highly recommended since this will lessen the likelihood of nutritional deficiencies. Anyone contemplating a switch from a normal to a vegetarian diet would be well advised to read authoritative reference material on the subject, written by qualified nutritionists, or to consult a registered dietitian.

Special diets and supplements

Swimmers are always looking for an edge—something that will give them an advantage. Since the difference between winning and losing can often be measured in fractions of a second, no athlete wants to feel that he or she did not try everything possible to achieve his or her best performance. Manipulating the diet and taking extra quantities of various vitamins and minerals seem to be relatively harmless methods to make the body work at its best. But do these efforts really help?

As noted earlier, vitamins are essential for normal body function. Unfortunately, swimmers have no way to judge their vitamin levels until they become deficient. Only then do the rather unpleasant symptoms appear. The characteristic sores and loss of vision associated with a deficiency in vitamin B_2 (riboflavin), for example, are a rare event in our society and unheard of among swimmers and other athletes. Most evidence suggests that, on the average, swimmers consume equal or greater amounts of vitamins than the recommended daily allowance. Some swimmers have, however, been found to take less than 50% of the recommended amount for these vitamins, based on the number of calories they were eating. One explanation for the low levels may be that the swimmers studied were vegetarians or ate diets low in animal products such as meat, cheese, milk, and eggs, which are the principal sources of vitamin B_6, B_{12}, and panothenic acid.

There have been a number of studies that found increased endurance with very large doses of vitamins C, E, and B-complex, but there are far more studies demonstrating that vitamins in excess of the recommended daily allowance will not improve performance in either strength or endurance activities. Experts generally agree that popping vitamins will not make up for a lack of talent or training or give swimmers an edge over their competition.

As a matter of fact, too much of a good thing can be harmful. Extremely large doses of vitamins A and D may produce some undesirable effects. Overdoses of vitamin A, for example, may cause a loss of appetite, loss of hair, enlargement of the liver and spleen, swelling over the long bones, and general irritability — scarcely ideal conditions for any athlete. These symptoms, however, have never been reported in swimmers, even in those taking 2—3 times the recommended daily allowance for these vitamins.

All in all, it appears that the recommended daily allowance for the various vitamins is about optimal for normal body operations, though possibly on the conservative side. Certainly, there is no convincing evidence to prove that vitamin pills taken to supplement a balanced diet will improve athletic performance. Extra doses of vitamins may be of some value if, for some reason, you wish to increase the vitamin content of your urine, since that is where most of the excess ends up. Perhaps that is why it is said that swimmers produce the most expensive urine in the world.

Minerals are the diet supplement next most widely used by athletes. Though swimmers do sweat during training, the amount of water and minerals lost from the body is small, even when the water temperature is fairly warm. The mineral content of the diet can easily replace the small losses experienced during training and competition. Even without mineral supplements, the body can get all it needs from the natural minerals in food.

Since iron-deficiency anemia is known to impair endurance performance, it is important to distinguish between true anemia and the plasma volume dilution associated with repeated days of training in warm weather. Training tends to increase the volume of plasma more than the number of red blood cells, producing a drop in hemoglobin concentration with no apparent effect on oxygen transport or endurance. Plasma water changes dramatically with both acute and chronic exercise, whereas the number of red cells remains relatively constant. Thus, changes in plasma volume can alter the concentration of red blood cells and hemoglobin, giving the false impression of anemia or an excess of blood cells.

Several studies have reported that between 36 and 82% of female swimmers are anemic or iron-deficient. In light of this high frequency of iron deficiency in females, it seems logical to suggest that they include iron-rich foods in their diets. In addition, swimmers suspected to be anemic or iron-deficient should be tested for serum ferritin, a measure of the body's iron stores and a method of determining the athlete's need for extra dietary iron. Iron supplementation should, however, be directed by a physician, since prolonged administration of iron can cause iron overload — a potentially serious condition.

Dieting to lose fat

Many swimmers wish to lose body fat while continuing to train hard. Unfortunately, to lose excess fat the body must be forced to rely more heavily on its fat reserves for energy, while taking in little fuel. This results in a caloric deficit and a gradual reduction in the body's fat weight. Though such a diet—exercise regimen may accelerate the rate of fat loss, it fails to allow for adequate replacement of muscle and liver glycogen stores. As a result, the athlete may feel heavy and is easily fatigued, able to train only at a relatively slow pace and with a reduced total work output.

During periods of voluntary weight loss the individual must take care to obtain the essential vitamins and minerals while consuming fewer than the required calories. Malnutrition among these individuals may occur when they consume foods low in these necessary ingredients. Under such extreme conditions it may be helpful to use vitamin and mineral supplements.

Attempts to lose weight should be scheduled for periods when the swimmers are not preparing for competition. During those periods they can afford to perform lower-intensity exercise for longer periods, thereby placing fewer demands on the body's limited carbohydrate stores. Though exercise aids in losing weight, the only known way to insure the removal of body fat is partial starvation. Too bad it isn't as easy or as enjoyable to get rid of body fat as it is to put it on!

The precompetition meal

Although a precompetition meal makes only a minor contribution to the immediate energy used during swimming, it may insure a normal level of blood sugar, and will help the swimmer to avoid the sensations of hunger and weakness. The diet plan should insure that the stomach and upper bowel are empty at the time of competition. Food and fluid intakes prior to competition should not leave the swimmer with the sensation of fullness. The diet should include food that swimmers are familiar with, and are convinced will make them win.

It is also important that swimmers do not eat anything with a high sugar content in the hour before competition or intense training. Such sugar feedings will increase blood glucose and insulin levels. In some individuals, the body overreacts and produces more insulin than is needed. This results in a very sharp decrease in the blood sugar level during the onset of exercise, causing the athlete to become hypoglycemic. This condition may induce fatigue and limit the swimmer's ability to train.

It has been suggested that a liquid precompetition meal is less likely to result in nervous indigestion, nausea, vomiting, and abdominal cramps. Such feedings are commercially available and have, in general, been found to be useful both before and between events. As with any precompetition feeding, however, they should not be taken within the final hour before the race. In some competitions, where the swimmer must perform in multiple preliminary and final events, it is often difficult to find time to feed the swimmer. Under these circumstances a liquid feeding that is low in fat and high in carbohydrate may be the only alternative.

Ergogenic aids

Ergogenic aids are substances that improve perform-

ance above that expected. Although some attention has already been given to the role of food supplements in athletic performance, this section will focus on those substances taken by swimmers to enhance performance. Is it possible to manipulate the diet to improve performance? The answer is a qualified yes, since it is easier to demonstrate that a poor diet will impair performance than it is to show that any select food will make an individual swim faster. Nevertheless, numerous attempts have been made to find a "magic food" to enhance performance.

Is it necessary for swimmers who are training for strength and muscle bulk to increase their normal dietary intake of protein? At one time it was thought that the muscle consumed itself as fuel for its own contractions, and that protein supplementation was essential to prevent the muscles from wasting away. It is now recognized that little protein is consumed as fuel for muscular work. If fats or carbohydrates are available, they are selected in preference to proteins as sources of energy. The factors that are responsible for building muscle size are complex and unaffected by the intake of extra amounts of protein. As a result, eating large amounts of protein will not cause the muscles to retain and incorporate the protein into additional tissue. Most of the excess is simply excreted from the body.

Does protein supplementation improve swimming performance? Even with heavy physical training or work, where energy expenditure may exceed 20.9 MJ (5000 kcal·day^{-1}), the diet consumed should provide adequate total protein if the proportion of protein in the total energy consumed is maintained. Early studies observed little or no difference in performance between diets which were low, normal and high in protein. Regardless of the amount of protein in the diet, no differences between diets were found for strength, endurance, serum protein, erythrocyte count or hemoglobin content.

In general it is agreed that a protein intake of 1 g·kg^{-1}·day^{-1} may be inadequate for the diets of swimmers in training. A small increase (+0.2 g·kg^{-1}·day^{-1}) in dietary protein may be helpful during the early stages of training to support increases in muscle mass, myoglobin, enzyme activities and red blood cell formation. The optimal intake during this period may be as low as 1.2 g·kg^{-1}·day^{-1}. However, it has been suggested that weight lifters or swimmers engaging in heavy strength training may need as high as 2 g·kg^{-1}·day^{-1}, though the exact protein requirements for these athletes remain debatable.

Carbohydrates to enhance performance

Early studies demonstrated that when men ate a diet containing a normal amount of carbohydrates— about 55% of total calories—their muscles stored approximately 100 mmol glycogen per kg muscle. Diets low in carbohydrate—less than 15% of calories—resulted in storage of only 53 mmol·kg^{-1}, whereas a rich-carbohydrate diet produced a muscle glycogen content of 205 mmol·kg^{-1}. When these men were asked to exercise to exhaustion at 75% of their maximal oxygen uptake, their exercise times were proportional to the amount of glycogen present in the muscles before the test. Carbohydrate in the diet has a direct influence on muscle glycogen stores and the ability to train and compete in endurance events.

As shown in Fig. 5.1, athletes who train intensely and eat low-carbohydrate diets (40% of total calories) often experience a day-to-day decline in muscle glycogen. When the same subjects consume high-carbohydrate diets (70% of total calories) of equal total caloric content, muscle glycogen replacement is nearly complete within the 22 h separating the training bouts. In addition, the swimmers perceived the training as much less difficult when muscle

glycogen was maintained than when it was lowered with training.

When swimmers eat only as much food as they desire, *ad libitum*, they often underestimate their caloric needs, failing to consume enough carbohydrate to compensate for that used during training or competition. This discrepancy between glycogen use and carbohydrate intake may explain, in part, why some swimmers become chronically fatigued and need 48 h or longer to recover completely from an exhaustive workout. It is suggested that individuals who train intensely on successive days should consume a diet rich in carbohydrates.

Since simple and complex carbohydrates are digested at different rates, one might anticipate differences in the rate and quantity of glycogen formation following their intake. Tests of this theory, however, are inconclusive. Men who were fed diets composed principally of either simple sugars or starches (70% of calories) for 2 days following exhaustive exercise revealed no significant difference in muscle glycogen formation for the two diets, although there was a trend toward greater glycogen storage when the men consumed starch. Recent studies, on the other hand, have shown that simple carbohydrates facilitate glycogen storage to a greater extent than do complex carbohydrates. In light of these conflicting reports, the preferential use of either simple or complex carbohydrates for muscle glycogen

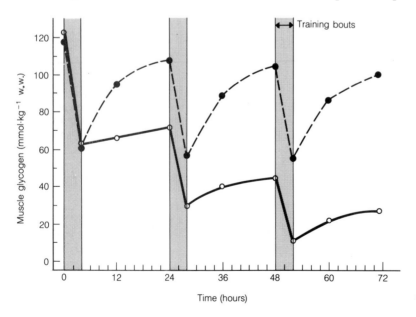

Fig. 5.1 Muscle glycogen content of the vastus lateralis (thigh) during 3 successive days of heavy training (2-h sessions) with diets whose caloric compositions were 40% carbohydrate (○) and 70% carbohydrate (●). From Costill & Miller (1980).

replacement is unclear, but probably does not have any practical importance.

In the preceding discussion we have established that different diets can markedly influence muscle glycogen stores and that the endurance needed for hard training depends on the muscle's glycogen content. While loading the muscles with extra quantities of glycogen may be valuable to the marathon runner, this process has been shown to have only minimal influence on performance in swimming events which last for less than a few minutes. Muscle glycogen depletion is not a common cause for fatigue and exhaustion in most swimming events, since normal levels may be adequate for the relatively short events of competitive swimming.

In order to insure an adequate muscle glycogen content before a major swimming competition, it is suggested that the swimmer should simply reduce the training intensity and eat a carbohydrate-rich diet in the 48−72 h before competition. This plan results in muscle glycogen values that are nearly twice those seen in untrained individuals — quite sufficient for any major competitive event.

Summary

It is generally agreed that nutrition can influence the swimmer's performance in training and competition. The preceding discussion has examined the essential nutrients. It was concluded that the optimum diet for swimmers, as for nonswimmers, must contain adequate quantities of water, calories, proteins, fats, carbohydrates, minerals, and vitamins in the proper proportions. A well balanced diet appears to provide the basis for energy production during swimming. Current evidence has shown that swimmers can perform well on a vegetarian diet, providing they make a careful selection of foods containing a balance of the essential amino acids, and adequate sources of vitamin A, riboflavin, vitamin B_{12}, vitamin D, calcium, iron, and sufficient calories. Finally, the precontest meal and feedings between events should be light, taken at least 2 h prior to the contest, and should be composed of foods that are easily digested. A liquid precontest meal appears to have many advantages over solid food.

Does food have special ergogenic qualities, or can you alter what you eat to improve performance? While it appears that most swimmers consume sufficient quantities of protein, fat, and carbohydrate, additional supplementation has little additional benefit. There is, however, evidence to indicate that carbohydrate loading can increase the storage of muscle glycogen, which may be helpful during periods of intensified training, or when the swimmer must compete in multiple events over several days. Various vitamins and minerals have been proposed as ergogenic aids. From the available research, it appears that the B-complex vitamins, and vitamins C and E, may have ergogenic properties, but the evidence is not conclusive.

Recommended reading

Bergström, J., Hermansen, L., Hultman, E. & Saltin, B. (1967) Diet, muscle glycogen, and physical performance. *Acta Physiol. Scand.* **71**:140−150.

Costill, D.L., Hinrichs, D., Fink, W.J. & Hoopes, D. (1988) Muscle glycogen depletion during swimming interval training. *J. Swim. Res.* **4**:15−18.

Costill, D.L. & Miller, J. (1980) Nutrition for endurance sport: carbohydrate and fluid balance. *Int. J. Sports Med.* **1**:2−14.

Dairy Council Digest (1980) *Nutr. Hum. Perform.* **51**:13−17.

Farrell, P.M. & Bieri, J.G. (1975) Megavitamin E supplementation in man. *Am. J. Clin. Nutr.* **28**:1381−1385.

Foster, C., Costill, D.L. & Fink, W.J. (1979) Effects of preexercise feedings on endurance performance. *Med. Sci. Sports* **11**:1−5.

Haymes, E.M. (1983) Proteins, vitamins, and iron. In Williams, M.H. (ed.) *Ergogenic Aids in Sport.* Champaign, Illinois: Human Kinetics, pp. 27−55.

Ivy, J.L., Costill, D.L., Fink, W.J. & Lower, R.W. (1979) Influence of caffeine and carbohydrate feedings on endurance performance. *Med. Sci. Sports* **11**:6−11.

Piehl, K. (1974) Time course for refilling of glycogen stores in human muscle fibers following exercise-induced glycogen depletion. *Acta Physiol. Scand.* **90**:297−302.

Sherman, W.M., Costill, D.L., Fink, W.J. & Miller, J.M. (1981) Effects of exercise−diet manipulation on muscle glycogen and its subsequent utilization during performance. *Int. J. Sports Med.* **2**:1−15.

Smith, N.J. (1976) *Food for Sport.* Palo Alto, California: Bull Publishing.

Williams, M.H. (1976) *Nutritional Aspects of Human Physical and Athletic Performance.* Springfield, Illinois: Charles C. Thomas.

Young, D.R. (1977) *Physical Performance, Fitness and Diet.* Springfield, Illinois: Charles C. Thomas.

Section 2

Mechanical Aspects

of Swimming

Chapter 6

Propulsion and resistance

Competitive swimming is a unique sport because athletes compete while suspended in a fluid medium. They propel their bodies by pushing against that fluid rather than a solid substance. The water offers less resistance to swimmers' propulsive efforts than is afforded by the solid surfaces that athletes exercise against on land. On the other hand, water offers considerably greater resistance to swimmers' forward movements because it is 1000 times more dense than air. It is no wonder, therefore, that the efficiency for swimming is lower than for any other sport.

Increasing that efficiency is as important as proper training where improving the performances of competitive swimmers is the concern. Increased efficiency can be attributed directly to the ability of swimmers to generate propulsive force while reducing the resistance of the water to their forward motion. Some of the most important factors involved in reducing resistance and increasing propulsive force will be discussed in this chapter.

Resistance

Water resists the movements of objects through it. The term used to describe the resistance of fluids is *drag*. One irrefutable rule concerning drag is that it will always be exerted opposite the direction in which the swimmers' bodies are moving. The increase in drag force has to do with the pattern of water flow around swimmers changing from laminar to turbulent.

Laminar and turbulent water flow

Water consists of molecules which tend to flow in smooth unbroken streams until they encounter some solid object that interrupts their movement. The smooth flow of water molecules has been termed

laminar while interrupted flow is called *turbulent*. The information in Table 6.1 summarizes these two characteristics of water flow.

Laminar flow has the least resistance associated with it because the water molecules are traveling in the same direction and at a uniform rate of speed. They are packed one on top of the other like laminated sheets of plywood, hence the term used to describe their pattern of flow.

When these laminar streams encounter solid objects, like swimmers' bodies, the molecules rebound wildly in all directions. Some of the water molecules will be pushed down and others up. Still others will be pushed forward. A portion of the water will be carried along with the swimmer for a short period due to friction between the water and the swimmer's body. This random motion of water molecules is an example of turbulent water flow. It is visible as white water at the surface and as air bubbles around swimmers' limbs under the water.

Water molecules that have become turbulent will intrude on other laminar streams. When they do so, they collide with the molecules in those streams, causing them to rebound in random directions as well. These random molecules then intrude on still more laminar streams in an ever-widening pattern of turbulence.

The swirling water increases the pressure in front of the swimmer relative to the pressure behind, where the flow is more laminar. This large pressure differential between front and rear is what holds swimmers back. Laminar and turbulent flow are illustrated in Fig. 6.1.

Table 6.1 Two characteristics of water flow

Laminar	Turbulent
Undisturbed streams of water molecules	Wildly mixed movements of water molecules in random directions
This type of water has the least amount of resistive drag	Characterized by white water and a large increase of resistive drag

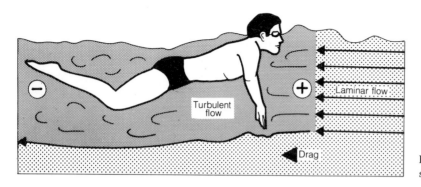

Fig. 6.1 Laminar and turbulent flow in swimming.

The drag encountered by this swimmer will be directly proportional to the amount of turbulence created. When water is mildly turbulent, only a few laminar streams are disturbed and the amount of resistive drag will be less. When the pattern of turbulence is great, a large number of laminar streams are affected and the retarding effect will be greater.

Turbulence, once it has been created, will continue downstream until laminar flow is re-established, which occurs some distance behind the section of water through which the swimmer is passing. Swimmers must open "holes" in the water for their bodies to go through. These holes do not fill in immediately after the body has passed through them. Accordingly, the area behind swimmers becomes a

kind of partial vacuum where only a small number of water molecules are swirling wildly. These whirling molecules, called *eddy currents*, have been indicated by the swirling water around the swimmers' legs in Fig. 6.1. Even though they are turbulent, the pressure of eddy currents is low because only a small number of water molecules are swirling. In effect, swimmers are being pushed back by the high pressure area in front of their bodies and pulled back by the low pressure area behind them.

The area of eddy currents will be larger and require longer to fill in when the pattern of turbulence is great. Consequently, the retarding effect on the swimmer's forward speed will be greater. Conversely, when the pattern of turbulence is less the area where eddy currents are present will fill in more rapidly.

The effect of size, shape and speed on resistive drag

There are three factors that determine the amount of resistance swimmers encounter. They are:
1 the space they take up in the water;
2 the shape they present to the water;
3 their speed of movement.
Descriptions of each have been provided in the next few sections.

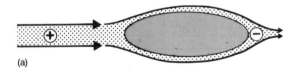

(a)

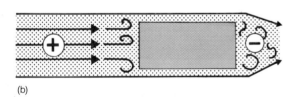

(b)

Fig. 6.2 The effect of shape on resistive drag. The object in (a) has a good shape for moving through the water; it is tapered at both ends. The shape of the object in (b) is not good. It has too many square corners that interrupt the backward flow of water.

The effect of shape

A tapered shape will produce the least amount of drag in the water (Fig. 6.2). Both of the objects in this figure have exactly the same surface area but one is tapered at both ends while the other is rectangular.

The object in Fig. 6.2a, because it is tapered at

both ends, allows the direction of water molecules to change gradually as they pass around it. This results in only a small amount of turbulence being created. The tapered front end causes a minimum of disturbance to the water flow because the molecules closest to the object can slide around it. Although they will be pushed to the side somewhat, they are able to continue moving forward as the object becomes progressively wider. Consequently, they disturb only a small number of adjacent streams and the pattern of turbulence is minimized. The tapered rear end diminishes the area of eddy currents behind the object by allowing the water to fill in quickly.

The rectangular shaped object in Fig. 6.2b presents a large, flat surface to the streams of water molecules in front of it. These molecules cannot change directions gradually or continue to move forward around the object. Instead, they rebound away in random directions when they come in contact with the flat surface. This causes them to intrude on a large number of adjacent streams, producing a wide pattern of turbulence that greatly increases the pressure in front of the object. The square rear end of the object keeps the streams separated for a longer time after passage of the object. This creates a larger area of eddy currents, considerably reducing the pressure behind the object. Consequently, the increased pressure differential between the front and rear of the rectangular object will exert a much greater retarding effect on its forward motion.

The shapes of boats, cars, airplanes and other objects that travel through air and water have evolved over the years into tapered shapes like the one in Fig. 6.2a. Unfortunately, the bodies of swimmers cannot remain in a static bullet-shaped position as they move through the water. They change positions constantly, presenting a variety of different shapes to the oncoming water flow. In comparison to slower swimmers, faster swimmers maintain the most streamlined shape possible as they assume these various positions. Ways to streamline swimmers' bodies will be discussed later in this chapter.

The effect of space (size)

Drag will be increased when swimmers take up more space in the water because they interrupt the flow of a greater number of water molecules. The space they occupy has both horizontal and lateral components. The horizontal component concerns the depth of their bodies. Swimmers disrupt fewer streams when they remain nearly level from head to feet. The lateral component refers to the space they occupy from side to side. Swimmers who wiggle from side to side will interrupt more streams of water than those who do not.

The effect of horizontal alignment is illustrated in Fig. 6.3. The two swimmers are exactly the same size but their bodies are oriented differently to the water so that the bottom swimmer takes up more space than the top one. The top swimmer is horizontal and streamlined. As you can see, he moves through a much smaller column of water than the bottom swimmer. That swimmer's body position is inclined downward from front to rear so that he encounters a much larger column of water as he moves forward. The bottom swimmer will encounter more drag simply because he must push his body forward against more water. With few exceptions, swimmers should try to remain as horizontal as possible when they move through the water.

The need to create large propulsive forces does not permit athletes to stay perfectly horizontal as they swim down the pool, however. As mentioned earlier, their body positions are constantly changing throughout each stroke cycle. Freestyle and backstroke swimmers must roll their bodies from side to side to gain propulsive force while breaststroke and

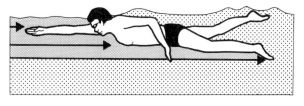

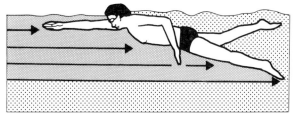

Fig. 6.3 The effect of the space objects take up in the water on resistive drag.

butterfly swimmers need to move their bodies up and down in an undulating manner for the same reason. Even though these motions increase drag, they increase propulsion to a greater extent. Consequently, to swim fast, athletes must balance the need to stay horizontal with the need to apply propulsive force. Swimmers can move their bodies around too much in their desire to apply propulsion and, by doing so, increase drag relatively more than they increase propulsion. By the same token, overdoing their attempts to remain horizontal can reduce propulsion more than it reduces drag. Suggestions for striking the proper balance between these two aspects of swimming propulsion have been provided in the chapters on each competitive stroke.

The effect of speed

The other major factor that influences drag is the speed of swimmers through the water. The effect of speed on drag may seem academic since it would be foolish for an athlete to swim slowly and lose races simply to reduce resistive drag. However, this effect does apply to competitive swimming. It demonstrates the wisdom of pacing races. An athlete who swims the first half of a race at a slower speed than an opponent will not be required to expend as much energy to overcome drag. If swimmers are nearly equal in ability, the one who paces the early part of the race may be able to win by finishing faster than a more fatigued competitor.

Types of drag

Experts have defined three categories of drag that affect swim performance. They are *form*, *wave* and *frictional drag*.

As its names implies, form drag is caused by the form or orientation of swimmers' bodies to the water they are moving through. It is a function of both the space swimmers take up in the water and the shapes their bodies assume. Wave drag is caused by waves that swimmers create and frictional drag is due to the contact between the swimmers' skin and water molecules. These three categories of drag are described in the following sections.

Form drag

As the name implies, this category of resistive drag is a result of the *forms* that swimmers' bodies take while moving forward through the water. As mentioned, swimmers want to minimize the space they take up by remaining as horizontal as possible (except where up and down movements provide more propulsive force than resistance). They should orient their bodies so that all contours taper gradually backward while presenting the smallest possible surface area to the water in front. They should strike a compromise between kicking deep enough to propel their bodies forward but not so deep as to increase form drag unnecessarily. Their bodies should not wiggle from side to side, although they need to roll them from side to side to increase propulsive force. They must be conscious of good horizontal alignment in all competitive strokes and good lateral alignment in the front and back crawl strokes.

The illustrations in Fig. 6.4 contrast good and poor horizontal alignment for three of the four competitive strokes. Figure 6.5 showed the effects of good and poor horizontal alignments in the front crawl stroke.

The back crawl swimmer in the Fig. 6.4 on the right has poor horizontal alignment. She has her head too high and her hips too low. The back crawl swimmer on the left shows good horizontal alignment with his body nearly horizontal and his kick working only through the effective propulsive range. His head is maintained in a natural position although it is flexed slightly at the neck.

The butterfly and breaststroke present special cases where horizontal alignment is concerned. The effective production of propulsive forces requires a certain amount of body undulation in both strokes. While this undulation increases the frontal surface area presented to the water, the trade-off between increased drag and propulsive force is probably a good one, that is, unless swimmers undulate too much.

The breaststroke is unique. There is an ongoing controversy over the flat versus the wave style with both camps claiming their style produces the least amount of form drag. Swimmers undulate more in the wave style yet probably create less drag than flat-style swimmers. This is because they do not decelerate as much during their leg recoveries. Drag is higher in the breaststroke when swimmers are recovering their legs

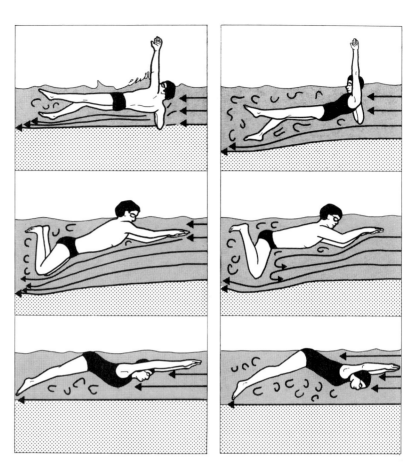

Fig. 6.4 A comparison of good and poor body positions in three of the four competitive strokes. For each stroke, the illustration on the left shows good alignment while the one on the right shows poor alignment.

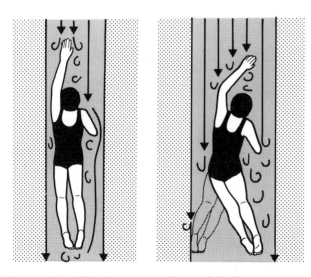

Fig. 6.5 The effect of excessive side-to-side body movements on drag in the front crawl stroke.

than during any other phase of the stroke cycle.

Figure 6.4 middle right shows a flat-style breaststroker recovering his legs. He is more horizontal than the wave-style swimmer on the left. Nevertheless, his flat position forces him to push his thighs down and forward against the water. With his hips at the surface, this is the only way he can keep his feet underwater as they recover forward. When fully recovered, his legs present a flat shape to the oncoming water that should increase drag considerably. This has been illustrated by the reversal in direction of the two streams of water molecules directly in front of the swimmers' thighs.

By lowering his hips, the wave-style swimmer on the left is able to recover his legs without flexing them at the hips. Consequently, he does not push his thighs forward and they present a more tapered shape that should produce less turbulence.

In butterfly, the swimmer on the left is undulating the desired amount to increase propulsive force while not so much as to increase form drag disproportionately. This is not true of the butterfly swimmer on the right. She is kicking too deep and driving her head down too far when her arms enter the water. Accordingly, she takes up more space in the water during this phase of the stroke and she presents a shape that is too near the perpendicular. This will reverse the flow of water causing turbulence and a large increase of form drag.

As mentioned earlier, excessive side-to-side movements of swimmers' bodies can disturb their lateral alignment in the front and back crawl strokes. Figure 6.5 shows top views of front crawl swimmers. The one on the left is streamlined while the swimmer on the right is wiggling excessively from side to side. That swimmer is entering her hand across the midline of her body which causes her hips to swing out toward that arm while her feet swing out in the opposite direction. These side-to-side movements will increase the turbulence around her body.

The backstroke swimmer on the right in Fig. 6.6 is also overreaching and his body will, likewise, swing from side to side. The swimmer on the left keeps her body aligned laterally by not overreaching on the entry and also by rolling her body from side to side.

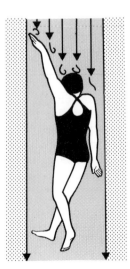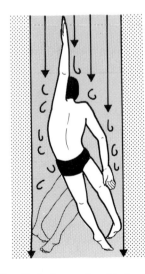

Fig. 6.6 Underneath view of the effect of excessive side-to-side body movements on resistive drag in the back crawl stroke.

Body roll

Rolling from side to side can reduce the tendency for the bodies of front crawl and backstroke swimmers to come out of lateral alignment. Early swimming experts mistakenly believed that swimmers would encounter less drag by maintaining their body in a flat position at the surface. That seemed a logical conclusion, except for the fact that swimmers in the front and back crawl strokes really don't have a choice between rolling and swimming flat. Their choice is to roll or wiggle. This is because, in both strokes, one arm is always sweeping down through the water while the other is traveling up. Swimmers' bodies, because they are suspended in the water, will naturally rotate from side to side following the movements of the arms. If they try to maintain a flat body position, the competing rotational forces from their arms will thrust their suspended trunks in lateral directions and they will wiggle from side to side.

Wave drag

Turbulence at the surface of the water is the cause of this form of drag. We are all aware that some pools, because of poor construction or inadequate lane lines, have more waves than others. Waves of this origin are beyond the control of competitors and are, perhaps, negligible to the outcome (but not the time) of the race since they should affect all swimmers equally. Swimmers do have some control over the waves they produce with their movements through the water, however.

Those movements create bow waves that press back against their bodies, slowing their forward speed. Bow waves are created by the heads and trunks of swimmers as they move forward, to the side or up and down. They are also produced by the recovery movements of their arms and legs. Their limbs push forward against the water causing it to become turbulent. This increases the pressure in front which, in turn, produces a backward force against their bodies that reduces their forward speed rapidly and markedly.

Figure 6.7 shows one way in which the recovery movements of competitive swimmers can increase drag. The freestyle swimmer is smashing his arm into the water on the recovery. A swimmer who

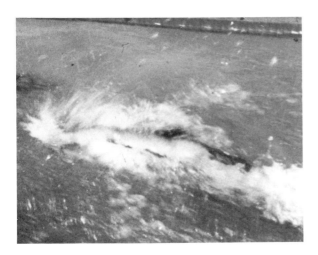

Fig. 6.7 A freestyle swimmer creating wave drag with his recovery movements.

pushes his hands and arms forward through the water in this manner will have his speed reduced by 30% within 1/16 of a second. This reduction in forward speed, when multiplied by several strokes per pool length, can have a devastating effect on performance.

Backstroke and freestyle swimmers frequently make a similar mistake when they push the backs of their hands forward during their entry into the water. It is far better for their hands to enter on their sides. This will reduce the frontal surface area presented to the water.

Frictional drag

Swimmers have practiced the ritual of shaving-down before major competitions for over three decades. During that time, experts have disagreed as to whether the reductions in time that accompanied this procedure were due to psychological, kinesthetic or physiological phenomena. Most felt that the latter explanation was the least likely of the three. There is now physiological evidence that the effect is due to a reduction in frictional drag.

Friction between swimmers' skin and the water causes them to carry some of the molecules along with them. These molecules collide with others immediately in front of them and rebound off in random directions. Those molecules intrude into adjacent streams causing a widening pattern of turbulence that increases drag.

The main factors influencing the amount of frictional drag swimmers encounter are their surface area, their velocity, and the roughness of their body surface. Swimmers have no control over surface area, and their speed can only be controlled to the extent that they pace early portions of their races. That leaves surface smoothness as the source of frictional drag most amenable to reduction.

Obviously, smooth surfaces cause less friction than rough surfaces, hence a possible reason for shaving down. Sharp and coworkers (1988; Sharp & Costill, 1989) have presented evidence suggesting this procedure does reduce frictional drag. They tested a group of swimmers before and after shaving down. There were 9 days between test periods. The swimmers completed identically paced submaximal swims during both tests. The researchers measured blood lactate concentrations to determine the effort of the paced swims. They also measured stroke length.

When shaved, the swimmers completed their paced swims with significantly lower blood lactate values and greater stroke lengths. Average blood lactate values for the group during the identically paced swims were 8.48 mmol·l^{-1} before and 6.74 mmol·l^{-1} after shaving. Average stroke length increased from 2.07 m per stroke cycle before shaving to 2.31 m per stroke cycle afterward. The increase in distance per stroke was presumed due to reduced frictional drag.

A tethered swim was used in another phase of the study by Sharp and Costill (1989). They assessed the energy cost for this test by measuring oxygen consumption during several incremental stages of work. They compared the results before and after shaving for the experimental group. Results were also compared for a group of swimmers who did not shave down between tests. The experimental group of swimmers showed similar reductions of blood lactate and increases in stroke length on the paced swims as had the swimmers in the earlier study. Members of the control group did not improve on either measure.

Although they improved on the free swims, the shaved swimmers did not reduce their energy cost during the tethered swimming tests. This would seem to rule out better kinesthetic feel for the water and, consequently, more efficient stroke mechanics as a reason for their improvements on the paced swims.

The subjects should have decreased their oxygen consumption at various work efforts during the tethered swims if they had been swimming more efficiently after shaving-down. On the other hand, since they were not moving through the water during the tethered swims, the effect of frictional drag was negligible. Thus, by a process of elimination, less frictional drag seemed to be the logical cause for the reduced effort on the paced swims after shaving-down.

In the final phase of their study, Sharp and Costill (1989) measured the rate of deceleration following a push-off for a group of swimmers before and after they shaved down. They used a special device called a velocity meter for this purpose. It measured swimmers' linear velocity by calculating the resistance to a harness device they wore as they traveled down the pool.

In this study, the swimmers pushed off the wall while wearing the harness and glided out until their velocities fell below $1 \text{ m} \cdot \text{s}^{-1}$. Their rate of decline was measured between $2 \text{ m} \cdot \text{s}^{-1}$, the usual velocity shortly after pushing off, and $1 \text{ m} \cdot \text{s}^{-1}$. The rate of decline was significantly more rapid before shaving. Apparently, the frictional drag on the swimmers' bodies was lower after shaving, consequently they did not decelerate as quickly. The results of these studies suggest that it would be wise to continue shaving-down when good performances are desired.

Propulsion

In our present state of knowledge, we do not know what laws of motion competitive swimmers apply to propel their bodies through the water. There are many theories but none have been conclusively proven. This last statement may have surprised you because many experts accept Bernoulli's theorem as the basis for swimming propulsion. Although this is certainly the prevailing theory at the moment, it is probably not the principal physical law swimmers apply to propel their bodies forward. While Bernoulli's theorem may contribute to some small extent, the primary propulsive mechanisms swimmers utilize are probably based on Newton's third law of motion. This is the law of action−reaction, which can be paraphrased as follows: *when swimmers push water*

back they will accelerate their bodies forward with a force of equal magnitude.

Perhaps the principal reason for rejecting Newton's law of action−reaction in favor of Bernoulli's theorem was the landmark study by Brown and Counsilman (1971). They showed that swimmers stroked diagonally rather than straight backward, causing us to search for another explanation for swimming propulsion. We settled on Bernoulli's theorem. Unfortunately, we misinterpreted Newton's action−reaction principle to mean that swimmers must push their arms and legs directly back in order to push water back. We failed to realize that they could accelerate water back very effectively while stroking in diagonal directions.

The basis for propulsion, according to Bernoulli's theorem, is that swimmers' hands act like foils. When water flows over them it travels faster over the knuckle side than under the palm. This in turn creates a pressure differential between the palm and knuckle sides that produces a lift force. When this lift force combines with the drag force acting on the hand they produce a resultant force that propels the swimmer's body forward.

While it is very likely that lift and resultant forces are produced when swimmers stroke diagonally, the magnitude of those forces is probably related more to the angles of attack of swimmers' hands and their resulting backward displacement of water than it is to any acceleration of fluid flow over their knuckles. If that were not the case, swimmers would have no need to angle their hands as they moved them through the water. They could simply utilize their foil shape to produce lift and resultant forces in accordance with Bernoulli's theorem. However, research and personal observations have shown that swimmers generate more propulsive force when they move their hands through the water at certain precise angles of attack (Maglischo, 1986; Maglischo et al., 1986, 1987a,b).

Figure 6.8 shows one way in which swimmers can displace water back with the diagonal sweeps of their hand. A freestyle swimmer is shown, from an underneath view, at mid-stroke, sweeping his hand in under his body. The swimmer's hand is sweeping in, back and up under his body, as indicated by the solid black arrow. (The upward direction cannot be seen due to the limitations inherent in displaying the movement in only two dimensions.) The relative flow

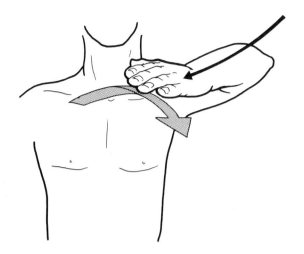

Fig. 6.8 A method for displacing water backward with diagonal stroking motions.

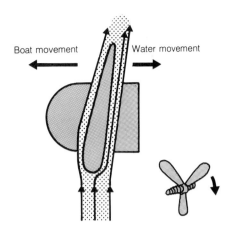

Fig. 6.9 An example of propeller propulsion.

of water takes place in the opposite direction: that is, it is traveling out, forward and down. That direction is indicated by the shaded arrow as it approaches the thumb-side of the swimmer's hand. Notice that his hand is angled (pitched) in so that the thumb-side is slightly higher than the little-finger-side. This angle causes water to be displaced back as his palm passes through it from thumb- to little-finger-sides. The backward force imparted to the water, in accordance with Newton's third law of motion, produces a counterforce of equal magnitude that should propel his body forward.

As mentioned earlier, both Bernoulli's theorem and Newton's action−reaction principle probably contribute to swimming propulsion. The role played by the latter physical law is probably considerably greater, however. Bernoulli's theorem is a needlessly complex method for describing the production of propulsive forces (Koehler, 1987). On the other hand, the concept of using sculling motions to displace water back and propel the body forward is much easier to comprehend and probably describes more accurately the most important propulsive mechanisms used by swimmers. It is not unlike the way that rotating propellers accelerate boats forward.

Outboard motors make use of a rotating propeller that has two or three blades inclined back from their leading to trailing edges: an example is shown in Fig. 6.9. Although they rotate in circular paths, the leading edge of each blade can displace water back as it passes through from leading to trailing edges. In doing so, the propeller can drive a boat forward. Notice from Fig. 6.9 how the angle of the propeller blade imparts a backward force to the water passing underneath it. This produces the counterforce that propels the boat forward.

Swimmers seem to use their hands like rotating propeller blades within a single armstroke. Their hands form a new blade each time they change directions.

Figure 6.10 shows a front crawl swimmer using her hands and arms like rotating propeller blades. In (a), she sweeps her hand and arm in under her body at mid-stroke. This motion is like the sweep of one of the blades on the rotating propeller shown. She "changes blades" in (b) by changing the direction and orientation of her hand as she sweeps it out and up during the final third of her underwater armstroke. The probable reason why swimmers change the directions their hands are moving two or more times during each underwater armstroke is probably related to the concept that more propulsion can be gained by accelerating slow-moving water backward. Once the swimmer accelerates water back it gains momentum and she must accelerate the speed of her hands to continue pushing against that water. At some point the energy required to accelerate the water back will become counterproductive. Consequently, once she has accelerated the water back sufficiently with one sculling motion, she changes the direction her hand is

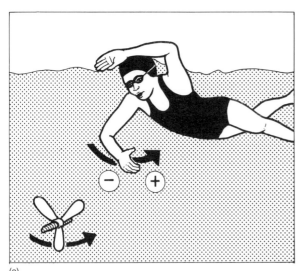

(a)

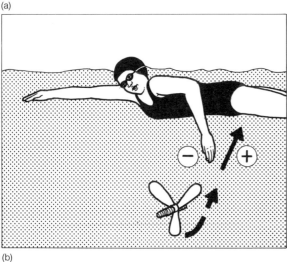

(b)

Fig. 6.10 Similarities between the hand movements of swimmers and the rotating blades of a propeller. (a) The swimmer is sweeping her hand in, up and back. (b) She is now sweeping her hand out, up and back.

moving so that a new leading edge can penetrate different and previously undisturbed streams of water molecules.

She gains at least two advantages from doing this. The first is that she does not need to use as much force to accelerate her limbs since the water she is pushing against was not moving initially. The second advantage is that she can increase the length of the propulsive phases of her strokes.

Direction, angle of attack, and velocity

There are three very important aspects of limb movements that determine the effectiveness of swimming propulsion—direction, angle of attack, and velocity. These are summarized in Table 6.2. An understanding of swimming propulsion requires a thorough knowledge of their effects.

Limb direction

The best way to visualize the direction of the propelling movements swimmers make with their arms and legs is through stroke patterns. These patterns can be expressed in two ways—relative to the water and relative to the swimmer's body. Patterns drawn relative to the water help us understand how the movements of swimmers' limbs affect the movement of water. They provide the most accurate representation because, in the final analysis, it is the effect swimmers' limbs exert on the direction of water flow that determines the amount of propulsive force they can produce.

The second way to depict stroke patterns is relative to swimmers' moving bodies. Patterns drawn in this manner are good for teaching stroke mechanics. They provide an excellent vehicle for communicating the directions of stroking motions to swimmers. Athletes tend to visualize their stroking motions relative to their bodies. Consequently, they will learn faster when the motions are presented in this way. For now, we'll concentrate on patterns that were drawn relative to the water because they can communicate the mechanisms of propulsion best.

Front, side and underneath patterns for the four competitive strokes are shown in Fig. 6.11. These

Table 6.2 Three aspects of limb movement that are important to swimming propulsion

1 Direction: determined from stroke patterns

2 Angle of attack: determined from the inclination of swimmers' hands and feet

3 Velocity: determined from hand and foot speeds

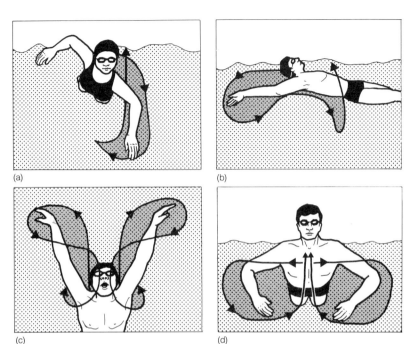

Fig. 6.11 Armstroke patterns for the four competitive strokes that have been drawn relative to the water. (a) Front view of the front crawl stroke; (b) side view of the backstroke; (c) underneath view of the butterfly; (d) front view of the breaststroke.

patterns were drawn from films of world-class athletes while they were swimming at competition speeds. The patterns shown describe, for one underwater armstroke, the movements of the swimmer's middle finger relative to a fixed point in the pool.

Notice that in all four competitive strokes, the swimmers' hands are traveling in predominantly lateral and vertical directions. Obviously, world-class swimmers would not be using these sculling motions if they were not propulsive. As you can see from the side views, there is also some backward motion in these stroke patterns. The backward movements are probably needed to insure that optimum amounts of water are displaced back. We can learn the directions the limbs should move in each competitive style by studying the similarities in the stroke patterns of world-class swimmers.

Angle of attack

The angle of attack is the angle formed by the inclination of the hand and arm (or leg and foot) to the direction it is moving. A two-dimensional angle of attack for the hand of a freestyle swimmer is shown from a side view in Fig. 6.12. He is completing the

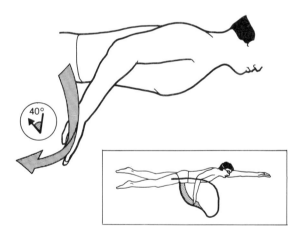

Fig. 6.12 Side view of a freestyle swimmer showing how the angle of attack of the hand is measured during the final sweep of the hand up to the surface.

final upward sweep of his hand to the surface. His hand is traveling up and back. It is also pitched up, from fingertips to wrist, at an angle of approximately 40°.

The hands, when used in this manner, can be likened to hydrofoils to understand the forces they create. The motions of foils through fluids are identified by their leading and trailing edges. In the example shown in Fig. 6.12, the wrist edge of the swimmer's hands is the leading edge because it is the first part to encounter undisturbed streams of water as it sweeps up. The little-finger-side is the trailing edge because it is the last part of the hand-foil to have contact with the water it passes through. Identifying these edges is important in understanding how swimmers displace water back with their stroking movements. While the palm and rear portion of the arm are always the underside of the hand-foil in swimming propulsion, the leading edge can be the fingertips, wrist, thumb-side or little-finger-side at various times during the underwater armstrokes of the four competitive styles. In certain cases, as in Fig. 6.12, the elbow can also serve as the leading edge.

Unfortunately, angles of attack can only be shown in two dimensions. Consequently, the 40° angle of inclination shown in Fig. 6.12 does not represent the three-dimensional angle of attack the swimmer is actually using during this phase of the stroke. The direction of motion and the inclination of the hand must be assessed from two views that encompass all three planes of motion before an accurate angle of attack can be calculated.

The angle of attack has great significance to the production of propulsive forces. Propulsion will be diminished if it is too great or too small. Information gained from studying foils suspended in wind tunnels supports this observation. Figure 6.13 shows why propulsive forces increase or decrease with changing angles of attack. Swimmers' hands have been sub-stituted for airfoils to show the application of this information to swimming propulsion. The hands are shown from an underneath view as though they were sweeping in under a swimmer's body at mid-stroke. The hands are sweeping in with angles of attack of 0, 40, 70 and 90°.

The amount of lift force is minimal when the angle of attack is 0°. This is because, as shown in Fig. 6.13, swimmers' hands pass through the water without displacing it back to any great extent. Consequently, there is only a small counterforce to propel them forward. This is shown by the small pressure dif-ferential between the palm and knuckle sides of the swimmer's hand. Propulsive force is increased con-siderably when the angle of attack approaches 40°.

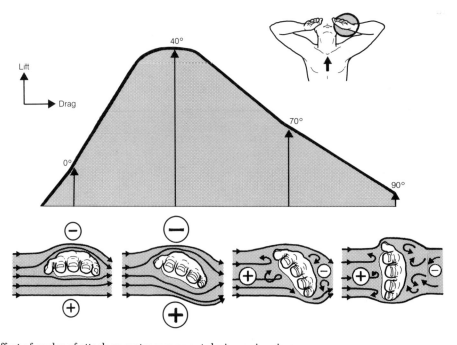

Fig. 6.13 The effect of angles of attack on water movement during swimming.

At this angle, a considerable amount of backward force is imparted to the water as it passes under the swimmer's palm from the leading (thumb-side) to trailing (little-finger-side) edges. This angle of attack is probably very close to the ideal that swimmers should use when sweeping their hands under their bodies.

Propulsive force is again reduced considerably when the angle of attack approaches the perpendicular. The palm presents a surface that is too flat when it is pitched at 70°. Consequently, the effect of the leading edge is lost as water strikes the palm in many places at once. This causes the speed of some water molecules to be slowed in their trip under the palm while other molecules rebound back. In both cases, they collide with the molecules behind them, setting off a chain reaction that creates a large amount of turbulence. In addition, the layer of water molecules passing over the top of the hand will break away and become turbulent. These molecules cannot make the large change of direction required to follow the contour of the hand from leading to trailing edges when the angle of attack is so near the perpendicular. Only a small amount of water will be displaced back as a result of this random turbulence.

The effect is even more devastating when the hand is perpendicular to its direction of movement. In this case, the hand acts like a paddle. There is no leading or trailing edge, only the large flat surface of the palm pushing several streams of water molecules to the side simultaneously. When the hand is moving fast this action is like throwing a bucket of water against a wall. That is, some of the molecules will squirt wildly away from the hand in random directions. A good portion of those remaining will have their motion reversed, causing a counterforce that will push the swimmer's body to the side in the opposite direction.

This angle of attack can be effective for propulsive purposes when swimmers' hands are traveling back. Indeed, this is the principal method some swimmers use to propel their bodies. It is not the method preferred by world-class athletes, however. If it were, their stroke patterns would show more backward motion and less movement in lateral and vertical directions.

It should be clear from the previous discussion that swimmers should use angles of attack that are between 20 and 60° during most phases of their underwater armstrokes (and perhaps during kicking).

The meaning of air bubbles behind the hands and feet

Many coaches have noticed that world-class swimmers have fewer air bubbles around their limbs when they stroke than do swimmers of lesser achievement. Air bubbles indicate turbulence and a concomitant loss of propulsive force. They signal that swimmers are using the wrong combination of direction and angle of attack in a particular phase of a stroke.

It is normal for air bubbles to appear around the hands and arms of all swimmers between the entry and catch positions of the butterfly, backstroke and front crawl. However, when this turbulence remains after the propulsive phases of the strokes begin, it suggests that swimmers are stroking incorrectly. Most likely they are probably using an angle of attack that is almost perpendicular to the directions their hands are moving. In other words, the swimmers are using their hands like paddles rather than propellers. In order to correct the problem, they must change the direction their limbs are moving, their angles of attack, or both.

Although it is interesting to speculate concerning the optimum angles of attack for swimming propulsion, the concept may be more academic than practical. As you have seen, swimmers stroke in semi-circular patterns. Consequently, they must adjust the orientation of their hands each time they change directions so the most effective angles of attack can be maintained during each phase of the underwater armstrokes. Accordingly, the swimmers' sensation is one of constantly changing angles of attack, even though they may simply be rotating their hands to attain the same angle in a new direction that was used during a previous stroke phase.

The final component of propulsive force, the speed or velocity of limb movements, will be discussed below.

Limb velocity

Counsilman and Wasilak (1982) were the first to investigate the relationship between limb velocity and swimming speed. They made us aware that the best swimmers accelerated their hands from the beginning to the end of their underwater armstrokes. Later research by Schleihauf (1984) showed that this concept was accurate but oversimplified. The swimmers did not accelerate their hands steadily from start to finish. Rather, hand speed was accelerated in pulses, decreasing and then increasing with each major change of direction during the underwater armstroke.

A typical hand velocity pattern is shown for a freestyle swimmer in Fig. 6.14. The velocities displayed are those taking place in diagonal directions during the underwater stroke of the swimmer's right hand. As such, they are three-dimensional, having backward, sideward, upward and downward components. They should be interpreted as representing hand velocity in any single direction, such as backward or upward. The tip the swimmer's middle finger was used as the reference for hand velocity. He was swimming 50 yards at 100-yard speed.

The curved line at the top of Fig. 6.14 shows the changing hand velocities throughout one underwater stroke cycle. The speed of the left hand decreases after entry until it is traveling only 1.8 m·s^{-1} (6 feet·s^{-1}) at the catch. Hand velocity increases to 3 m·s^{-1} (10 feet·s^{-1}) during the first propulsive sweep, as his hand comes under his body. This is followed by another increase to 5 m·s^{-1} (8 feet·s^{-1}) while he sweeps his hand toward the surface. His left hand then decelerates as he releases pressure on the water and slides it out into the recovery.

His right hand, which entered the water earlier, sweeps down to the catch with its velocity decreasing to 1.8 m·s^{-1}. It then accelerates to 4 m·s^{-1} while he sweeps it in under his body. It decelerates slightly to 3.4 m·s^{-1} during the transition to the next propulsive sweep. His hand then accelerates to a maximum velocity of nearly 6 m·s^{-1} (17 feet·s^{-1}) during this sweep. Notice that accelerations and decelerations of his forward speed correspond very closely to these changes in hand velocities.

This hand velocity pattern is representative of patterns used in the remaining three competitive strokes. In all cases, the swimmers accelerate and decelerate their hand in pulses corresponding to each major change of direction during the stroke cycle. They slow during each change of direction and then accelerate throughout the succeeding movement. The maximum velocities attained by the hands are dependent upon the swimming speed.

There is probably a precise relationship between hand speed and angle of attack that should be used during each phase of the four underwater armstrokes. Apparently, swimmers consciously maintain some submaximal hand velocity until the final portion of the armstroke. The fact that the swimmer in Fig. 6.14 accelerates his hand speed to only 3 m·s^{-1} during the sweep under his body provides support for the concept of optimal hand velocities. He was obviously capable of accelerating it to velocities of 6 m·s^{-1} or

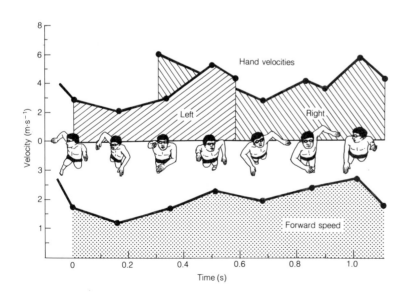

Fig. 6.14 A typical hand velocity pattern for the front crawl stroke.

more, as indicated by the final propulsive sweep. This means that he chose intuitively to use some optimum, rather than maximum, hand velocity at mid-stroke.

Importance of the catch to swimming propulsion

The catch is that point in the underwater armstroke where propulsion begins. Most swimmers mistakenly believe that it should take place immediately after their hands enter the water or, in the case of breaststroke, immediately after they begin sweeping out. This belief has resulted in perhaps the most common stroke problem in competitive swimming—the dropped elbow.

Actually, in all strokes, the catch is made when the arms are approximately one-third of the way through their underwater stroke. Swimmers require this length of time to get their arms in position to displace water backward.

Figure 6.15 shows when swimmers begin to apply propulsive force during the front crawl. The swimmer is Matt Biondi, winner of five gold medals in the 1988 Olympic Games and world record holder for 100-m freestyle. The graph shows the propulsive force being produced during one underwater armstroke. That force is expressed in kilograms on the vertical axis. Time in tenths of a second is displayed on the horizontal axis. A side-view stroke pattern is also supplied at the top of the graph. That pattern is marked in tenths of a second so you can compare the phase of the armstroke to the propulsive force being produced. The calculations were made from film when Biondi was swimming at 100-m speed.

The graph demonstrates that he does not begin to apply propulsive force with his right arm for approximately 0.30 s after it has entered the water. At that time, he has completed approximately one-third of his underwater armstroke.

Swimmers follow a similar plan in the other competitive strokes. They wait until their arms are sufficiently deep enough to press back against the water. Coaches frequently refer to this position of the arms as having a high elbow, because swimmers' elbows are always above their hands when it is attained. Swimmers should not attempt to apply propulsive force until their arms are in this high-elbow position. Any attempt to do so will only reduce their forward speed. Their arms will be facing out or down instead of back and they will not be able to

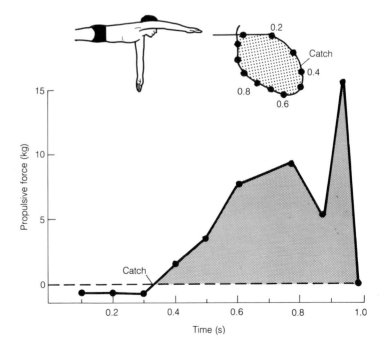

Fig. 6.15 A propulsive force graph for the front crawl stroke. The subject is Matt Biondi, world record holder and 1988 Olympic gold medallist in the 50- and 100-m freestyle. He is swimming at 100-m speed. The method for calculating propulsive force was that developed by Schleihauf *et al.* (1988).

displace water backwards. In turn, this will waste effort and decelerate their forward speed. Photos of high-elbow catch positions will be shown for each stroke in the following chapters.

The four sweeps common to all competitive strokes

After studying films and video tapes for several years it became clear that the propulsive arm movements of competitive swimmers could be reduced to four basic sweeps. The rules governing a particular stroke sometimes cause these sweeps to appear different from one to the next because the swimmers' arms must travel in somewhat different directions. However, when the manner in which they displace water back is examined, the nature of certain sweeps are remarkably similar from one stroke to the next. The purpose of this section will be to describe how these basic sweeps can be used to displace water backward in each competitive stroke.

The four basic arm sweeps have been termed outsweep, downsweep, insweep and upsweep. Their functions are summarized in Table 6.3. A description of each has been provided in the following sections.

Outsweep

The outsweep is the initial underwater movement in the breaststroke and butterfly. The underneath view in Fig. 6.16 shows a butterfly swimmer completing this sweep. It is not a propulsive movement but instead is used to move swimmers' hands and arms into position for the catch where the first propulsive sweep begins.

Table 6.3 Four basic arms sweeps used by competitive swimmers

---

1 Outsweep: the initial underwater sweep in the butterfly and breaststroke

2 Downsweep: the initial underwater sweep used in the front crawl and backstroke

3 Insweep: the second sweep used in all competitive strokes

4 Upsweep: the final sweep of the front crawl and butterfly

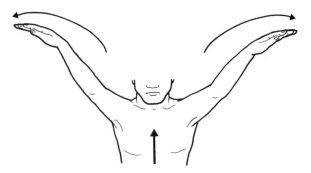

Fig. 6.16 The outsweep.

The outsweep is performed in the following manner. Immediately after their hands enter the water in butterfly (and during the last portion of the underwater recovery in breaststroke), swimmers sweep their arms out in a curvilinear path until they are outside the width of their shoulders where the catch is made. The palms of their hands should be facing down as the outsweep begins and they remain in this position until the movement is nearly completed. In this way, the hands can be slipped through the water at an angle of attack near 0° until the arms are in position to apply propulsive force. The palms should be rotated out and back as the arms near the end of the outsweep, so they are pitched out and back at the catch.

Swimmers' hand velocities decelerate after the entry until they are barely moving at the catch. The first propulsive sweep, the insweep, follows the outsweep in butterfly and breaststroke.

Downsweep

Front crawl swimmers use the downsweep (Fig. 6.17) to begin their underwater armstrokes. It is also used by backstrokers who favor a deep catch. Both swimmers in Fig. 6.17 are at the catch position following the downsweep of their respective strokes.

Like the outsweep, the downsweep is not a propulsive movement. Its major purpose is to position the hand and arm for the propulsive sweeps that follow.

The downsweep is executed as follows. After entering the water, the hand should be directed down in a curvilinear path that ends with a catch. The wrist

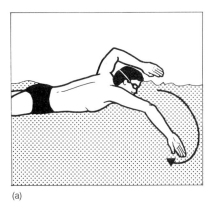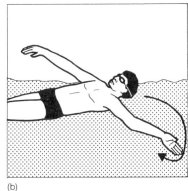

Fig. 6.17 The downsweep in (a) front crawl, and (b) backstroke.

(a)   (b)

should be flexed to initiate the downsweep followed by flexion at the elbow so the water is behind the arm and hand at the catch. The hand should be rotated slightly out and back as it travels toward the catch. The catch should be made when the elbow is above the hand, not before. The hand will be approximately 40–60 cm (15–24 in) deep at that time.

A word of caution should be voiced here. Stroke patterns show that the hand also slides out during the downsweep. Swimmers should not emphasize this direction, however. It is a byproduct of shoulder roll and will occur naturally. It is easy to overdo this facet of the movement if it is stressed.

Hand speed should decelerate gradually from the entry until, as with the outsweep, the hand is barely moving at the catch.

Insweep

The insweep follows the downsweep in freestyle and backstroke. It follows the outsweep in butterfly and breaststroke. It is the first major propulsive sweep in all of the competitive strokes, except the backstroke. In that stroke, the corresponding movement is termed an upsweep because swimmers are supine and their arm moves upward more than inward during this motion. Nevertheless, the manner in which propulsion is generated during the upsweep of the backstroke is identical to the insweep in all respects but direction. The way that water can be displaced during this sweep was described earlier, and illustrated in Fig. 6.8.

The insweep begins at the catch. From that point, swimmers sweep their hands down, in, and then up until the hands are under their bodies at or slightly beyond the midline.

Their arms, which were flexed slightly at the elbows when the catch was made, continue bending during this sweep until they are flexed nearly 90° at the end of the insweep. Their palms are gradually rotated in throughout the sweep until they are pitched in and up when it has been completed. Swimmers' hands should accelerate smoothly, but moderately, from the catch to the end of the insweep.

Underwater films show that some world-class freestyle swimmers sweep their hands beyond the midlines of their bodies. Other swimmers with equally impressive times sweep their hands in only to the midline while still others barely sweep their hands under their bodies at all. There are two possible explanations why swimmers use these differing insweep styles. The first may be that some use the insweep more effectively than others. These swimmers sweep their hands to the midline or beyond because they can generate a great deal of propulsive force for a long period of time during this movement. Conversely, those swimmers who do not gain very much propulsive from this movement may intuitively abbreviate the insweep so they can move on to a more propulsive motion.

The second reason some swimmers sweep their hands under their bodies more than others may have to do with the width of their hands at the beginning of the insweep. Swimmers who have their hands well outside shoulder width when the insweep begins may utilize the sweep over an adequate distance before their hand reaches the midline. On the other hand, swimmers who begin the insweep with their hand inside the width of their shoulders may have to sweep across the midline to utilize the full propulsive potential of this movement.

This same information applies to butterfly and breaststroke swimmers. Some butterflyers sweep their hands into the midline while other do not. Although all breaststroke swimmers sweep their hands into the midline, some release pressure on the water before their hands travel in very far, while others apply force until their hands are almost together. It is generally a good idea to teach swimmers to sweep their hands into the midline. All swimmers should not be forced to stroke in this way, if it does not seem to be beneficial.

The ways that breaststroke and butterfly swimmers execute the insweep will be described in the chapters on those strokes. The corresponding movement in the backstroke, the upsweep, will be described in the chapter where the mechanics of that stroke are discussed.

Upsweep

The upsweep follows the insweep in the front crawl and butterfly strokes. There are also corresponding movements in the backstroke which will be described in Chapter 9.

The upsweep begins at the completion of the insweep and continues until the swimmer's hand approaches the thigh. It is a semi-circular sweep of the hands, out, up and back toward the surface of the water. The hand is rotated out rapidly so it is pitched out and back during most of the upsweep. The outward angle of attack can best be seen from Fig. 6.18b. The upsweep ends when the swimmer's hand approaches the thigh. At that point, the swimmer releases pressure on the water and rotates the palm inward as the recovery begins.

Hand speed slows during the transition from insweep to upsweep. It is then accelerated rapidly throughout the remainder of this motion. Swimmers' hands generally reach their fastest speeds near the end of this sweep.

There is a misconception that the arm is also extended rapidly at the elbow during the upsweep. Actually, the amount of extension is moderate with the arm remaining flexed at the elbow throughout the propulsive phase of this motion. This probably permits the forearm to participate in displacing water backward. If the arm was extended too rapidly, it would be pushing up against the water at too great an angle of attack. It is only after pressure on the water is released and the recovery begins that some swimmers extend their elbows.

Butterfly swimmers should execute the upsweep in a similar manner to freestylers. Contrary to popular belief, they do not extend their arms completely during this motion either. Some extend their arms, but only during the first portion of the recovery.

The success of the upsweep is, in large part, due to swimmers' ability to keep the hands hyperextended at the wrists during the final portion of this movement. If

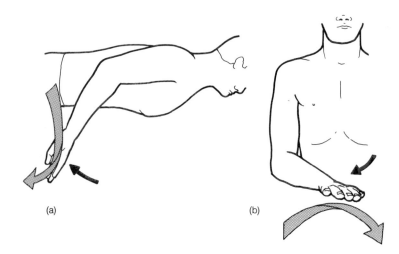

(a)   (b)

Fig. 6.18 The upsweep as used in the front crawl stroke. (a) Side and (b) underneath views show how water can be displaced back by the out-and-up sweep of the hand during this phase of the underwater armstroke.

they do this, they can displace water back with the palm even after the orientation of the forearms is no longer adequate for this purpose. This is particularly true of butterfly swimmers. One of the most common mistakes swimmers make during this sweep is to push the hand up and back toward a flexed position. When they do this the hand has a nearly perpendicular orientation to the water. At this angle of attack the hand will push water up rather than back and forward speed will be reduced. Swimmers should be coached to keep their hand facing back as long as possible during the upsweep.

Figure 6.18 illustrates how water can be displaced back during the upsweep. The wrist and little-finger-side of the hands are the leading edge and the thumb-side and fingertips the trailing edge during the upsweep because the hand is moving up and out in a diagonal path. Two views of this movement have been displayed to aid readers in comprehending the three-dimensional nature of the propulsive movements.

The underneath view (Fig. 6.18b) shows how water can be displaced back in the first portion of the upsweep, as the swimmer's hand is coming out from underneath his body. He sweeps it out and back in the direction of the solid black arrow. His hand is pitched out and back. The leading edge is the little-finger-side and the trailing edge is the thumb-side. The water, which was traveling under his palm in the opposite direction, is displaced back by the angle of attack of his hand.

The side view (Fig. 6.18a) illustrates how water can be displaced back by the final upward portion of this movement. The swimmer's arm is traveling up and back in the direction of the solid black arrow. His hand is pitched back and slightly up. The propulsive contributions of swimmers' forearms are probably more evident here than in the other sweeping movements. The leading edge of the swimmer's hand—arm-foil is probably the elbow and the trailing edge is his fingertips. The shaded arrow shows how water can be displaced back from leading to trailing edges as it passes down the underside of the swimmer's forearm and across his palm from wrist to fingertips.

The kick: propulsive or not?

Many of us believed, mistakenly, that the kick was not an important propulsive agent in the freestyle,

backstroke and butterfly strokes. The principal argument advanced was that the feet and legs were not moving back in these strokes. Consequently, the legs were thought to exert only stabilizing forces with their up-and-down kicking motions. That belief should be re-examined in light of the discovery that diagonal sweeps of the arms are propulsive.

It seems reasonable to assume that the water can be displaced back by up and down movements of the legs just as it can be displaced back by vertical movements of the arms. Figure 6.19 shows how the downbeat of the dolphin kick probably produces propulsive force during butterfly swimming. The solid black arrow depicts the direction the swimmer's feet move during the downbeat of this kick. They travel almost directly down. With his knees bent and his toes pointed up, the swimmer's lower legs take on the characteristics of a hydrofoil. His knees are the leading edge and his toes the trailing edge of that foil. Flexion at the knees provides an angle of attack that allows the anterior portions of his lower legs to displace water back in the direction of the shaded arrows as they pass down through it.

Freestyle swimmers probably propel their bodies forward in a similar manner, with the downbeats of their flutter kicks. The corresponding movement is an upbeat in the backstroke and is probably also propulsive.

Summary

The purpose of this chapter has been to describe some important concepts of swimming propulsion. The

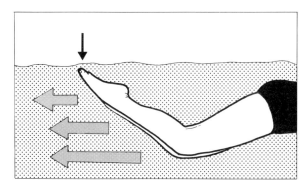

Fig. 6.19 Propulsion during the dolphin kick.

term *concepts* was used because there are no proven principles of propulsion, only theories.

In simplest terms, swimming fast is a matter of increasing propulsion while reducing the resistance of water to forward movement. *Drag* is the term commonly used when referring to water resistance.

Three categories of resistive drag have been identified. These are *form*, *wave*, and *frictional* drag. Form drag refers to the resistance to forward motion created by the space swimmers take up in the water and the shape their bodies present to the oncoming flow. In most cases, they should remain as horizontal and as tapered as possible from head to toes. Some undulating trunk movements are needed to apply propulsive force effectively in the butterfly and breaststroke. While these movements have the potential to increase form drag, they increase propulsive force relatively more, making the trade-off advantageous for increasing swimming speed. Swimmers should also roll their bodies from side to side when swimming the front and back crawl strokes. This will counteract the tendency for their bodies to swing from side to side as a result of the alternating lateral and vertical movements of their arms.

Swimmers can reduce wave drag by slicing their hands into the water while swimming the three competitive strokes where recoveries are made over the water. This technique will also reduce wave drag for breaststrokers who recover their arms over the water. Frictional drag can be reduced by shaving-down before important competitions and by wearing suits made of low-friction fabrics that are designed to fit like a second skin.

While pushing back against the water can propel swimmers forward, stroke patterns for the four competitive strokes show that they prefer to stroke diagonally. Obviously, the majority of their propulsive motions take place in lateral and vertical directions. The theory subscribed to in this text is that the most important propulsive principle they are applying is Newton's law of action—reaction, not Bernoulli's theorem. Swimmers are using their arms and legs like rotating propeller blades to displace water back with their diagonal sweeps. The term *sculling* is commonly used in reference to these diagonal movements. The term *sweep* has been used here because it expresses the nature of these movements best.

In addition to direction, two other very important aspects of propulsion are the *angle of attack*, or pitch, of the limbs and their *speed* as they sweep through the water. More water can be displaced back when swimmers rotate their hands somewhat in the direction they are moving. Propulsion will be reduced if they fail to rotate them sufficiently because water will pass by without being displaced back by any significant amount. Propulsive force will also be reduced if the hands are rotated in too much. In this case, the angle of attack will be so great that water will bounce off the limbs in random directions with very little being displaced back.

Each competitive stroke contains two or more distinct sweeping motions. That is, the hands make major changes in direction and pitch two or more times during each underwater armstroke.

Swimmers accelerate their hands in pulses during the various phases of each competitive stroke. Each pulse corresponds to a major directional change. The slowest pulses of limb velocity take place early in the underwater stroke cycle and the fastest velocities are reached in the final portions.

The propulsive movements of the arms can be reduced to four basic sweeps—*outsweep*, *downsweep*, *insweep*, and *upsweep*. The outsweep is the first movement in the underwater armstroke for butterfly and breaststroke swimmers. The downsweep performs the same function in the front crawl and backstroke. Neither of these sweeps is propulsive. They are used to position the arm to catch before applying propulsive force. The catch usually begins when swimmers' hands are approximately one-third of the way through their underwater movements.

The insweep is the first propulsive movement in the front crawl and butterfly. It is the only propulsive arm movement in breaststroke. A similar movement is termed an *upsweep* in backstroke because swimmers are in a supine position. The upsweep is the final propulsive motion in the front crawl and butterfly strokes.

The kick probably plays a larger role in propulsion than is popularly believed. The vertical and lateral movements of the legs can displace water back equally as well as it is pushed back by the vertical and lateral movements of the arms.

Recommended reading

Brown, R.M. & Counsilman, J.E. (1971) The role of lift in propelling swimmers. In Cooper, J.M. (ed.) *Biomechanics*. Chicago: Athletic Institute, pp. 179–188.

Clarys, J.P. (1979) Human morphology and hydrodynamics. In Terauds, J. & Bedingfield, E.W. (eds) *Swimming III*. Baltimore, Maryland: University Park Press, pp. 3–41.

Clarys, J.P. & Jiskoot, J. (1975) Total resistance of selected body positions in the front crawl. In Lewillie, L. & Clarys, J.P. (eds) *Swimming II*. Baltimore, Maryland: University Park Press, pp. 110–117.

Colwin, C. (1984) Fluid dynamics: vortex circulation in swimming propulsion. In Welsh, T.F. (ed.) *1983 ASCA World Clinic Yearbook*. Fort Lauderdale, Florida: American Swimming Coaches Association, pp. 38–46.

Colwin, C. (1985a) Essential fluid dynamics of swimming propulsion. In Leonard, J.L. (ed.) *ASCA Newsletter No. 1*. Fort Lauderdale, Florida: American Swimming Coaches Association, pp. 22–27.

Colwin, C. (1985b) Practical application of flow analysis as a coaching tool. *ASCA Newsletter* **September/October**:5–8. (Fort Lauderdale, Florida: American Swimming Coaches Association).

Counsilman, J. & Wasilak, J. (1982) The importance of hand speed and hand acceleration. In Ousley, R.M. (ed.) *1981 ASCA World Clinic Yearbook*. Fort Lauderdale, Florida: American Swimming Coaches Association, pp. 41–55.

Craig, A.B. Jr., Boomer, W.L. & Skehan, P.L. (1988) Patterns of velocity in breaststroke swimming. In Ungerechts, B., Wilke, K. & Reischle, K. (eds) *Swimming Science V*. Champaign, Illinois: Human Kinetics, pp. 73–77.

de Groot, G. & van Ingen Schenau, G.J. (1988) Fundamental mechanics applied to swimming technique and propelling efficiency. In Ungerechts, B., Wilke, K. & Reischle, K. (eds) *Swimming Science V*. Champaign, Illinois: Human Kinetics, pp. 17–29.

East, D.J. (1970) Swimming: an analysis of stroke frequency, stroke length and performance. *N.Z.J. Health, Phys. Ed. and Recr.* **3**:16–27.

Firby, H. (1975) *Howard Firby on Swimming*. London: Pelham Books.

Hay, J.G. (1986) The status of research on the biomechanics of swimming. In Hay, J.G. (ed.) *Starting, Stroking and Turning*. Iowa City, Iowa: Biomechanics Laboratory, University of Iowa, pp. 53–76.

Hay, J.G. & Thayer, A. (1986) Flow visualization of competitive swimming techniques: the tufts method (preliminary report). In Hay, J.G. (ed.) *Starting, Stroking and Turning*. Iowa City, Iowa: Biomechanics Laboratory, University of Iowa, pp. 201–210.

Hinrichs, R. (1986) Biomechanics of butterfly. In Johnston, T., Woolger, J. & Scheider, D. (eds) *1985 ASCA World Clinic Yearbook*. Fort Lauderdale, Florida: American Swimming Coaches Association, p. 94.

Hollander, A.P., de Groot, G., van Ingen Schneau, G.J., Kahman, R. & Toussaint, H.M. (1988) Contributions of the legs to propulsion in front crawl swimming. In Ungerechts, B., Wilke, K. & Reischle, K. (eds) *Swimming Science V*. Champaign, Illinois: Human Kinetics, pp. 39–43.

Holmer, I. (1974) Energy cost of the arm stroke, leg kick and the whole stroke in competitive swimming style. *J. Appl. Phys.* **33**:105–118.

Jiskoot, J. & Clarys, J.P. (1975) Body resistance on and under the water surface. In Lewillie, L. & Clarys, J.P. (eds) *Swimming II*. Baltimore, Maryland: University Park Press, pp. 105–109.

Koehler, J.A. (1987) *Bernoulli, bah or how aircraft fly*. Unpublished manuscript, University of Saskatchewan, Saskatoon, Saskatchewan.

Kreighbaum, E. & Barthels, K.M. (1985) *Biomechanics: A Qualitative Approach for Studying Human Motion*. Minneapolis, Minnesota: Burgess.

Letzelter, H. & Freitag, W. (1983) Stroke length and stroke frequency variations in men's and women's 100-m freestyle swimming. In Hollander, A.P., Huijing, P.A. & de Groot, G. (eds) *Biomechanics and Medicine in Swimming*. Champaign, Illinois: Human Kinetics, pp. 315–322.

Lighthill, J. (1969) Hydrodynamics of aquatic animal propulsion. *Annu. Rev. Fluid Mech.* **1**:413–446.

Luedtke, D. (1986) Backstroke biomechanics. In Johnston, T., Woolger, J. & Scheider, D. (eds) *1985 ASCA World Clinic Yearbook*. Fort Lauderdale, Florida: American Swimming Coaches Association, p. 95.

Maglischo, E.W. (1986) Sprint freestyle biomechanics. In Johnston, T., Woolger, J. & Scheider, D. (eds) *1985 ASCA World Clinic Yearbook*. Fort Lauderdale, Florida: American Swimming Coaches Association, p. 98.

Maglischo, C.W., Maglischo, E.W., Higgins, J. *et al.* (1986) A biomechanical analysis of the 1984 US Olympic swimming team: the distance freestylers. *J. Swimm. Res.* **2**:12–16.

Maglischo, C.W., Maglischo, E.W., Luedtke, D. *et al.* (1987a) The swimmer: a study of propulsion and drag. *SOMA* **2**:40–44.

Maglischo, C.W., Maglischo, E.W. & Santos, T.R. (1987b) The relationship between the forward velocity of the center of gravity and the hip in the four competitive strokes. *J. Swim. Res.* **3**:11–17.

Northrip, J.W., Logan, G.A. & McKinney, W.C. (1974) *Introduction to Biomechanic Analysis of Sport*. Dubuque, Iowa: W. C. Brown.

Ohmichi, H., Takamoto, M. & Miyashita, M. (1983) Measurement of the waves caused by swimmers. In Hollander, P.A., Huijing P.A. & de Groot, G. (eds) *Biomechanics and Medicine in Swimming*. Champaign, Illinois: Human Kinetics, pp. 103–107.

Pai, Y-C. (1986) A hydrodynamic study of the oscillation

motion in swimming. In Hay, J.G. (ed.) *Starting, Stroking and Turning*. Iowa City, Iowa: Biomechanics Laboratory, University of Iowa, pp. 145–150.

Persyn, U., de Maeyer, J. & Vervaecke, H. (1975) Investigation of hydrodynamic determinants of competitive swimming strokes. In Lewillie, L. & Clarys, J.P. (eds) *Swimming II*. Baltimore, Maryland: University Park Press, pp. 214–222.

Persyn, U., Van Tilborgh, L., Daly, D., Colman, V., Vijfvinkel, D.J. & Verhetsel, D. (1988) Computerized evaluation and advice in swimming. In Ungerechts, B., Wilke, K. & Reischle, K. (eds) *Swimming Science V*. Champaign, Illinois: Human Kinetics, pp. 341–349.

Plagenhoff, S. (1971) *Patterns of Human Motion*. Englewood Cliffs, New Jersey: Prentice-Hall.

Reischle, K. (1979) A kinematic investigation of movement patterns in swimming with photo-optical methods. In Terauds, J. & Bedingfield, E.W. (eds) *Swimming III*. Baltimore, Maryland: University Park Press, pp. 97–104.

Remmonds, P. & Bartlett, R.M. (1981) Effects of finger separation. *Swim. Tech.* **18**:28–30.

Rouse, H. (1946) *Elementary Mechanics of Fluids*. New York: Dover Publications.

Schleihauf, R. (1986) Biomechanics. In Johnston, T., Woolger, J. & Scheider D. (eds) *1985 ASCA World Clinic Yearbook*. Fort Lauderdale, Florida: American Swimming Coaches Association, pp. 88–93.

Schleihauf, R.E. Jr. (1978) Swimming propulsion: a hydrodynamic analysis. In Ousley, B. (ed.) *1977 ASCA World Clinic Yearbook*. Fort Lauderdale, Florida: American Swimming Coaches Association, pp. 49–86.

Schleihauf, R.E. Jr. (1979) A hydrodynamic analysis of swimming propulsion. In Terauds, J. & Bedingfield, E.W. (eds) *Swimming III*. Baltimore, Maryland: University Park Press, pp. 70–109.

Schleihauf, R.E. (1984) Biomechanics of swimming propulsion. In Johnston, T., Woolger, J. & Scheilder, D. (eds) *1983 ASCA World Clinic Yearbook*. Fort Lauderdale, Florida: American Swimming Coaches Association, pp. 19–24.

Schleihauf, R.E., Higgins, J.R., Hinrichs, R. *et al.* (1988) Propulsive techniques: front crawl stroke, butterfly, backstroke and breaststroke. In Ungerechts, B., Wilke, K. & Reischle, K. (eds) *Swimming Science V*. Champaign, Illinois: Human Kinetics, pp. 53–60.

Sharp, R.L. & Costill, D.L. (1989) Influence of body hair removal on physiological responses during breaststroke swimming. *Med. Sci. Sports Exerc.* **21**:576–580.

Sharp, R.L., Hackney, A.C., Cain, S.M. & Ness, R.J. (1988) The effect of shaving down on the physiologic cost of freestyle swimming. *J. Swim. Res.* **4**:9–13.

Toussaint, H.M. (1988) *Mechanics and Energetics of Swimming*. Amsterdam: Toussaint, H.M.

Toussaint, H.M., van der Helm, F.C.T., Elzerman, J.R., Hollander, A.P., de Groot, G. & van Ingen Schneau, G.J. (1983) A power balance applied to swimming. In Hollander, A.P., Huijing, P.A. & de Groot, G. (eds) *Biomechanics and Medicine in Swimming*. Champaign, Illinois: Human Kinetics, pp. 165–172.

Watkins, J. & Gordon, A.T. (1983) The effects of leg action on performance in the sprint front crawl stroke. In Hollander, A.P., Huijing, P.A. & de Groot, G. (eds) *Biomechanics and Medicine in Swimming*. Champaign, Illinois: Human Kinetics, pp. 310–314.

Wood, T.C. (1978) A fluid dynamic analysis of the propulsive potential of the hand and forearm in swimming. In Terauds, J. & Bedingfield, E.W. (eds) *Swimming III*. Baltimore, Maryland: University Park Press.

Chapter 7

Front crawl

Swimmers use an alternating armstroke and a flutter kick in the front crawl stroke. This stroke is more popularly known as the freestyle. The rules permit swimmers the freedom to choose any style for certain races. They almost always choose the front crawl stroke because it is the fastest method for completing the distance. Therefore, it has become synonymous with the term freestyle.

One stroke cycle consists of a right and left armstroke and a varying number of kicks. Several different kick rhythms are in use with regard to the timing between the arms and legs. The most prevalent styles are the six-beat, four-beat, two-beat, and two-beat crossover kick. The parts of the stroke have been described under the following headings.

1 The armstroke, including the directional sweeps, angles of attack, velocity changes, recovery and the timing of the two armstrokes of each stroke cycle.
2 The flutter kick.
3 The body position and breathing style.
4 The various rhythms between arms and legs in use today.

The armstroke

The underwater armstroke of the front crawl consists of three diagonal sweeps: downsweep, insweep, and upsweep. The entry and stretch and the release and recovery will also be described. Underwater sequence photos of an athlete swimming the front crawl are shown in Fig. 7.1. Surface views of the recovery and entry are displayed in Fig. 7.2.

Entry and stretch

Underwater views of the entry and stretch can be seen from a side view in Fig. 7.1c. The entry is made directly in front of the swimmer's shoulder with her elbow flexed slightly and her palm pitched out. In this way, she can slip her hand into the water on edge and her arm can follow, entering in nearly the same portion of water.

Wave drag will be produced on the entry, as the swimmer's hand pushes forward through the water. Entering in the streamlined manner as described should keep that resistance to a minimum.

Swimmers should be careful that the hand does not swing across the face during the entry. This will cause their bodies to wiggle from side to side. Instead, the hand should enter somewhere between the middle of the head and the tip of the same shoulder.

After it enters the water, the swimmer's arm is extended almost directly forward just beneath the surface. Her palm rotates down as she extends her arm forward. This phase of the armstroke can be seen from an underneath view (Fig. 7.1c). The swimmer is stretching her right arm forward. This phase of the armstroke has been termed a *stretch* rather than a glide because the arm does not stop moving forward.

Swimmers should not begin the propulsive phase of their armstroke immediately after the hand enters the water. As shown in Fig. 7.1, the other arm will be midway through its propulsive phase when the entry is made, so the efforts of the arm in front would interfere with those of the arm behind if any attempt was made to begin stroking with the former arm. The arm in front should be streamlined and maintained within the confines of the space taken up by the swimmer's partially submerged body during the stretch. This phase of the stroke should continue until the other arm finishes its propulsive phase. The next phase, the downsweep, should begin at that point.

Downsweep and catch

The downsweep is shown from a side view in Fig. 7.1. As indicated, it should begin immediately when the propulsive phase of the opposite arm has been completed. The arm in front should sweep down in a curvilinear path until the catch has been made. The swimmer gradually flexes her arm at the elbow during the downsweep to get it facing back at the catch. The catch takes place near the end of the downsweep when the swimmer's elbow has come up above her hand and her forearm and upper arm are facing back

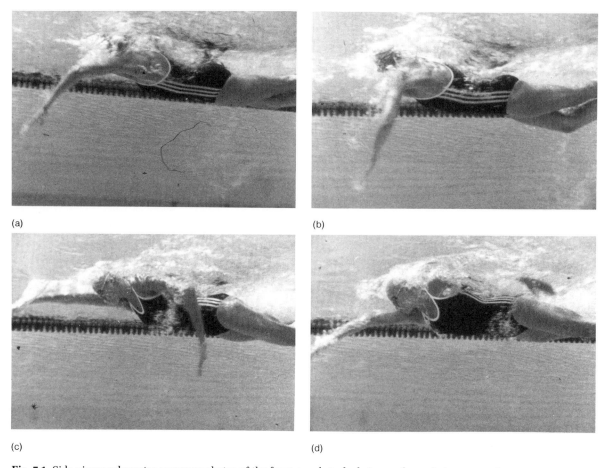

(a)

(b)

(c)

(d)

Fig. 7.1 Side-view underwater sequence photos of the front crawl stroke being performed at race speed.

against the water. The catch position appears in Fig. 7.1a and e.

The swimmer's hand also slides slightly outside the shoulder during the downsweep and the palm is rotated out slightly at the catch. These positions of the arm and hand place the swimmer in position to apply more propulsive force during the insweep that follows. As mentioned in Chapter 6, the outward movement of the hand is a natural after-effect that takes place as a swimmer's shoulder follows the arm during the downsweep. It should not be emphasized or it may become excessive.

Swimmers should not try to apply propulsive force until their arms are in this position. The arm must be facing back in order to displace water back during its diagonal sculling motions. The downsweep is not propulsive. Its primary purpose is to position the arm for the propulsive sweep that follows. If swimmers apply force before their arms have been positioned properly at the catch, they will simply push the water down and decelerate their forward speed.

The insweep

The insweep is shown in Fig. 7.1d and f. It is the first propulsive sweep of the front crawl armstroke. It is also a semi-circular motion, beginning at the catch and continuing until the swimmer's arm has traveled under the body to the midline or slightly beyond. The swimmer's arm, which was flexed slightly at the catch, continues bending throughout the insweep until it is flexed approximately 90° at the completion

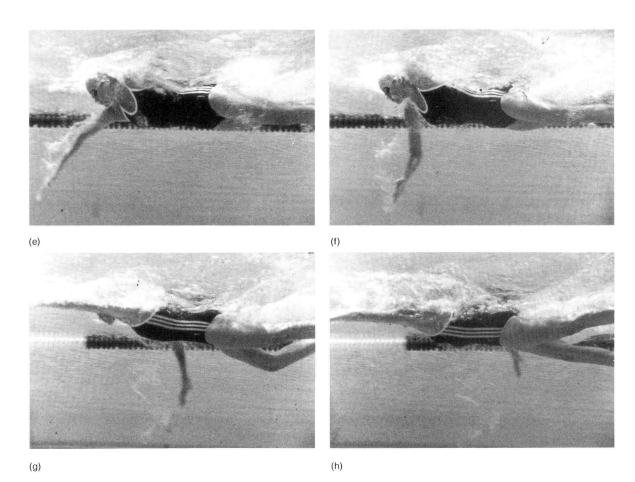

(e)

(f)

(g)

(h)

Fig. 7.1 (contd)

of this motion. The palm of the hand rotates in slowly during the insweep until it is facing slightly in and up when the movement ends.

Swimmers should accelerate their hands moderately from the beginning to the end of the insweep. Their hands are not traveling at maximum velocity, however. That effort should be saved for the next propulsive sweep.

Some swimmers sweep their hand in beyond the midline of their bodies while others complete the insweep somewhere between the outer border and the midline of their bodies. All swimmers should bring their hands at least under the midline of their bodies. This will put their arm in position to deliver more propulsion during the next sweep.

Sweeping the hand in beyond the midline of

the body is not necessarily a stroke defect. Those swimmers who use sculling movements effectively frequently stroke in this way. A word of caution is in order, however. Sweeping in beyond the midline may cause the hips to swing from side to side. It may be necessary to shorten the insweep if this happens.

Swimmers generally sweep the arm opposite their breathing side across their bodies more than they sweep in with the other arm. This is because most roll more to their breathing sides. Consequently, they need a longer insweep to rotate their bodies back toward the other side. While some propulsive force may be lost in rotating their bodies, the trade-off is beneficial because it places their bodies in better alignment for the most propulsive phase of the underwater armstroke—the upsweep.

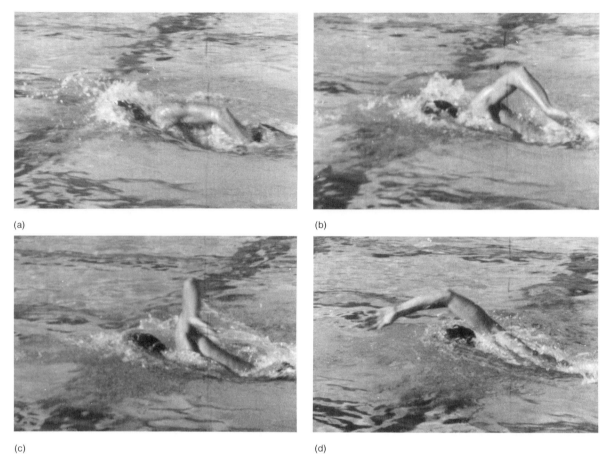

(a)

(b)

(c)

(d)

Fig. 7.2 Surface view of the front crawl arm recovery.

The upsweep

The upsweep is the second and final propulsive sweep of the front crawl stroke (Fig. 7.1). It begins at completion of the preceding insweep. The pitch is changed from in to out by rotating the hand out quickly and the swimmer sweeps the arm out, up and back toward the surface of the water. The upsweep ends when the swimmer's hand passes the thigh, not when the hand reaches the surface of the water. Swimmers' arms extend slightly during the upsweep but, contrary to popular belief, they do not extend completely. Hand speed accelerates to its maximum velocity during this movement.

Two mistakes that swimmers commonly make during the upsweep are to extend their arms completely, and to apply force to the surface of the

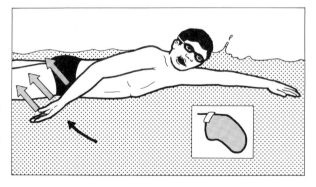

Fig. 7.3 Overextending the arm during the upsweep. The swimmer in this figure has extended his arm too much during the upsweep. This causes him to push the water up more than he is displacing it back.

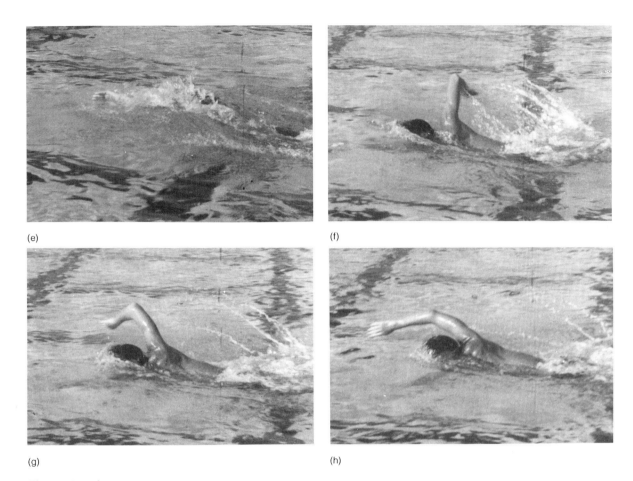

(e)

(f)

(g)

(h)

Fig. 7.2 (contd)

water. In both cases, the angle of attack of the hand and arm can become too great to be propulsive. Consequently, water is pushed up more than it is displaced back. Figure 7.3 shows the effect of these mistakes; the swimmer has his elbow nearly extended as it sweeps toward the surface. At that large angle of attack, it presents a flat surface to the water, creating turbulence and a deceleration of forward speed.

Release and recovery

Based on the statements in the previous section, the recovery obviously begins before the swimmer's hand leaves the water. It starts when the elbow comes above the surface during the preceding upsweep. At that point, she begins flexing her arm to start it moving forward while her hand is still underwater. The

release point can be seen underwater in Fig. 7.1d and from the surface in Fig. 7.2a.

The overlap between the end of the upsweep and the beginning of the recovery conserves angular momentum. It reduces the muscular effort required to overcome the backward inertia of the arm and start it moving forward. Pressure should be released as the swimmer's hand passes her thigh (her elbow will be out of the water by then). Her palm is turned in so her hand can travel on edge for the short distance to the surface. This will keep resistance to a minimum as the hand travels up.

After leaving the water, the arm should be brought forward for the next entry in the traditional high-elbow style. The surface-view sequence in Fig. 7.2 shows a swimmer executing a high-elbow recovery. He partially flexes the arm during the first half of the movement and extends it in the second half. Gradual flexion at his elbow allows the swimmer's arm to continue moving up and forward after it leaves the water. It also keeps his hand from swinging out too wide. Although the arm will naturally swing out and around to some extent, swimmers should make every effort to keep their arm moving directly forward. If the recovery is too low and wide, the excessive sideward movements of their arms will pull their bodies out of alignment.

The swimmer begins extending his arm forward for the entry once his hand passes his shoulder. The entry should be made while his arm is still slightly flexed so it creates minimal turbulence. The palm of his hand, which was facing in toward his body during the first half of the recovery, should be facing out as he reaches forward for the entry.

It is very important that swimmers' arms pass their shoulders with elbows high, as shown in Fig. 7.2. This puts the arm in the best position to enter the water with minimal turbulence.

Rolling the body from side to side is also very important to making a good recovery. Swimmers should roll toward the side of their recovering arm so that the shoulder of that arm is higher than the other. This makes it easier to maintain a high-elbow position and a nearly linear direction of movement as the arms travel through the air. Most swimmers recover their arm higher and more linearly on the breathing side and use a somewhat lower and more lateral swing over the water on the nonbreathing side. This is because they do not roll their body sufficiently toward the nonbreathing side. Consequently, the shoulder does not roll up as high on that side and the arm must swing out more during its path over the water. In addition, the arm usually creates more wave drag during the entry because the forearm and upperarm drag water forward after coming down behind the point where the hand entered. Some degree of asymmetry is always present between the arm recoveries on the breathing and nonbreathing sides. Nevertheless, the amount of roll to the nonbreathing side must be sufficient to complete the upsweep properly and to recover without disturbing lateral alignment or producing excessive turbulence at the entry.

The purpose of the recovery is to place swimmers' arms in position for another underwater stroke. This is an important, but nonpropulsive function. The goals of the recovery should be to get the arm over the water with the least disruption of lateral alignment, and to provide a short period of reduced effort for the arm, shoulder, and trunk muscles. Swimmers should try to relax the recovering arm during the recovery, using only enough effort to maintain it in the proper relationship with the other. When swimmers want faster turnover they should concentrate on stroking faster, not recovering faster. If they do this, the speed of their recovery will increase naturally to keep up with the speed of the stroking arm. Thus effort will not be wasted or alignment disrupted.

Timing of the arms

During the front crawl stroke, the two arms have precise relationships that are very important to fast swimming. Those relationships are shown in Fig. 7.1. The alternating movements of the arms must be coordinated with body roll and vice versa in order to facilitate the three sweeps and maintain the body in the most streamlined position possible during each stroke cycle. The most important event in this sequence is that the arm in front should enter the water when the other arm is midway through its insweep (Fig. 7.1). This will permit swimmers to roll their bodies toward the stroking side in preparation for the upsweep. Another important feature of this relationship is that the arm in front should not begin sweeping down until the other has completed its upsweep. While this last point is true of middle-distance and distance races, the relationship between the stretch and upsweep of the other arm changes somewhat when swimmers are sprinting.

Sprinters reduce the stretch and start the downsweep of one arm during the upsweep of the other. They do this so they can catch and begin the propulsive phase of the next armstroke almost immediately as the other arm releases pressure. This intensifies the energy cost of swimming because it increases the resistance in front as compared to stretching the front arm forward in a streamlined manner. It will, nevertheless, result in faster times for shorter distances. In middle-distance and distance races, swimmers choose to sacrifice speed and conserve energy by delaying the downsweep until the propulsive phase of the stroking arm has been completed.

The flutter kick

The flutter kick consists of alternating diagonal sweeps of the legs. Although the legs move somewhat laterally during the various kicking movements, their primary directions are up and down. Thus, the two primary kicking motions have been termed *upbeat* and *downbeat.*

Downbeat

The downbeat of both legs can be seen in Fig. 7.1. They move in an alternating rhythm so that the downbeat of one leg is taking place during the upbeat of the other.

The downbeat is a whip-like movement that begins with flexion at the hip followed by extension at the knee. A leg begins its downbeat before reaching the highest point in the previous upbeat. Swimmers begin flexing their leg at the hip as the leg passes the body on its way up to the surface. Consequently, swimmers' thighs will be starting down while their lower legs continue up. The continued upward motion of the lower leg is a passive movement that is not technically part of the preceding upbeat even though the leg continues on its upward path. When the flutter kick is done correctly, the lower leg should be relaxed so the pressure of the water below pushes it up into a flexed position when the swimmer starts pushing the thigh down. Shortly thereafter, the lower leg will follow the thigh, by extending down in a whip-like manner.

The pressure of the water pushing up on the swimmer's leg also pushes the foot into an extended position with toes pointed up (plantar flexed) and with the foot turned in (inverted). A better-than-average ability to point the toes (extend the feet) should be a decided advantage to swimmers in the flutter kick. It will enable them to maintain an angle of attack that permits the backward displacement of water for a longer portion of each downbeat.

Upbeat

At completion of the previous downbeat, the leg rebounds up toward the surface. The leg is extended at the knee and it swings up from the hip. Accordingly, most of the work of this movement is done by the gluteus maximus muscles that extend the leg at the hip. The leg is maintained in an extended position by the pressure of the water pushing down on it from above. That same water also pushes the swimmer's foot into a natural position where it is neither flexed nor extended. As mentioned previously, the upbeat actually ends when the swimmer's leg passes the body. That is when the thigh begins to flex at the hip for the next downbeat.

The water is largely responsible for positioning the legs during the flutter kick. In most cases, the muscles around the knees and ankles remain relaxed so the water can push the legs and feet into the proper positions during each phase of the kick. The only exception to this statement is during the final portion of the downbeat when the legs are extended vigorously at the knees and flexed at the ankles. Otherwise, muscles responsible for performing the work during the flutter kick are the ones that swing the thighs up and down from the hip joints.

Inexperienced swimmers often work against the natural positioning effects of water pressure by flexing their legs at the knees during the upbeat. They alternately flex and extend their lower legs without swinging their thighs very much from the hip joints. These swimmers generally push water forward with their lower legs during the upbeat. That action decelerates their forward speed during this phase and partially offsets the propulsion gained during the downbeat. The result, of course, is a reduction of overall forward speed.

Kick width

The flutter kick should be too shallow or too deep. The optimum width is probably between 50 and 80 cm (approximately 20–30 in). Cureton (1930) recommended a maximum width of 61 cm (24 in). Allen (1948) found that a kick width of approximately 30 cm (12 in) was superior to a narrower kick of 15 cm (6 in) for increasing propulsive force.

Obviously, swimmers should kick wide enough both to stabilize and to propel their bodies forward. Nevertheless, they should not kick too wide or they will increase form drag unnecessarily. The foot should probably reach the surface of the water during the upbeat. It may break the surface, but only slightly. Kicking up too high will simply push the swimmer's body down. At completion of the downbeat the foot should be just below the body line.

Lateral kicks

As indicated earlier, the legs kick diagonally. The lateral components of these kicks probably assist in body rotation and stabilization. Body rotation is facilitated and lateral alignment can be preserved if one leg is kicking in the same direction in which the swimmer's body is rolling. In the meantime, the other leg should be kicking in the opposite direction. That is, when the body is rolling to the right, one leg should kick diagonally down and to the right while the other kicks diagonally up and to the left. These movements should be reversed when the swimmer rolls the body toward the left side.

The usual practice of kicking with a board may be fine for improving leg endurance but it inhibits diagonal kicking. Accordingly, a large proportion of kicking drills should be done without a board so the kick can be used in combination with body rotation.

How propulsive is the flutter kick?

This has been debated for several years. Until recently, prevailing opinion denied the propulsive capabilities of the flutter kick. That belief has changed in recent years. It seems certain that the kick can contribute to propulsion. In Chapter 6 it was described how the legs can displace water back and propel swimmers forward. There is still some question as to the wisdom of expending the effort required to utilize the flutter kick for propulsion, however.

The most vigorous kicking rhythm used by successful sprint swimmers is the six-beat kick. A great majority of distance and middle-distance swimmers use a fewer number of beats per stroke cycle, however, presumably to save energy. Some very successful sprint swimmers have also used abbreviated kicking rhythms successfully. These swimmers have apparently chosen intuitively to sacrifice some propulsive force to save energy by doing less work with their legs.

Adrian et al. (1966) have provided the most compelling argument against vigorous kicking. They measured the oxygen consumption of 12 competitive swimmers while they were kicking only, pulling only and when swimming the full stroke. Kicking used four times more oxygen than pulling. The oxygen requirement was 24.5 liters when the subjects kicked at a

speed of 1 m·s^{-1} (3.5 ft·s^{-1}) as compared to a requirement of only 7 liters when they pulled at the same speed. These results have been supported by other researchers who found that kicking caused a considerable increase in the energy cost of swimming (Holmer, 1974; Charbonnier et al., 1975; Åstrand, 1978).

These data make a persuasive case for reducing the effort used in kicking, at least during middle-distance and distance races. Swimmers do not need all of the propulsive force they are capable of producing when they are pacing these races at some submaximal speed. The argument is not so strong where sprint events are concerned, however. It seems that the full propulsive potential of the legs should be utilized to produce the fastest possible speed in sprint races and during the final sprint in middle-distance and distance races. Why, then, have some sprinters been successful with two-beat and four-beat rhythms? Perhaps because factors such as body build, specific muscular weakness, specific joint flexibility, and various physiological capacities made it more efficient for them to use fewer kicks per stroke cycle.

In this regard, Persyn and his coworkers (1975) at the Leuven Institute in Belgium have reported the following results from a study of 62 national-level Belgian and Dutch swimmers. Six-beat kickers had larger vital capacities, greater inward rotating ability at the hips, larger hands, and greater triceps extension and shoulder extension strength. The legs of six-beat kickers also tended to sink more easily. Perhaps only swimmers with great respiratory capacity and excellent kicks can use six-beat kicks without becoming unduly fatigued. Other swimmers may be better advised to reduce their kicking efforts, unless needed to keep their legs from sinking.

Another possible explanation for the fact that some swimmers do not use six-beat kicks is that the demands of training forced them to develop abbreviated rhythms early in their careers. If this is true, we can only speculate whether they would have been faster using six-beat kicks.

The downbeat is probably the only propulsive phase of the flutter kick because swimmers can maintain an angle of attack with their legs that will displace water back during this phase. The upbeat is another story. Swimmers' legs travel up and forward during this time and they should be maintained in an extended position. Consequently the legs can only push water up while the angle of attack of the feet is too small to produce any significant amount of propulsive force. The probable purposes of the upbeat are to return the leg for another downbeat, and to counteract the tendency of swimmers' bodies to be pushed up or to the side by the movements of their arms. For this reason, the effort expended in performing the upbeat should be kept to a minimum.

Body position and breathing

As explained in Chapter 6, swimmers encounter less resistance when their bodies are in good horizontal and lateral alignment throughout the stroke cycle. The most likely time to upset these alignments is when they turn the head to the side to breathe; when they stroke their arms in under their bodies, and during arm recovery.

Horizontal alignment

The keys to good horizontal alignment are a natural head position, neither too high nor too low; a fairly straight back, and a narrow kick. The swimmers in Figs 7.1 and 7.2 have their bodies well aligned.

Front crawl swimmers' faces should be in the water. The waterline should be somewhere between the hairline and the middle of the head. When they breathe, they should roll, not lift, the head. The chins should be up just enough to permit swimmers to focus their eyes forward. They should not arch their backs excessively to achieve a high body position. The width of their kicks should be such that the feet barely reach the surface on the upbeat and are only slightly below the body on the downbeat.

What of the common observation that good sprinters ride high in the water? They seem to hydroplane over the water giving the impression that they are swimming with their heads up and backs arched. Sprinters ride high because their speed increases the drag under their bodies. That drag lifts them higher in the water. They do not arch their backs, nor should they. Even sprinters will ride lower in the water when they are swimming longer distances at slower speeds. There will be less drag under their bodies to push them up. Conversely, distance swimmers will ride higher when they sprint because the drag will be increased. Any attempt to augment this natural

hydroplane would be foolhardy. Some potential propulsive force would have to be sacrificed to press down on the water so swimmers could maintain a high body position.

Lateral alignment

The swimmer in Fig. 7.4 has his body in excellent lateral alignment. You could draw a straight line down the middle of his trunk, from his neck to his crotch, regardless of whether his body is rolled to the right or to the left. Swimmers maintain good lateral alignment principally by rolling their bodies from side to side in concert with the movements of their arms and shoulders.

Although it is possible to roll too much, most swimmers roll too little. Front crawl swimmers should roll at least 45° to each side (from a prone position). Most will roll more than 45° toward their breathing side.

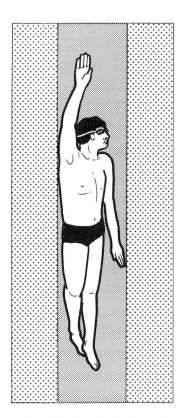

Fig. 7.4 An underneath view of a front crawl swimmer showing good lateral alignment.

Breathing

Head movements should be coordinated with body roll to reduce the tendency for swimmers to lift their heads for a breath. The swimmer rotates his face toward the surface as the arm on his breathing side is completing its upsweep. This is because his body is rolling to the right, enabling him to get his mouth above the surface without lifting his head or rotating it excessively. He actually breathes below the normal flat surface of the water in a cavity formed by the bow wave in front of his head.

The breath should be taken during the first half of the recovery and the swimmer's face should be returned to the water during the second half of the movement. The return should also be coordinated with body roll to the opposite side. This will put his face back into the water and his body in the best possible alignment during the most propulsive phase of that armstroke, the upsweep.

Competitive swimmers should never hold their breath while swimming races that are longer than 100 m. They should maintain a steady supply of oxygen by breathing once during each stroke cycle. Holding the breath will cause fatigue. (There are exceptions to this statement that will be explained in the section on alternate breathing.)

They should begin to exhale immediately after inhaling. However, they must time the exhalation so another breath is not needed before they are ready to begin the next stroke cycle. The exhalation is very slow at first with just enough air escaping from the mouth and, particularly, the nose to reduce thoracic pressure. This slow exhalation continues until the mouth is near the surface for the next inhalation. At that time, the remaining air should be exhaled rapidly to prepare for another inhalation. The exhalation should be completed as the mouth breaks the surface so they can inhale immediately.

The usual pattern is to breathe once during every stroke cycle and always to the same side. Some swimmers prefer a different style called *alternate breathing*.

Alternate breathing

This method has been used by many world-class swimmers, particularly females. The following advantages have been cited.

1 The stroke is more symmetrical. Alternate breathing encourages swimmers to roll their bodies equally to both sides. This increases body rotation and encourages a more effective armstroke.

2 Pulmonary diffusing capacity can be improved by restricted breathing.

3 Swimmers can watch competitors on both sides.

These reasons notwithstanding, the most compelling argument against alternate breathing is that the oxygen supply will be reduced in races. This, in turn, will cause swimmers to fatigue sooner. Alternate breathers inhale twice during every three stroke cycles, whereas conventional breathers inhale once every cycle. Consequently, most swimmers should be advised to breathe conventionally in all races beyond 100 m.

There are exceptions to the previous statement, however. In our experience, the strokes of some swimmers have improved so dramatically that they swam faster when they breathed alternately, in spite of a reduced oxygen supply. You can determine which swimmers, if any, fall into this category with a simple test procedure called *experimental swims*.

Have the swimmers complete a long set of repeats, 2000—3000 m in length. They should use alternate breathing on the even-numbered swims and conventional breathing on the odd-numbered repeats. It may be worthwhile for certain swimmers to consider using alternate breathing in races if they are consistently faster on the even-numbered swims.

There is one additional circumstance when alternate breathing could be recommended. That is for training young swimmers. Children may learn to swim more symmetrically by using alternate breathing when their strokes are evolving. Once they have developed high elbow recoveries and good propulsive sweeps with both arms, they may be able to breathe conventionally in longer races and still retain these desirable stroke techniques.

Timing of the arms and legs

The usual way of expressing the timing between the arms and legs is according to the number of kicks per stroke cycle. The most prominent patterns are the six-beat, two-beat and four-beat rhythms.

The six-beat kick

This rhythm incorporates three leg beats per arm-stroke or six beats per stroke cycle. Actually there are six kicks per armstroke because one leg is kicking up as the other is kicking down. However, it is common practice to refer to kick rhythms according to the number of downbeats only.

In this style, there is a downbeat coordinated with each of the three sweeps that make up an underwater armstroke. The downbeat of one leg corresponds to the downsweep of the arm on the same side. The insweep is accompanied by a downbeat from the opposite leg and the leg on the same side kicks down, once again, during the upsweep of that arm.

The coordination between arm sweeps and leg beats is so precise that the beginning and end of each downbeat coincides exactly with the beginning and end of the corresponding arm sweep. For this reason, it is tempting to recommend the six-beat rhythm as the best possible timing between arms and legs. Nevertheless, as stated earlier, many world-class swimmers have been successful at all distances using other rhythms.

The two-beat kick

In this style, swimmers complete two downbeats per arm cycle or one downbeat per armstroke. Each downbeat accompanies the insweep and upsweep of the arm on the same side as the leg that is kicking down. The opposite leg executes an upbeat at the same time. At the end of each beat, the legs hesitate in a spread position until the downsweep of the next armstroke has been completed. Then the downbeat of the leg on that side is completed during the insweep and upsweep of the arm.

The two-beat kick probably requires less energy than other kicking rhythms. That's why it is used by a great number of distance swimmers, particularly females. Females, because they are naturally more buoyant, probably do not need to kick to keep their legs afloat. Many males require faster rhythms to keep their legs from sinking. For this reason, males seem to prefer four-beat kicks and two-beat crossover rhythms.

Swimmers who use a two-beat kick tend to modify the timing of their arms from the style described earlier in this chapter. They do this to compensate for the fact that they are not kicking during the downsweep of their armstrokes. They do not use a long stretch after entry. Rather, they stretch their arm quickly and begin the downsweep sooner so they can make a quick catch when the other arm finishes its propulsive phase. Two-beat swimmers will enter one arm slightly later in relationship to the other to facilitate the short stretch. The entering arm will go into the water after the other has completed its insweep. By doing so, the stroking arm will complete its propulsive phase sooner after the entry. Consequently, the arm in front can begin sweeping down without creating a large amount of drag during the upsweep of the other.

A second modification that two-beat swimmers generally make is to shorten the insweep. They go from the catch to the upsweep with only a small insweep. This modification may be used because there is no kick from the opposite leg to counterbalance the insweep.

Another style of two-beat kick preferred by a significant number of male swimmers is the two-beat crossover kick.

The two-beat crossover kick

The difference between this and the previous rhythm is that the legs do not "hang" during the downsweep of each armstroke. Instead, the lower leg kicks up and in while the top leg kicks down over it, causing the legs to cross while swimmers sweep their arms down. The legs are then uncrossed in time to kick down during the insweep and upsweep of the armstroke, just as they did in the straight two-beat rhythm. The leg crossing over the top will always be the one corresponding to the arm that is stroking. That is, the right leg crosses over the left when the right arm is stroking. The reverse occurs when the left arm is stroking. The left leg crosses over the right. That same leg will be the one that kicks down during the armstroke.

This rhythm appears to be a compromise for swimmers whose legs tend to sink when they use a two-beat kick. It actually consists of four beats, two major and two minor downbeats of the legs. The two cross-beats probably aid in maintaining the legs near the surface. Additionally, crossing the legs probably helps in the maintenance of lateral alignment by preventing the hips from swinging laterally while swimmers are recovering their arms.

The four-beat kick

This rhythm is really a combination of the six-beat and two-beat styles. Swimmers use a two-beat timing during one armstroke and a six-beat on the other. They kick down once during the insweep and upsweep of one arm just as they would if they were using a two-beat timing. They execute three downbeats during the other armstroke in the same pattern they would use with a six-beat kick.

Many swimmers use the two-beat timing on their breathing side, perhaps to facilitate inhalation or because they do not sweep their arm under their body as much on that side.

Breathing patterns for freestyle competition

Most coaches recommend restricted breathing patterns for short races such as 25-, 50- and 100-m freestyle. The dilemma facing a swimmer is that breathing too often may reduce speed, whereas breathing too little will reduce the oxygen supply and cause fatigue. So it is important for sprint swimmers to determine how much speed is lost by breathing, and whether increasing speed or reducing fatigue is more important to success in these races. Some suggestions follow.

25- and 50-m races

These distances are too short for oxygen deprivation to limit performance. Accordingly, races of 25 m are usually swum without breathing. Even 8-year-old swimmers can be trained to swim these distances without breathing.

Some athletes, teenaged and older, can also race 50 m without breathing, although most take 1−3 breaths during the race. In a 1-breath pattern, swimmers breathe at approximately the 30-m mark. Pre- and early-teens are best advised to use a 2- or 3-breath pattern. The first breath should be taken approximately 5 m from the turn in short-course races. The remaining 1 or 2 are taken on the second length. In the 2-breath pattern the second should be taken about half the distance between the turn and finish. If

swimmers are using a 3-breath pattern, the second and third inhalations should be taken approximately one-third and two-thirds of the way to the finish.

The breaths can be taken at approximately the same positions in long-course races except, of course, that there is no turn. The first time they breathe should be at the 20-m mark, the second at approximately the 30-m mark and the third at 40 m.

Swimmers in 50-m events should experiment with 0-, 1-, 2- and 3-breath patterns to determine which produces the fastest time. The breaths probably contribute very little to muscle energy supply. Rather, they allow the expulsion of carbon dioxide, thereby reducing the distress caused by the build-up of that substance in their bodies.

Preteen and early-teen age-group swimmers (that is swimmers below the age of 16 years) may find all of these breathing patterns too difficult to use because it takes them longer to complete a 50-m race. Those swimmers should breathe during every second stroke cycle.

100-m races

Races of 100 m present a complex problem where breathing patterns are concerned. A compromise must be struck between increasing speed and delaying fatigue. Swimmers must be careful they do not restrict their breathing too much in the first half of the race. It requires several seconds for oxygen to get from the lungs to the muscles. Consequently, the air swimmers inhale during the first part of the race will be supplying oxygen to the muscles during later portions. If swimmers wait until they feel the need for a breath, the damage will be done. The small amount of time that may be added by breathing early in the race should be more than compensated for by increased speed in later portions.

The following breathing patterns are recommended for 100-m races. Swimmers should experiment until they find the one that suits them best.
1 Breathe every second cycle for the first quarter of the race and every cycle for the final three-quarters.
2 Breathe every second cycle for the first half of the race and every cycle thereafter.
3 Breathe every second cycle for the entire race.

Many swimmers prefer to breathe during every stroke cycle in 100-m races. They should not be discouraged from doing so unless one of the above patterns proves superior. Regardless of the pattern preferred, swimmers should always swim the final 5–10 m without breathing so they can finish as fast as possible.

Longer races

At distances of 200 m and longer, experts generally agree that swimmers should breathe once each stroke cycle after the first 10 m of the race. Any increase in drag or decrease in propulsive force occasioned by frequent turning of the head will be more than compensated for by the increased oxygen supply.

Recommended reading

Adrian, M., Singh, M. & Karpovich, P. (1966) Energy cost of the leg kick, arm stroke and whole stroke. *J. Appl. Phys.* **21**:1763–1766.

Allen, R.H. (1948) *A study of the leg stroke in swimming the crawl stroke.* Master's thesis, State University of Iowa.

Alley, L.E. (1952) An analysis of water resistance and propulsion in swimming the crawl stroke. *Res. Q.* **23**:253–270.

Åstrand, P.-O. (1978) Aerobic power in swimming. In Eriksson, B. & Furberg, B. (eds) *Swimming Medicine IV.* Baltimore, Maryland: University Park Press, pp. 127–131.

Bachman, J.C. (1969) A comparison of hand positions in swimming freestyle. *Swim Tech.* **6**:72–73.

Bachrach, W. (1924) *The Outline of Swimming.* Chicago: Bradwell.

Bucher, W. (1975) The influence of the leg kick and the arm stroke on the total speed during the crawl stroke. In Lewillie, L. & Clarys, J.P. (eds) *Swimming II.* Baltimore, Maryland: University Park Press, pp. 180–187.

Charbonnier, J.P., Lacour, J.P., Rigffal, J. & Flandrois, R. (1975) Experimental study of the performance of competitive swimmers. *J. Appl. Phys.* **34**:157–167.

Counsilman, J.E. (1955) Forces in swimming two types of crawl stroke. *Res. Q.* **26**:127–139.

Cureton, T.K. (1930) Relationship of respiration to speed efficiency in swimming. *Res. Q.* **1**:66.

Firby H. (1975) *Howard Firby on Swimming.* London: Pelham Books.

Healey, J.H. (1970) *A comparative study to determine the relationship between plantar flexion at the ankle joint and success in selected skills in swimming.* Unpublished doctoral dissertation, University of Utah, Salt Lake City, Utah.

Hendrickson, C.B. (1949) *Effect of development of foot flexibility on learning the flutter kick.* Unpublished master's thesis, University of Wisconsin, Madison, Wisconsin.

Hollander, A.P., de Groot, G., van Ingen Schneau, G.J., Kahman, R. & Toussaint, H.M. (1988) Contributions of the legs to propulsion in front crawl swimming. In Ungerechts, B., Wilke, K. & Reischle, K. (eds) *Swimming Science V.* Champaign, Illinois: Human Kinetics, pp. 39–43.

Holmer, I. (1974) Energy cost of the arm stroke, leg kick and the whole stroke in competitive swimming style. *J. Appl. Phys.* **33**:105–118.

Kemper, H.C.G., Clarys, J.P., Verschuur, R. & Jiskoot, J. (1983) Total efficiency and swimming drag in swimming the front crawl. In Hollander, A.P., Huijing, P.A. & de Groot, G. (eds) *Biomechanics and Medicine in Swimming.* Champaign, Illinois: Human Kinetics, pp. 199–206.

Lawrence, L. (1969) The importance of the freestyle leg kick. *Int. Swimmer* **5**:11–12.

Maglischo, E. (1984) A 3-dimensional cinematographical analysis of competitive swimming strokes. In Johnston, T., Woolger, J. & Scheider, D. (eds) *1983 ASCA World Clinic Yearbook.* Fort Lauderdale, Florida: American Swimming Coaches Association, pp. 1–14.

Maglischo, E.W. (1986) Sprint freestyle biomechanics. In Johnston, T., Woolger, J. & Scheider, D. (eds) *1985 ASCA World Clinic Yearbook.* Fort Lauderdale, Florida: American Swimming Coaches Association, p. 98.

Maglischo, C.W., Maglischo, E.W., Higgins, J. *et al.* (1986) A biomechanical analysis of the 1984 US Olympic swimming team: the distance freestylers. *J. Swim. Res.* **2**:12–16.

Miyashita, M. (1975) Arm action in the crawl stroke. In Lewillie, L. & Clarys, J.P. (eds) *Swimming II.* Baltimore, Maryland: University Park Press, pp. 167–173.

Onusseit, H.F. (1973) Two-beat versus six-beat; which kick is best. *Swim. Tech.* **9**:41–43.

Persyn, U., De Maeyer, J. & Vervaecke, H. (1975) Investigation of hydrodynamic determinants of competitive swimming strokes. In Lewillie, L. & Clarys, J.P. (eds) *Swimming II.* Baltimore, Maryland: University Park Press, pp. 214–222.

Robertson, D.F. (1960) *Relationship of strength of selected muscle groups and ankle flexibility to the flutter kick in swimming.* Master's thesis, State University of Iowa, Iowa City, Iowa.

Schleihauf, R.E. Jr (1974) A biomechanical analysis of freestyle. *Swim. Tech.* **11**:88–96.

Schleihauf, R.E., Gray, L. & DeRose, J. (1983) Three-dimensional analysis of hand propulsion in the sprint front crawl stroke. In Hollander, A.P., Huijing, P.A. & de Groot, G. (eds) *Biomechanics and Medicine in Swimming.* Champaign, Illinois: Human Kinetics, pp. 173–183.

Schleihauf, R.E., Higgins, J.R., Hinrichs, R. *et al.* (1988)

Propulsive techniques: front crawl stroke, butterfly, backstroke and breaststroke. In Ungerechts, B., Wilke, K. & Reischle, K. (eds) *Swimming Science V*. Champaign, Illinois: Human Kinetics, pp. 53–60.

Toussaint, H.M., van der Helm, F.C.T., Elzerman, J.R., Hollander, A.P., de Groot, G. & van Ingen Schneau, G.J. (1983) A power balance applied to swimming. In Hollander, A.P., Huijing, P.A. & de Groot, G. (eds) *Biomechanics and Medicine in Swimming*. Champaign, Illinois: Human Kinetics, pp. 165–172.

Watkins, J. & Gordon, A.T. (1983) The effects of leg action on performance in the sprint front crawl stroke. In Hollander, A.P., Huijing, P.A. & de Groot, G. (eds) *Biomechanics and Medicine in Swimming*. Champaign, Illinois: Human Kinetics, pp. 310–314.

Chapter 8

Butterfly

The arms stroke simultaneously in the butterfly and there are two dolphin kicks during each stroke cycle. The parts of the butterfly stroke will be described under five sections.

1 The armstroke.
2 The dolphin kick.
3 Timing between arms and legs.
4 Body position.
5 Breathing.

The armstroke

The butterfly armstroke consists of three diagonal sweeps and a recovery. The sweeps used are the outsweep, including the entry and catch, the insweep, and the upsweep. The underwater armstroke is pictured from a side view in Fig. 8.1. The recovery is shown from a surface view in Fig. 8.2.

The outsweep, entry, and catch

These phases of the armstroke are shown from the surface in Fig. 8.2. The underwater movements of the arms can be seen from a side view in Fig. 8.1.

The swimmer's hands should enter the water at shoulder width or slightly wider. The palms of the hands should be facing out so they slide into the water on edge (Fig. 8.2).

After entering the water, the hands should sweep out and down until the arms are outside the shoulders and facing back against the water. That is the catch position where arm propulsion begins (Fig. 8.1b). The hands may be facing out slightly when beginning the outsweep or they can be facing down. Regardless of their position at the start, the palms should rotate out during the outsweep until they are facing out and back

when the catch is made. Hand speed will decelerate until the arms are barely moving at the catch. The outsweep is not a propulsive movement. It should be a gentle, stretching motion. Its purpose is to place the hands in position for the propulsive insweep that follows.

Swimmers should flex the arms gradually as they near the catch position to aid in getting them facing back. Any attempt to apply propulsive force before the hands and arms are facing back and aligned in this way will only decelerate forward speed by pushing water out or down.

The insweep

The insweep is shown in Fig. 8.1. It is the first of two propulsive sweeps in the butterfly armstroke. The arms sweep down, in and up in a semi-circular movement that is accomplished by continued flexing at the elbows after the catch. The insweep ends when the swimmer's hands are almost touching under the body. The arms will be flexed approximately 90° at the elbows at this time (Fig. 8.1d).

The hands, which were pitched out and back at the catch, are gradually rotated in during the insweep until they are pitched in and up when they come together under the body. Hand speed accelerates moderately during the movement.

Not all swimmers bring their hands together under the body during this movement. Some terminate the insweep earlier. The best method is not known at this time, since world-class butterfly swimmers have used both styles. Hand width at the end of the outsweep is one factor that probably determines how far the hands sweep under the body. Swimmers who catch wide naturally start their insweeps with their hands further apart. Consequently, they may be able to utilize the propulsive potential of the insweep without bringing their hands very close together under their bodies. It is also possible that swimmers who have an affinity for sculling use the insweep over a longer distance. On the other hand, those who do not, terminate the movement earlier to get on to the upsweep.

The upsweep

The upsweep is shown in Fig. 8.1. It begins as the hands are coming together near the end of the

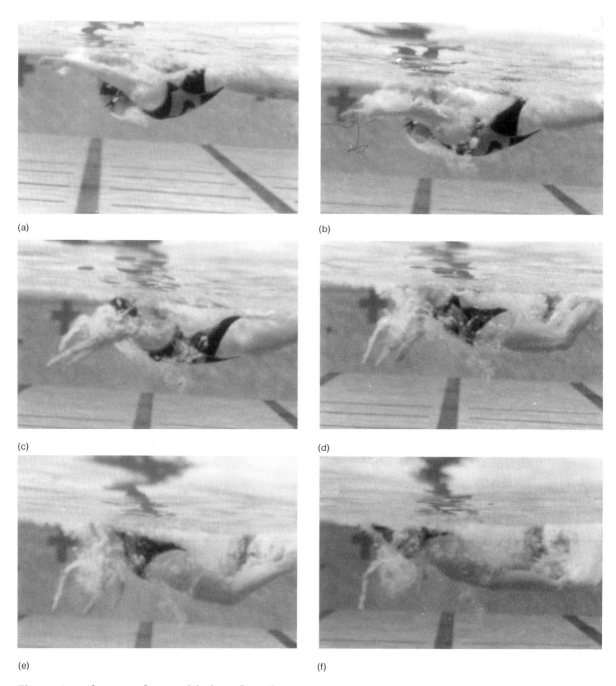

(a)

(b)

(c)

(d)

(e)

(f)

Fig. 8.1 An underwater side view of the butterfly stroke.

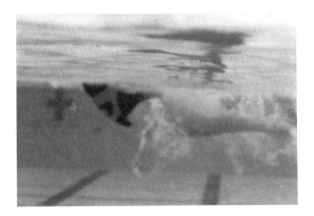

(g)

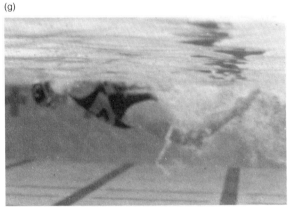

(h)

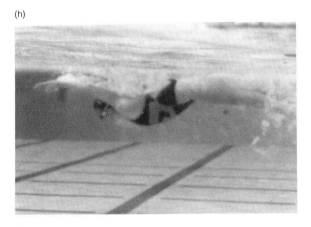

(i)

Fig. 8.1 (contd)

preceding insweep. They circle out and back and sweep up toward the surface of the water. The hands rotate out quickly so they are pitched out and back during the upsweep. Hand speed slows during the transition from insweep to upsweep. After that, the hands accelerate until they release pressure on the water. The release takes place when the swimmer's hands pass the thighs. The recovery begins at this time. The swimmer's arms will extend slightly during the upsweep. However, they will remain flexed somewhat until the release takes place.

Release and recovery

The release and beginning of the recovery are shown from underwater in Fig. 8.1h. The above-water portions of the recovery can be seen in Fig. 8.2.

As described, the release occurs before the swimmer's hands reach the surface and before the arms are completely extended. The release is made as the hands pass the thighs. At that time, the swimmer turns the palms in so the hands can slide up and out of the water, on edge, with a minimum of resistance.

The arms, which were extended slowly earlier during the upsweep, extend rapidly after the release so that they leave the water circling up, out and forward. They travel over the water until the entry is made. The arms may be completely extended or slightly flexed during the first half of the recovery. It is recommended that swimmers flex their arms slightly during the second half of the recovery to make the transition from entry to outsweep with a minimum of effort. The arms will be traveling in during the final portion of the recovery but their direction must change to out after they enter the water. That change can be facilitated if the arms are flexed slightly before entering the water. This permits them to be extended after the entry, which assists in starting the hands out even while the arms are traveling in.

The swimmer's hands should remain on the sides during the recovery, facing in during the first half and out during the second half. The recovery should be quick, but not rushed. Swimmers must have time to get their legs positioned for the downbeat of the first kick before their arms enter the water. The arms should be relaxed as much as possible so the muscles can rest during the recovery. Swimmers should let the momentum of the upsweep carry their arms through

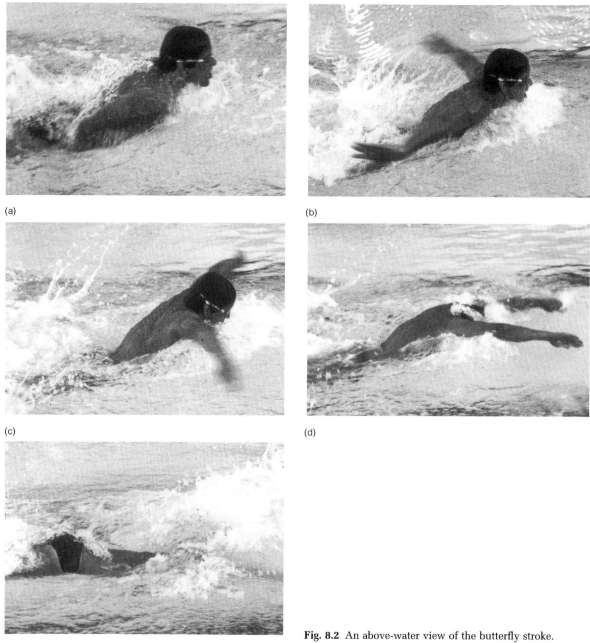

(a)

(b)

(c)

(d)

(e)

Fig. 8.2 An above-water view of the butterfly stroke.

the first half of the recovery. In the second half, they should use only enough muscular effort to effect the change of direction to forward that is required to make the entry.

Although the recovery is low and lateral, the arms should be carried high enough to remain clear of the water or they will drag forward through it and increase wave drag. The swimmers should raise their shoulders out of the water slightly in order to allow their arms space to recover without dragging. Butterfly swimmers have traditionally been taught to keep their shoulders in the water during the recovery. To the contrary, films show that the majority of world-class swimmers in this stroke have their shoulders out of the water during the recovery. Of course, it is possible to lift the shoulders too high out of the water. When the upward movement exceeds the forward motion, a swimmer's trunk and legs will drop deeper in the water. They must keep their shoulders moving forward as well as up during the recovery to prevent this from happening.

The dolphin kick

The *dolphin kick* is the term used for the leg movements in butterfly because they move as one unit like the tail (fluke) of a dolphin. The underwater photos in Fig. 8.1 show the dolphin kick. It is a series of wave-like motions that start in the lower back and travel down the length of the swimmer's legs and consist of an upbeat and a downbeat. There are two dolphin kicks per armstroke. The first takes place when the swimmer's hands enter the water and sweep out and the second kick is executed when the hands sweep out and up toward the surface at the end of the underwater armstroke. The downbeat of the first kick probably accelerates the body forward. The primary purpose of the second kick is probably to prevent the hips from being pulled down as the arms sweep up. The upbeats of both kicks are probably not propulsive for the reasons described in the Chapter 6.

The upbeat

Like the flutter kick, the dolphin kick is a whip-like motion where one beat begins when the other is nearing completion. The upbeat is shown in Fig. 8.1.

It begins as the legs are nearly extended during the

downbeat of the preceding kick. The downbeat of the lower legs starts a rebound-like reaction that pushes the swimmer's thighs up (Fig. 8.1a). After completing the downbeat, the legs continue sweeping up in an extended position until they are at the same level as the hips. The next downbeat begins at this time.

The work of lifting the legs is done by the muscles that extend the hip joints — the *gluteus maximus*. Water pressure from above maintains the swimmer's legs in an extended position during the upbeat. It also pushes the feet into a natural position midway between extension and flexion. Swimmers should not bend their legs at the knees during the upbeat.

The downbeat

The downbeat of the first kick, which is the larger of the two kicks in each stroke cycle, is shown in Fig. 8.1. It is a whip-like action that begins with flexion at the hips, followed by extension of the knees, and finally, flexion at the ankles. This kick is initiated by flexing the hips as the swimmer's feet pass above the level of the body (Fig. 8.1d). At the point, she begins pressing her thighs down. The water pressure, which is now pushing up from underneath, causes the legs to bend and pushes her feet up into an extended and pigeon-toed position (plantar flexed and inverted). Shortly after her thighs begin moving down, the swimmer vigorously extends her lower legs to complete the downbeat.

A better-than-average ability to extend the feet at the ankles is probably essential to an effective dolphin kick. Barthels and Adrian (1974) concluded that this was more important than strength. Butterflyers should be able to extend their feet 70–85° from the vertical.

Good dolphin kickers spread their knees at the beginning of the downbeat and then bring them together at the end. This probably serves two purposes: the feet can be pitched in and up more when the knees are apart, and the feet will remain pitched in and up longer if the thighs are rotated in as the legs extend.

Although one of the primary functions of the dolphin kick is to elevate and submerge the hips, swimmers must be careful that these up-and-down movements are not excessive. The hips should flow up and over the surface during the first downbeat when the kick has been performed properly. They should fall just below the surface on the subsequent upbeat. Excessive up-and-down hip movements will increase form and wave drag.

Timing of the armstroke and kick

The fact that there are two kicks to each armstroke was mentioned earlier. The downbeat of the first kick should be executed during the entry and outsweep of the arms while the downbeat of the second coincides with the upsweep of the underwater armstroke. This explanation, although correct, is an oversimplification of the complex timing between the arm and leg movements in this stroke.

The proper relationships between these two kicks and the armstroke can be seen most clearly in Fig. 8.1. The downbeat of the first kick should begin just as the swimmer's hands enter the water. In this way, it will counteract the drag produced by the arms as they move forward into the water. The downbeat continues during the outsweep and should be completed just before the catch is made (Fig. 8.1a).

The following upbeat takes place during the insweep of the arms. This movement improves streamlining during this propulsive phase of the armstroke while getting the legs in position for the next downbeat.

The downbeat of the second kick should be executed in time with the upsweep of the arms (Fig. 8.1e and g). The next upbeat takes place during the arm recovery. This action performs the same functions as the upbeat of the first kick. It brings the legs up near the surface so the body is streamlined when the swimmer is decelerating rapidly. It also places the legs in position for the downbeat of the next kick.

For a long time experts have debated whether one of the dolphin kicks in each stroke cycle should be emphasized more than the other. Those who believe in such emphasis refer to the two kicks as major and minor. It may not be wise for swimmers consciously to put more effort into one kick than the other. Differences in body position, not effort, cause the first kick to be longer and more propulsive. The swimmer's head is down during this downbeat, and the hips can travel up and forward for a longer distance. This, in turn, permits her to kick down for a longer time (Fig. 8.1i). The upbeat that follows will also be longer in order to bring the hips down in alignment with the body (Fig. 8.1a–c). The upbeat of the first kick appears to involve not only the legs and hips but the lower back as well. Extension of the swimmer's spine brings the legs up and lowers the hips.

On the other hand, the second kick appears to be more knee-oriented. Elevation of a swimmer's shoulders and trunk prevents her from flexing the hips as much when the kick is executed. The next upbeat, the one that coincides with the arm recovery, is also shorter because the trunk is elevated and the legs cannot sweep up for as long a distance without pushing the head and shoulders down.

Body position

It is useless to talk of one body position for the butterfly because a swimmer's body is constantly changing positions throughout each stroke cycle. However, there are three positions that the body assumes during each cycle that play an important role in reducing drag.

1 The swimmer's body should be as level as possible during the most propulsive phases of the armstroke. Those phases are the insweep and the upsweep (Fig. 8.1). This is accomplished by bringing the legs up during the insweep and by not kicking too deep during the upsweep.

2 The hips should travel up and forward through the surface during the first downbeat (Fig. 8.1). If the hips do reach the surface, the kick has not been sufficiently propulsive, nor has it served the function of streamlining the body.

3 The force of the second kick should not be so great that it pushes the swimmer's hips above the surface (Fig. 8.1). That will interfere with the arm recovery.

Up-and-down movements of the swimmer's body should not be excessive. The effect of this mistake was illustrated in Fig. 6.6. Excessive undulation increases the space swimmers take up in the water and, consequently, the resistance of that water to forward movement. Swimmers should not push the hips up excessively high and they should not dive the heads excessively deep.

Adequate undulation occurs when:

1 the head drops just below the arms as the hands enter the water (Fig. 8.1);

2 the hips rise just enough to break the surface on the first downbeat of the legs;

3 the hips and legs are not deep enough in the water when they complete the downbeat of the second kick.

Breathing

The correct sequence for breathing is shown from the surface in Fig. 8.2. Since many of the head movements take place under the surface, some of the underwater photos in Fig. 8.1 will also be referred to.

The head movements necessary for bringing the swimmer's face above the surface for a breath begin during the outsweep of the armstroke. Swimmers will be looking down when the arms enter the water but should begin raising the head toward the surface during the outsweep or they will have to delay breathing until too late in the stroke cycle (Fig. 8.1a and d). They continue looking up and the head approaches the surface during the insweep of the arms. The face should break through the surface of the water during the upsweep of the arms (Fig. 8.2a). Swimmers should inhale while completing that movement and during the first half of the arm recovery (Fig. 8.2a and b). The face should drop back into the water during the second half of the recovery (Fig. 8.2c and d).

If the lifting of the head is delayed during the outsweep, the swimmer will have to delay starting the arm recovery until the head reaches the surface. This is the usual cause of the hitch in the strokes of some butterflyers when the hands are about to leave the water.

Butterfly swimmers usually do not breathe during every stroke cycle when they race. The usual advice is to breathe once during each two armstrokes in 100-m events. This is referred to as a 1-and-1 breathing pattern. This pattern is thought to be a good compromise between the need to take in oxygen and the desire to maintain a horizontal body position. Some coaches also recommend this breathing pattern for 200-m events. However, there are others who feel a 1-and-1 pattern does not supply enough oxygen for the longer race. They recommend patterns where breaths are taken during two or three consecutive stroke cycles before a nonbreathing stroke is completed. These breathing frequencies are referred to as 2-and-1 and 3-and-1 patterns. The extra breathing strokes increase oxygen consumption while the

periodic nonbreathing strokes allow swimmers to regain horizontal alignment.

Although breathing patterns of 1-and-1, 2-and-1 and 3-and-1 have been recommended almost universally, many butterfly swimmers disregard them and breathe during every stroke cycle. This pattern is used most frequently in 200-m races, although some successful butterfly swimmers have also used it in the 100-m event. There are so many successful swimmers using a variety of breathing patterns that it is impossible to know which is best for each event. One thing is certain, however. Swimmers should select a breathing pattern and keep to it from the beginning to the end of a race. They should not breathe whenever they feel the need. If swimmers restrict their breathing too much early in the race, it may cause them to fatigue severely at a later point in the event.

Each butterfly swimmer should determine his or her most effective breathing pattern by using a form of the experimental drill described in Chapter 7. The drill can be performed as follows. Swim a set of 12 or more 50- to 100-m butterfly on a short-to-medium rest interval. Alternate breathing methods from one repeat to the next, using 3-and-1, 2-and-1, and 1-and-1, and vary stroke patterns. Repeat this drill over several days, discarding the patterns that are clearly less effective, until you find the one that is consistently faster for the swimmer. That pattern should be used in competition. If there is no difference in speed between certain patterns, the pattern that provides the greatest oxygen supply should be used.

Breathing to the side

Some butterfly swimmers breathe to the side. It is believed that the energy cost of lifting the head can be reduced if the face is rotated to the side, as in the front crawl. It is also felt that this helps to maintain good horizontal alignment because the act of lifting the head tends to submerge the hips. This reasoning is faulty because it overlooks an important difference between the butterfly and front crawl. Front crawl swimmers can roll the body to bring the face above the surface. A butterflyer must rotate the head with the body in a prone position. The range of motion in the neck is usually too little to get the mouth out of the water *unless* the head is elevated above the surface. Consequently, a butterflyer who breathes to the side must lift the head and shoulders out of the water as much or more than a swimmer who breathes to the front. Thus, breathing to the side is not recommended.

Recommended reading

Barthels, K.M. & Adrian, M.J. (1971) Variability in the dolphin kick under four conditions. In Lewillie, L. & Clarys, J.P. (eds) *First International Symposium on Biomechanics in Swimming, Waterpolo and Diving Proceedings*. Brussels: Université Libre de Bruxelles, Laboratoire de L'Effort, pp. 105–118.

Barthels, K. & Adrian, M.J. (1974) Three dimensional spatial hand patterns of skilled butterfly swimmers. In Clarys, J.P. & Lewillie, L. (eds) *Swimming II*. Baltimore, Maryland: University Park Press, pp. 154–160.

Cavill, M.J. (1972) *A mathematical and cinematographical analysis of propulsive effects in the dolphin butterfly*. Unpublished master's thesis, University of Wisconsin, Madison, Wisconsin.

Crist, J.M. (1979) An analytical comparison between two types of butterfly pull patterns: the crossover and the keyhole. *Swim. Tech.* **15**:110–117.

Hinrichs, R. (1986) Biomechanics of butterfly. In Johnston, T., Woolger, J. & Scheider, D. (eds) *1985 ASCA World Clinic Yearbook*. Fort Lauderdale, Florida: American Swimming Coaches Association, p. 94.

Jensen, R.K. & McIlwain, J. (1979) Modeling lower extremity forces in the dolphin kick. In Terauds, J. & Bedingfield, E.W. (eds) *Swimming III*. Baltimore, Maryland: University Park Press, pp. 137–147.

Persyn, U., Vervaecke, H. & Verhetsel, D. (1983) Factors influencing stroke mechanics and speed in swimming butterfly. In Matsui, H. & Koybayashi, K. (eds) *Biomechanics VII-B*. Champaign, Illinois: Human Kinetics, pp. 833–841.

Schleihauf, R.E., Higgins, J.R., Hinrichs, R. *et al.* (1988) Propulsive techniques: front crawl stroke, butterfly, backstroke and breaststroke. In Ungerechts, B., Wilke, K. & Reischle, K. (eds) *Swimming Science V*. Champaign, Illinois: Human Kinetics, pp. 53–60.

Ungerechts, B.E. (1983) A comparison of the movements of the rear parts of dolphin and butterfly swimmers. In Hollander, A.P., Huijing, P.A. & de Groot, G. (eds) *Biomechanics and Medicine in Swimming*. Champaign, Illinois: Human Kinetics, pp. 215–221.

Chapter 9

Backstroke

Like the front crawl, the back crawl stroke consists of an alternating armstroke and a flutter kick. Unlike the crawl, however, swimmers are on their backs. This forces them to stroke to the sides rather than underneath the body. The back crawl stroke is discussed under five headings.

1　The armstroke.
2　The flutter kick.
3　Timing of the arms and legs.
4　Body position.
5　Breathing.

The armstroke

Side-view photos of the underwater armstroke are displayed in Fig. 9.1. Surface views of the arm recovery are shown in Fig. 9.2.

The back crawl armstroke consists of four sweeps and a recovery. For purposes of explanation, the sweeps have been termed first downsweep, first upsweep, second downsweep, and second upsweep.

First downsweep

The first downsweep of the right arm can be seen in Fig. 9.1a–c. The swimmer's arm enters the water fully extended and directly in front of his shoulder. His palm is facing out to the side. After his arm enters the water, he sweeps it down and out to the catch position. That is when his hand is at nearly its deepest and widest point. Figure 9.1c shows the catch position for the swimmer's right arm.

A common mistake made by many swimmers is to begin pushing against the water immediately after the arm enters the water. They must be cautioned to wait until they reach the catch position. The arm cannot be positioned to displace water back until they are near

the end of the downsweep. Any attempt to apply force before then will only push water down and decrease forward speed.

The swimmer in Fig. 9.1 rotates his palm down near the end of the first downsweep until it is facing down and back at the catch. His arm is flexed slightly at the elbow in preparation for the propulsive sweep that follows, when the catch is made.

The first downsweep is not propulsive. Its primary purpose is to place the swimmer's arm in position to apply propulsive force. It may also play a role in supporting his head and shoulders while his opposite arm is recovering over the water.

First upsweep

Figure 9.1c–e shows this phase of the armstroke. The first upsweep is the first propulsive phase of the underwater armstroke. It begins at the catch. From there, the swimmer sweeps his arm up and back in a semi-circular path until it is flexed approximately 90° and opposite his chest when the sweep ends. His hand rotates up and in while it is being brought toward the surface (Fig. 9.1e). His hand speed accelerates throughout the movement but it should not reach its maximum velocity until the end of the next sweep.

Figure 9.3 shows how swimmers displace water back during the first upsweep. The thumb-side is the leading edge of the swimmer's hand-foil and the little-finger-side is the trailing edge. This angle of attack, together with the upward direction in which the arm is moving, causes the relative flow of water to change from down to back. That directional change is illustrated by the shaded arrow representing water passing under the swimmer's palm from thumb- to little-finger-sides.

Second downsweep

The swimmer in Fig. 9.1 is performing the second downsweep in f and g for the right arm and l and m for the left. It begins as his hand passes the peak of the preceding upsweep. After that, his arm sweeps back and down in a semi-circular path until it is completely extended and well below his thigh. His hand, which was pitched up at the end of the upsweep, is rotated down during this sweep. It should be facing down toward the bottom of the pool when the sweep is

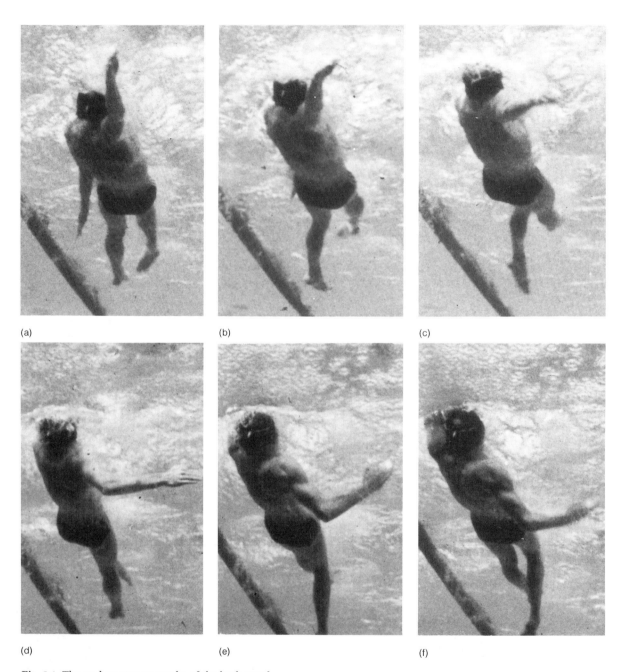

(a)   (b)   (c)

(d)   (e)   (f)

Fig. 9.1 The underwater armstroke of the back crawl.

completed. The swimmer's fingertips should *remain facing to the side* throughout the first downsweep (Fig. 9.1f and l).

Swimmers should not rotate their fingers up when they start this movement; this was mistakenly taught in the 1970s. However, underwater films have clearly shown that the majority of world-class swimmers keep their fingers pointed to the side. Sweeping the hands down with the fingers facing up will place swimmer's forearms at the wrong angle of attack.

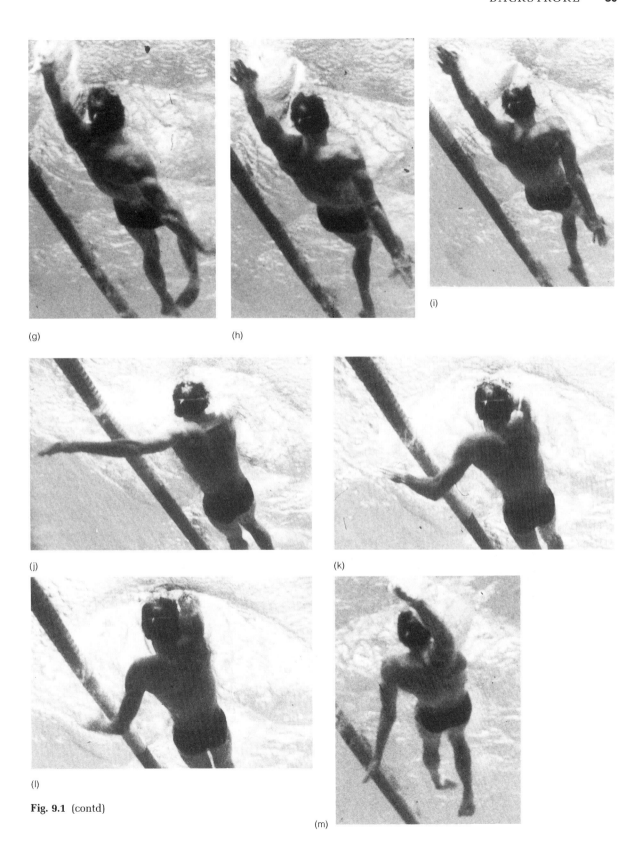

(g)

(h)

(i)

(j)

(k)

(l)

(m)

Fig. 9.1 (contd)

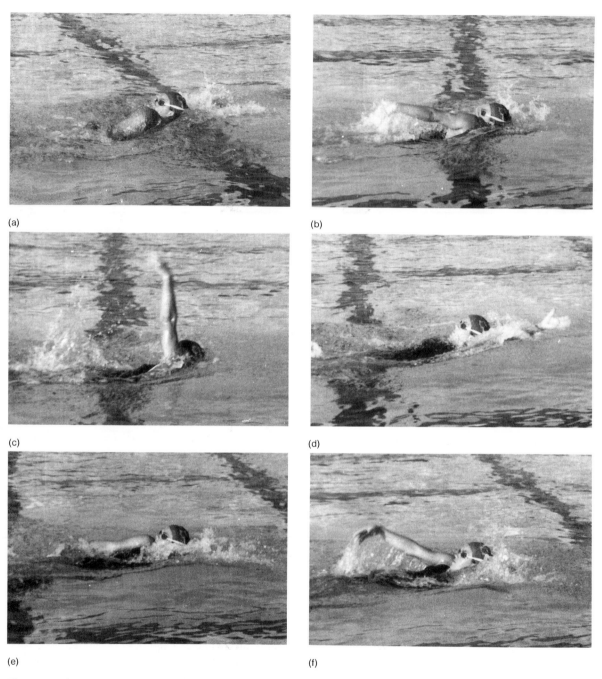

(a)

(b)

(c)

(d)

(e)

(f)

Fig. 9.2 Surface view of the back crawl arm recovery.

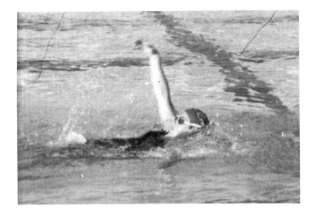

(g)

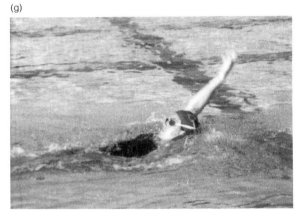

(h)

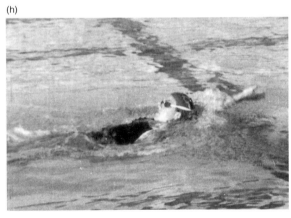

(i)

Fig. 9.2 (contd)

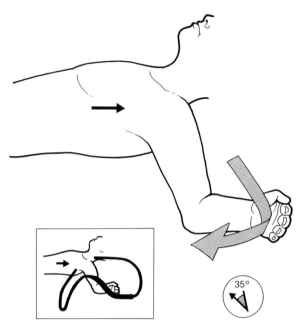

Fig. 9.3 The method for achieving propulsion during the first upsweep.

Hand speed should decrease during the transition to the second downsweep and then accelerate throughout the movement until the swimmer's hand is traveling at its maximum speed when the sweep ends.

Swimmers have traditionally been taught to sweep the arm in toward the thigh during this downsweep. Contrary to this method, it is more effective to sweep the arm straight down and back, or even out somewhat. These methods permit swimmers to position their forearms so they can displace water back longer during the course of the movement. It also positions their arm for the next propulsive sweep.

The proposed propulsive mechanism for the second downsweep is illustrated in Fig. 9.4. With the hand pitched down and out and traveling down, the leading edge of the swimmer's hand-foil is the little-finger-side. The thumb-side is the trailing edge. This combination of direction and angle of attack accelerates water back as his hand passes down through it. The shaded arrow shows how the relative direction of water flow changes from up to back as it passes under the swimmer's palm from the little-finger- to thumb-side. The counterforce should accelerate him forward.

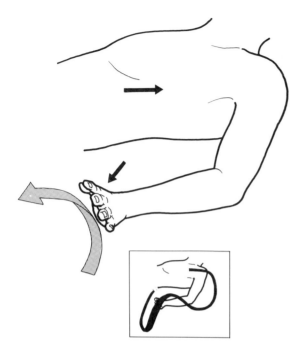

Fig. 9.4 The method for generating propulsion during the second downsweep.

back and slightly up. Their fingertips should be pointing down (Fig. 9.1h). Hand velocity will decrease slightly during the transition from second downsweep to second upsweep. It then accelerates, reaching maximum velocity as this movement is completed. Figure 9.5 illustrates how swimmers can displace water back during this sweep.

The wrist edge of the hand becomes the leading edge and the fingertips the trailing edge of the swimmer's hand. With this combination of direction and angle of attack, the relative flow of water will be displaced from down to back, in the direction of the shaded arrow, as it passes under the swimmer's palm from the wrist to little-finger edges.

Not all swimmers use the second upsweep for propulsion. Some simply begin recovering their arms after the second downsweep has been completed. This is not surprising since few, if any, have been taught to use this sweep for propulsion. It is surprising that several world-class backstroke swimmers are gaining propulsion from this motion without any awareness they are doing so.

Swimmers who wish to use it should make wide

Second upsweep

The description of this motion as a propulsive sweep may come as a surprise. Experts have believed for many years that the propulsive phase of the underwater armstroke ended when the second downsweep was completed. New information shows that swimmers can generate propulsive force as they bring their arms toward the surface (Luedtke, 1986).

The technique for making a propulsive second upsweep appears in Fig. 9.1h and i. It is very similar to the upsweep of the front crawl stroke except, of course, that the swimmer is in a supine, rather than prone, position.

From the end of the preceding downsweep, swimmers sweep their hand up, back, and in until it reaches the rear of the thigh. The recovery begins at that point. The hand starts traveling forward as well as up after it reaches the thigh and no more propulsion can be gained.

They should hyperextend their hands at the wrist during the second upsweep so their palms are facing

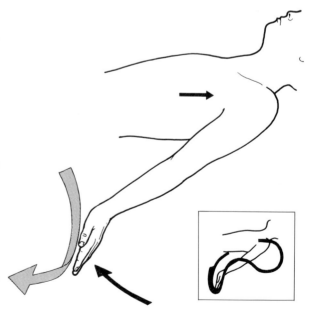

Fig. 9.5 The method for displacing water back during the second upsweep.

second downsweeps. This places their arm in position to displace water back during the second upsweep. Those who do not should direct the second downsweep in toward their thigh so they can begin their recovery immediately after sweeping the arm down.

It is not possible to state with certainty that the wide stroke is superior to the narrow stroke because world-class swimmers are using both at the present time. We believe, however, that it is potentially superior and that the majority of world-class swimmers will be using the wide stroke in years to come.

The release, recovery and entry

Figure 9.1 shows an underwater view of the release and the first portion of the recovery. A surface view appears in Fig. 9.2.

As stated earlier, swimmers should release pressure on the water when their hand approaches the lower portion of the thigh as they complete the second upsweep. At that time, they turn their palm in toward their body and slide their hand up out of the water on edge. This reduces the surface area of the hand and prevents a large increase of resistance during its upward movement. Swimmers' hands should leave the water thumbs first, not little finger first, as some experts have suggested (Fig. 9.2f). Hand speed should decelerate markedly at the release. Continued upward rolling of their shoulders assists them in lifting their arm out of the water with minimal effort.

After leaving the water, the arm should travel up and forward over the water until the entry is made. The recovery should be made high and overhead, not low and to the side. This will reduce any tendency for the arm to pull the swimmer's hips and legs out of lateral alignment.

The palm should be facing in during the first half of the recovery and out during the second half. The change from in to out is made as the hand passes its highest point and starts down for the entry.

The recovery should be made quickly but gently. Swimmers' hands and arms should be relaxed as much as possible so that the muscles rest between underwater armstrokes.

As mentioned earlier, the entry is made with the arm extended and directly forward of the shoulder (Fig. 9.2i). The hand should be facing out so it can slice into the water without causing excessive turbulence.

Timing of the arms

The arms stroke in an alternating, windmill fashion during this stroke. The recovering arm should enter the water when the stroking arm has completed its second downsweep. The downsweep of the front arm should begin while the rear arm is executing the second upsweep. In this way, propulsion can be maintained until the front arm has had time to sweep down to the catch position.

Differences in the stroke patterns of backstroke swimmers

The major differences in the styles used by backstroke swimmers fall into two categories: swimmers who use a deep catch versus those who prefer a shallow catch, and those who use a narrow stroke versus those who use a wide stroke. The wide stroke was recommended earlier as being potentially superior to the narrow style. Nevertheless, swimmers should not be forced to use this style. It is in the developmental stage. We will learn whether it can stand the test of time once it has been taught to a larger number of swimmers.

From a theoretical point of view, the deep catch should also be more effective than a shallow stroke. A deep catch makes a long propulsive upsweep more likely. However, some swimmers are not good scullers while others do not have adequate ability to hyperflex their shoulders (reach their arms back and down) to use these techniques effectively. When they try, they end up rolling excessively, pushing down on the water during the first downsweep, or sweeping their hands up and down over long distances at the wrong angle of attack.

Backstroke swimmers who are poor scullers or those who have relatively inflexible shoulders probably do not sacrifice propulsive force with a shallow downsweep and short upsweep because they could not have performed these skills well initially. Consequently, the net result may be that they gain more propulsion with a wide catch and short upsweep than they could with the deep catch and long upsweep. There are several world-class backstrokers who have used this style over the years.

Obviously, all swimmers should not be forced to use the deep catch even though it may be superior from a theoretical point of view. The decision as to which style to use may depend upon a particular swimmer's sculling skills and the range of motion in his or her shoulder joints.

The best technique for most backstroke swimmers may be a compromise between the two styles. They should sweep their hand down and out approximately equal amounts during the first downsweep. This should allow an effective catch for all but the most inflexible swimmers. That catch should be followed by an upsweep of moderate length directed back as well as up.

The flutter kick

The flutter kick for the back crawl stroke is very similar to the one used in the front crawl. It consists of alternating diagonal thrusts of the legs. There are some slight differences between the kicks in the two strokes that are worth mentioning, however. The underwater mechanics can be seen in Fig. 9.1. The two major movements in this kick, the upbeat and downbeat, are described below.

The upbeat

The upbeat is a whip-like extension of the leg that begins with flexion at the hip, followed quickly by extension at the knee, ending with partial flexion of the foot (the toes kick up and through the surface). The upbeat of the swimmer's right leg can be seen in Fig. 9.1a−f.

The upbeat begins as the foot passes below the buttocks during the preceding downbeat. At that point, the swimmer flexes at the hip and starts her thigh moving up (Fig. 9.2e). In the meantime, the lower leg and foot have been relaxed so the water pressing down from above pushes the leg into a flexed position at the knee while also pushing the foot down into an extended and pigeon-toed position (plantar flexed and inverted). This position of the foot is shown in Fig. 9.1g.

The thigh continues up until it passes above the hip. At that point, the swimmer extends his leg rapidly at the knee, sweeping it diagonally up toward the surface. That movement continues until the leg is completely extended just below the surface of the water.

Swimmers' legs will be flexed more during the upbeat in this stroke than in the corresponding downbeat of the front crawl stroke (approximately 10° more). This puts the legs into an excellent position for delivering propulsive force. The same amount of knee flexion is not possible in the front crawl because it would put the lower legs and feet above the surface of the water.

The downbeat

The downbeat of the leg is a rebound-like action that begins as it completes the previous upbeat. Figure 9.1a−c show the downbeat of the swimmer's left leg.

His thigh starts traveling down in a rebound-like action as he completes the preceding upbeat. Once that upbeat has been completed, his entire leg sweeps down. It is maintained in an extended position until it passes below his body line. His foot is in a natural position, midway between flexion and extension. The pressure of the water pushing up from underneath his legs and feet keeps them in this position. The downbeat ends when the swimmer's leg passes below his body during its downward path. At that point, he begins flexing his thigh at the hip to start the next upbeat.

The upbeat is probably a propulsive movement because the swimmer's leg and foot can be positioned to displace water back during most of it. The downbeat, on the other hand, is probably not propulsive. The extended position of the swimmer's leg provides a perpendicular angle of attack that should only be useful for pushing water down. Consequently, swimmers should not use great force or unnecessary speed during the downbeat.

Timing of the arms and legs

Backstrokers, almost without exception, use a six-beat timing where there are six upbeats (and downbeats) of the legs during each stroke cycle, or three upbeats per armstroke. These beats are synchronized with the first three sweeps of the armstroke in much the same way as was described for the front crawl stroke (Chapter 7). The fourth sweep—the second upsweep—will be taking place while the other arm is executing its first downsweep. The coordination of arms and legs with six-beat timing can be seen in Fig. 9.1. The sequence is as follows.

1 The right leg kicks up (and the left down) during the first downsweep of the right arm while the left arm is completing its second upsweep (Fig. 9.1a–c).
2 The left leg kicks up (and the right down) during the first upsweep of the right armstroke (Fig. 9.1c–e).
3 The right leg kicks up, once again (and the left down) during the second downsweep of the right armstroke (Fig. 9.1f–i).

A similar but opposite sequence of arm and leg movements is repeated during the left armstroke.

The similarity between the timing of this stroke and the six-beat timing of the front crawl lends additional support to the theory that six-beat timing may be the most efficient method for both strokes. This statement is at least true for distances of 200 m and less.

The kick also performs a stabilizing function, maintaining the swimmer's body in alignment. Swimmers should kick diagonally up and down in time with the roll of their bodies.

Body position

Backstrokers have more problems maintaining lateral alignment than athletes in other strokes. This is because their arms are moving alternately and tend to swing out to the side as they recover over the water. Some also have a tendency to sit in the water, with their hips down and heads up, which upsets their horizontal alignment.

The swimmer in Fig. 9.1 has good horizontal alignment. His body is nearly horizontal with the surface of the water although he pikes at the waist slightly. This small bend enables him to keep his thighs from breaking through the surface of the water during the upbeat of his kick. Viewed from the surface, the back of a backstroke swimmer's head should be resting in the water with the waterline passing just under his ears. The chin should be tucked slightly with the eyes focused back and up (Fig. 9.2). Swimmers should not arch their backs nor should they bend excessively at the waist.

Swimmers in this stroke must also keep their bodies from swinging from side to side. Good lateral alignment is shown from an underneath view in Fig. 9.6. The swimmer's hips and legs remain within shoulder width at all times, even though she is rolling from side to side.

Where lateral alignment is concerned, the best

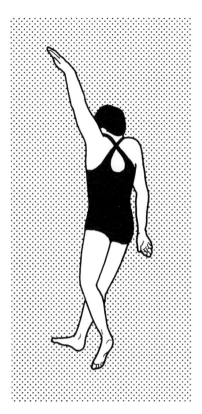

Fig. 9.6 An underneath view of a backstroke swimmer showing good lateral alignment.

preventive measure is for swimmers to roll their bodies in harmony with the movements of their arms. The alternate action of the arms in the back crawl causes one arm to be moving down when the other is traveling up. It is very important for swimmers to roll their bodies in the same directions their arms are moving if they want to prevent their hips and legs swinging from side to side. While it is possible to roll too much, it is far more common for backstrokers to roll too little. Backstroke swimmers should roll approximately 45° to each side. They should roll to the right as their right arm enters the water and sweeps down and they should also roll to the left when their left arm enters the water and sweeps down. Their bodies will be pulled out of alignment if these rolling movements are not timed properly, or if swimmers roll their shoulders while trying to keep their hips flat. Their entire bodies should roll as a unit—shoulders, hips and legs. Any body part that fails to roll in time with the others will be pulled out of alignment. The only exception to these statements concerns the head. It should remain in a stationary position with eyes focused up and back. The roll should be from shoulders to toes.

Another important function of body roll is to facilitate the arm recovery. When swimmers roll their bodies in the direction of their entering arm, the opposite shoulder will come out of the water so that the recovery of that arm can be made without pushing a large amount of water forward.

Breathing

Unlike swimmers in the other competitive strokes, backstrokers' faces are not submerged during part of each stroke cycle. Consequently, they do not need to inhale and exhale at specific times. Nevertheless, some coaches feel it is more efficient to establish a breathing rhythm. They recommend inhaling during one arm recovery and exhaling on the other. This advice may not be necessary, because with their faces above the water where they can breathe any time they want, backstrokers may naturally develop other rhythms that suit them better. Regardless, teaching a swimmer to inhale on one arm recovery and exhale on the next will probably not do any harm. The breathing rate they will use should be sound from a physiological point of view.

Trained athletes strike a compromise between the rate and depth of breathing by taking between 30 and 50 breaths per minute during strenuous exercise (Åstrand & Rodahl, 1977). Most backstroke swimmers complete 30–40 stroke cycles in 100-m races that require in the neighborhood of 60 s to complete. Therefore, inhaling on one armstroke of each cycle would allow them to breathe at this optimum rate.

Recommended reading

Åstrand, P.-O. & Rodahl, K. (1977) *Textbook of Work Physiology*. San Francisco: McGraw-Hill.

Luedtke, D. (1986) Backstroke biomechanics. In Johnston, T., Woolger, J. & Scheider, D. (eds) *1985 ASCA World Clinic Yearbook*. Fort Lauderdale, Florida: American Swimming Coaches Association, p. 95.

Persyn, U., De Maeyer, J. & Vervaecke, H. (1975) Investigation of hydrodynamic determinants of competitive swimming strokes. In Lewillie, L. & Clarys, J.P. (eds) *Swimming II*. Baltimore, Maryland: University Park Press, pp. 214–222.

Pfeifer, H. (1984) Some selected problems of technique and training in backstroke swimming. In Cramer, J.L. (ed.) *How to Develop Olympic Level Swimmers*. Helsinki: International Sports Media, pp. 160–179.

Schleihauf, R.E., Higgins, J.R., Hinrichs, R. *et al.* (1988) Propulsive techniques: front crawl stroke, butterfly, backstroke and breaststroke. In Ungerechts, B., Wilke, K. & Reischle, K. (eds) *Swimming Science V*. Champaign, Illinois: Human Kinetics, pp. 53–60.

Chapter 10

Breaststroke

The breaststroke is the slowest of the competitive strokes. Although breaststroke swimmers are able to generate more force during the propulsive phases than athletes in the other swimming strokes, they also decelerate markedly each time they recover the legs in preparation for a kick. This consequently reduces the average velocity per stroke considerably below that of other styles.

More than any of the other competitive strokes, the breaststroke is undergoing style changes at an accelerated rate. Experts disagree about the efficacy of swimming the stroke with a relatively flat body position versus an undulating style that resembles the butterfly body position. A recent rule change has resulted in more swimmers using the undulating style. The rule change permits swimmers to drop the head underwater during portions of each stroke cycle. This has allowed swimmers to move the body more freely. The undulating style that is currently most popular has been termed the *wave stroke*. Many world-class breaststrokers have adopted this style or other styles that involve undulation. The undulating style will be described in this chapter as it is considered to be the best way to swim the stroke, for several reasons, and these reasons will be discussed.

The breaststroke is described under the following four headings.
1 The armstroke.
2 The kick.
3 Timing of the armstroke and kick.
4 Body position and breathing.
The underwater pulldown that is permitted after the start and after each turn is also been described.

The armstroke

The breaststroke armstroke can be seen in the underwater side-view photos of Fig. 10.1. A surface view of the breaststroke appears in Fig. 10.2. For descriptive purposes, the different phases of the armstroke have been termed the outsweep, the insweep, and the recovery.

The outsweep

The swimmer can be seen executing the outsweep in Fig. 10.1a−c. The outsweep begins as the swimmer's legs come together to complete the propulsive phase of the kick. The swimmer sweeps the arms out to the catch position. The catch is made when the hands are outside shoulder width and facing back against the water. The catch position can be seen in Fig. 10.1c.

The swimmer's arms are extended during most of the outsweep. However, they flex slightly in preparation for the propulsive phase of the stroke when nearing the catch position. The hands should be facing down when the outsweep begins. They rotate out as they near the catch until they are pitched out and backward when the outsweep has been completed.

The outsweep is not propulsive; consequently, swimmers should sweep the hands out slowly and gently.

The insweep

The insweep is the propulsive phase of the armstroke (Fig. 10.1c−e). Once the catch has been made, the swimmer executes a large semi-circular sweep with the arms. They sweep downward, inward and then up until they are together under the head. The insweep should end just before the swimmer's hands come together. Starting at the catch, the arms continue to flex at the elbows until they are flexed more than 90° when the insweep has been completed. The palms, which were pitched out, are gradually rotated inward throughout the sweep. Hand velocity should accelerate steadily throughout the movement until the swimmer's hands are traveling at maximum speed when they come together.

The recovery

The swimmer is shown completing the arm recovery in Fig. 10.1g−i. This is one of the most controversial phases of the stroke cycle, of which some elements will be mentioned in the following description.

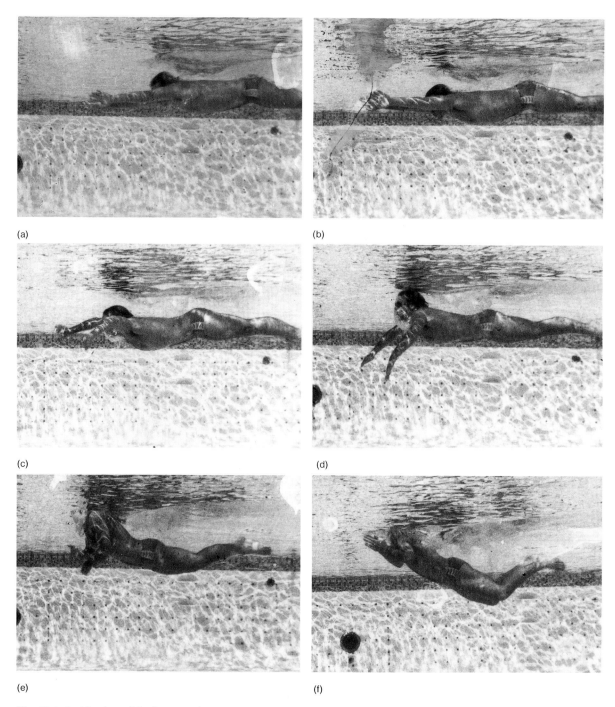

Fig. 10.1 A side view of the breaststroke.

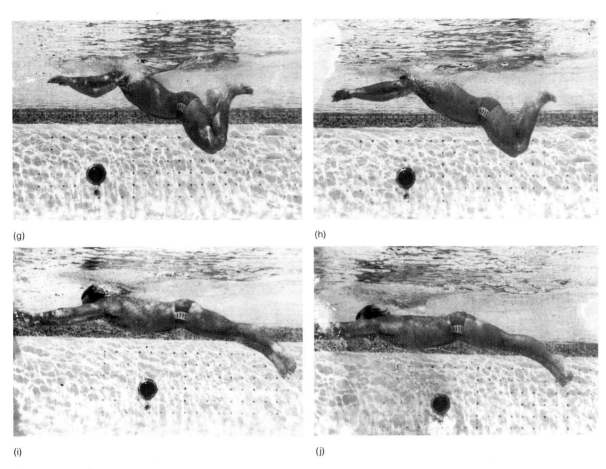

(g)

(h)

(i)

(j)

Fig. 10.1 (contd)

The arm recovery begins when the swimmer's hands are approximately halfway through the inward movement. Pressure on the water is released at this time. The swimmer continues to flex the arms, however, bringing them up under the chin before extending them forward for the next armstroke.

The swimmer then squeezes the elbows down and in shortly after the recovery begins. This will help change the direction in which the arms are traveling from inward to forward. The palms were rotating in during the previous insweep. They continue traveling in this direction until they are facing up as the hands come under the chin (Fig. 10.1f). They then rotate down to a prone position as the arms are extended forward (Fig. 10.1g).

Some breaststroke swimmers prefer to recover the arms over the water while others keep them underneath. Both styles have been used by successful athletes, consequently it is not possible to recommend one method over the other at this time. It is also impossible to state with any certainty that swimmers who recover over the water encounter less resistive drag. All swimmers who attempt to recover in this style drag the arms through the water somewhat. It remains to be determined whether the wave drag they produce is less resistive than the drag created when recovering the arms underwater.

Swimmers who prefer to recover underwater should make every effort to streamline the arms as they extend them forward. This can be accomplished by

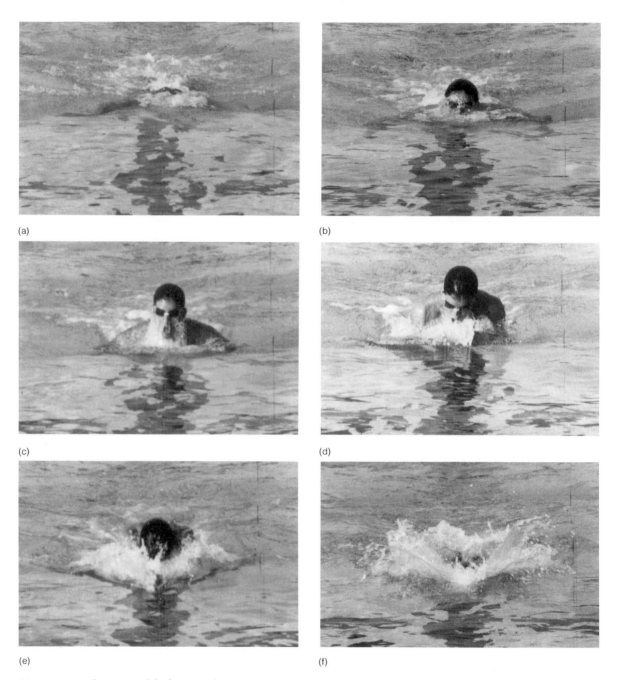

(a)

(b)

(c)

(d)

(e)

(f)

Fig. 10.2 A surface view of the breaststroke.

keeping the arms close together and by putting the hands together so they resemble an arrowhead. The arms should recover just under the surface. An underwater recovery that is excessively deep will produce greater resistive drag. Additionally, this may cause the swimmer to waste time sweeping the hands upward during the subsequent upsweep.

Coaches frequently debate whether swimmers should rotate the palms up during the recovery. Underwater films and video tapes have shown that many excellent breaststroke swimmers use this technique. At first glance this seems to be a superfluous motion because it cannot possibly be propulsive. However, this movement is probably a follow-through motion that is the natural after-effect of a good insweep. The swimmer's palms should rotate inwardly as they release pressure at the end of the insweep. Consequently, the inertia will continue them rotating in and up through the first portion of the recovery. Swimmers who prevent the palms from rotating upward will have to terminate the insweep prematurely to avoid the inward inertia caused by the hands.

Hand speed should decelerate during the recovery so that the swimmer's arms are moving slowly as they sweep out for the catch. Many swimmers are being instructed to accelerate the hands forward during the recovery in a style that has been termed a *lunge*. Accelerating the arms in this way should increase resistance and is therefore not recommended. The lunge probably results from the interrelationship between arm recovery, body undulation and the beginning of the propulsive phase of the kick. A discussion of these relationships has been included in the section on body position, below.

The kick

The leg action in this stroke has evolved from a wide, circling wedge kick, to a shorter, snappy whip kick. Initially, the whip kick was thought to be superior because water could be pushed back by extending the legs and using the soles of the feet like paddles. We realize now, however, that the feet, like the arms, also scull in circular paths. The kick style used by most present-day breaststrokers is actually a combination of the wedge and whip styles. Breaststroke swimmers

separate the legs and squeeze them together, but only to a limited extent. They do not spread the legs nearly as wide as did the old-style wedge-kick swimmers. There are five phases of the kick.

1 Recovery.
2 Outsweep.
3 Insweep.
4 Lift.
5 Glide.

The insweep is the only propulsive phase of the kick. The kick can be seen in Fig. 10.1.

The recovery

The swimmer's legs are in the recovery phase in Fig. 10.1e−g. After completing the propulsive phase of the armstroke, the lower legs are brought forward until they are very near the buttocks. The lower legs travel forward because of flexion at the knees, *not* at the hips. The lower legs have less mass and therefore will not push as much water forward during recovery. The thighs, on the other hand, are much larger, therefore if swimmers push them down and forward when they recover the legs, the retarding effect will be such that they will almost come to a complete stop.

Swimmers must drop the hips and incline the body down from head to hips in order to recover the legs without flexing at the hips. That is the only way they can keep the feet underwater. This is, perhaps, the most important reason why many skilled breaststroke swimmers raise the head and shoulder out of the water.

The toes of the swimmer in Fig. 10.1 are pointed back (feet extended) and the lower legs are held close together during leg recovery. The lower legs should be aligned inside the hips throughout the recovery to reduce form drag. The feet travel almost directly forward, rather than up and forward. The knees separate slightly during the recovery to keep the lower legs and feet inside the confines of the body. The knees should not separate very much outside the width of the shoulders, however.

The forward speed of swimmers will decelerate to its lowest point during the leg recovery. For this reason, the legs should be brought up quickly, but *gently*. The feet should begin sweeping out as they approach the buttocks, signaling the next phase of the kick—the outsweep.

The outsweep

In Fig. 10.1g and h the swimmer is sweeping the legs outward. This is not a propulsive phase of the kick. The purpose is to place the feet in position for the propulsive insweep that follows. At that point, the swimmer begins circling the feet outward as they approach the buttocks. They continue out until they are outside the hips and facing back against the water. That is the catch position (Fig. 10.1h).

The swimmer's legs should be flexed at the knees as much as possible so they pass very close to the buttocks. This will permit a higher position, resulting in a longer insweeping action. The feet should be plantar flexed and rotated outward at the ankles just prior to the catch. A high degree of ankle flexibility in these planes is a decided advantage in breaststroke swimmers because it enables them to place the feet in a position to displace water back earlier during the kick. Swimmers should perform special flexibility exercises to increase ankle flexion and rotation ability if they lack flexibility in these directions.

Swimmers should flex the thighs at the hip slightly during the outsweep. This statement may seem to conflict with one that was made earlier. There is, however, no contradiction. Swimmers should keep the hip flexion to a minimum during the recovery phase. However, they will need to flex the hips somewhat during the outsweep in order to deliver an optimum amount of force in the next phase of the kick. Although flexing at the hips will increase drag, it increases propulsive force even more because both the hip and knee extensor muscles will be working during the insweep that follows.

The difference between this technique and the one used by flat-style breaststrokers concerns the time course and amount of flexion. Flat-style breast-strokers begin flexing the hips during the recovery. Consequently, they flex them for a longer period of time and to a greater extent. Swimmers who use this style of recovery will flex the thighs quickly and only a small amount just before starting the propulsive phase of the kick. Thus, they will decelerate less than flat-style breaststrokers while gaining additional propulsion over swimmers who do not flex the legs at the hips.

The velocity of swimmers' feet should decelerate during the outsweep until the feet are not moving

much faster than the body when the catch is made. The propulsive phase — the insweep — will begin at that point.

The insweep

The insweep has two phases. The first portion could more correctly be called a downsweep because the swimmer's feet are traveling downward more than inward at this time. It is only during the final portion that they sweep in. This phase of the kick is described as one motion with two parts, because swimmers feel it as one continuous sweep of the legs.

The insweep begins at the catch and continues until the legs are completely extended and nearly together behind the swimmer. It is a semi-circular movement in which the legs sweep out, back, down, and in. The legs should be extended at the hips and the knees until they are completely straight at the end of this phase. The feet should be rotated down and in until the soles face each other. Figures 10.3 and 10.4 illustrate how propulsion is produced during both the down and in portions of the insweep.

The feet should be facing out and rotated down slightly as they sweep down in the first portion of the insweep. In this position, the leading edges of the

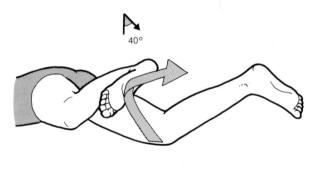

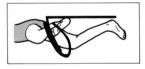

Fig. 10.3 Propulsion is produced during the downward portion of the insweep of the breaststroke kick. The illustration shows how water can be displaced backward by the combination of direction and angle of attack during the first downward portion.

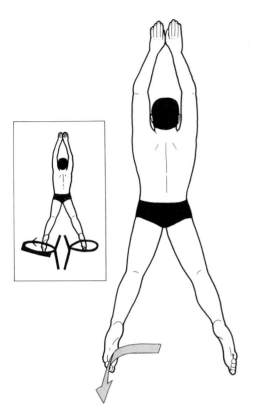

Fig. 10.4 Propulsion generated during the inward portion of the insweep of the breaststroke kick.

feet are the big-toe-sides and the trailing edges are the little-toe-side. The shaded arrow in Fig. 10.3 illustrates how the relative direction of water can be changed from up to back as the swimmer's feet pass down and back through it from leading to trailing edges. The slight downward angle of attack of the feet changes the direction of water flow to back as it passes underneath the soles from big- to little-toe-sides.

The first portion of the insweep continues until the swimmer's legs are extended. This is the most propulsive phase. As the legs extend, the direction of the feet changes from down to in as they execute the second portion of this movement. The feet sweep across the water until they come together. The in-sweep ends just before the swimmer's feet come together. At this time, the swimmer releases the pressure on the water and begins to lift the legs toward the surface. The probable way in which swimmers can

propel the body forward by accelerating water back is shown in Fig. 10.4.

In this position, the big-toe-side continues to function as the leading edge of the foot-propeller and the little toe remains the trailing edge as the feet sweep in. This combination of direction and angle of attack should cause the relative flow of water to change from out to back as the swimmer's feet travel through it from leading to trailing edges.

The angle of attack of the feet is a very important and misunderstood feature of this phase of the insweep. The feet should remain flexed at the ankles so that the swimmer's toes are pointing toward the bottom. The soles of the feet should be facing *in*, not up. Swimmers are commonly taught to extend the feet back and lift the legs to the surface during this phase. This causes the soles of the feet to push up against the water, which will decelerate the forward speed. Swimmers should not point the toes back and lift the legs until the insweep has been completed.

A swimmer's hips will dolphin up slightly when they perform the insweep correctly. This happens because the legs sweep down as well as in. The downward movement exerts a drag force that elevates the hips. Swimmers should not try to eliminate this slight dolphin motion as they will sacrifice some propulsive force.

As in all things, it is possible to overdo the dolphin action. If swimmers concentrate only on elevating the hips, the feet will be directed down too much and forward propulsion will be lessened. The dolphin action should be a natural aftermath of a correct kick. Swimmers should not make a conscious effort to elevate the hips. By the same token, they also should not try to keep them from moving upward. The velocity of the feet should increase steadily throughout the insweep, reaching a peak just before they release pressure on the water to begin the lift.

The lift

The swimmer in Fig. 10.1j can be seen lifting the legs toward the surface after completing the insweep. The lift is a continuation of the circular sweep that began with the insweep. The legs do not stop moving when the propulsive phase ends. Instead, they continue in and up until they are together and in line with the swimmer's trunk. The speed of the feet decelerates during the lift until the legs have stopped moving. They are now being pulled along by the armstroke.

Some believe the lift is a propulsive phase of the kick. This, however, is doubtful, as the swimmer's legs will be moving up and forward at a very large angle of attack during the lift. As a result they will push water up and forward, which should decelerate, rather than accelerate, forward speed. For this reason, the swimmer should lift the legs gently, using this motion only for the purpose of streamlining the legs behind.

The glide

The glide position takes place during the propulsive phase of the armstroke. This phase of the kick appears in Fig. 10.1a−d. Once the swimmer's legs are in line with the body, they are held close together in a streamlined position during the propulsive phases of the armstroke. The legs and feet are completely extended with the toes pointing downward.

Timing of the armstroke and kick

There are three styles of breaststroke timing advocated by the various swimming experts — continuous, glide and overlap. When continuous timing is used, the armstroke begins after the legs come together. In glide timing there is a short interval between the completion of the kick and the beginning of the armstroke, during which swimmers coast or glide along. In overlap timing the armstroke begins before the propulsive phase of the kick has been completed.

The majority of coaches agree that glide timing is the least effective of the three because swimmers decelerate from the time the propulsive phase of the kick ends until the propulsive phase of the armstroke begins. (Remember this statement — it will be important later in this section.) Those who prefer continuous timing believe the gap between applications of force by the legs and arms is eliminated by this method. The fallacy in this belief is that the outsweep of the armstroke is not propulsive. Consequently, swimmers who use continuous timing will also decelerate during the interval between the time they complete the propulsive phase of the kick when the arms sweep out to the catch position.

Overlap timing is the best method for eliminating, or

at least reducing, the period of deceleration between the propulsive phase of the kick and the propulsive phase of the armstroke. Swimmers should begin sweeping the arms out as the legs complete the last portion of the insweep. This will allow them to catch and begin propelling the body forward with the arms almost immediately after the propulsive phase of the kick has been completed.

Body position and breathing

These two factors go hand in hand and therefore will be discussed in the same section.

Body position

As with the butterfly stroke, it is useless to talk of one body position for an undulating style of breaststroke. There are three phases of the stroke cycle where the swimmer's body must be in the most streamlined position possible.

1 *Propulsive phase of the kick.* The body must be as horizontal as possible during the propulsive phases of the armstroke and kick. The trunk should be nearly horizontal with hips near the surface, shoulders in the water, and arms nearly extended during the propulsive phases of the kick. It will also improve streamlining if the head is underwater and between the extended arms, now that the rules permit this technique.

2 *Propulsive phase of the armstroke.* The trunk should be horizontal with hips near the surface and legs in line with the body during the propulsive phases of the armstroke. Although the swimmer is traveling toward the surface for a breath, the face should remain underwater until the propulsive phase of the armstroke is nearly completed.

3 *Leg recovery.* The trunk should be inclined down from head to knees during the leg recovery and the swimmer should not flex the legs at the hips until the outsweep of the legs has begun.

Breathing

Breaststroke swimmers should breathe once during each stroke cycle, regardless of the race distance. Breathing is such an integral part of the rhythm of this stroke that it aids rather than interferes with propulsion. Swimmers seem to lose the rhythm when they do not breathe. The swimmer in Fig. 10.2 demonstrates the proper breathing sequence from the surface. The underwater movements of the head involved in bringing the head to the surface for a breath can be seen in Fig. 10.1.

Swimmers should look down with the head tucked between the arms as they extend the arms forward prior to beginning the armstroke. They should begin to lift the face toward the surface when the arms start to sweep out (Fig. 10.1a). This is a very important point, for if they delay lifting the face until the catch is made, much of the force from the early portion of the insweep will be used for that purpose rather than for propulsion. Swimmers would have to turn the palms down during the first portion of the insweep and push down on the water to lift the head to the surface. This would sacrifice some propulsive force and decelerate the forward motion.

The head should be on the surface when the swimmer makes the catch with the hands (Fig. 10.1c). Following this, the downward movements of the arms will help lift the face so that the mouth breaks through the surface as the arms release pressure on the water and start to recover. The swimmer should inhale while recovering the arms forward. The head should be lowered into the water between the arms during the last portion of the arm recovery (Fig. 10.1a and i)

The interrelationship between the leg recovery and head drop is an important determinant of success in the undulating style of breaststroke. There are two very important techniques that should be used.

1 Swimmers should keep the heads and shoulders above the surface until the legs have been recovered and the outsweep of the kick begins. This will keep the hips submerged so that the legs can be recovered forward without flexing at the hips. Lowering the head and shoulders too early will cause the hips to be pushed upward toward the surface.

2 How swimmers recover the arms is also important to maintaining this position. They should recover them forward at the surface of the water to aid in maintaining the shoulders high until the leg recovery has been completed.

The underwater armstroke

Breaststroke rules permit the swimmer to take one underwater stroke immediately after the start of the race and one after each turn. When they complete that stroke, the head must break the surface of the water before the hands reach the widest part of the next armstroke. This underwater armstroke can be very powerful, so swimmers should practice this until they can perform it well. Many races are lost because of poor underwater armstrokes.

The underwater armstroke is similar to an exaggerated butterfly armstroke. It consists of an outsweep, insweep and upsweep. There are also two glides, one before the stroke begins and one after it has been completed. The second glide is followed by a kick to the surface. Sequence photos of the underwater armstroke can be seen in Fig. 10.5.

First glide

After the push-off or dive, the swimmer holds a streamlined position until the speed begins to decelerate (Fig. 10.5a). The arms should be together and stretched tightly overhead during the glide. Placing one hand over the other helps to maintain this position. The head is held between the arms and the body does not sag, nor is it piked at the waist. The legs are held tightly together with the toes extended back.

Outsweep to catch

The swimmer performs the outsweep shown in Fig. 10.5b−d. The outsweep begins when the swimmer slows from near race speed during the glide. At that point, the swimmer sweeps the arms out to the side until they are outside the shoulders. The swimmer should also sweep the hands up so that they are above the head when the catch is made. The upward sweep will place the arms in position to execute a longer and more propulsive insweep. The catch is made when the arms are facing back against the water (Fig. 10.5d).

The arms begin flexing at the elbows as they near the end of the outsweep so they can make a smooth transition to the insweep. The palms were facing down when the outsweep began. They should be rotated out slowly as the arms sweep out until they are pitched out and back at the catch.

The outsweep of the arms is not propulsive. Swimmers should *not* be encouraged to push water

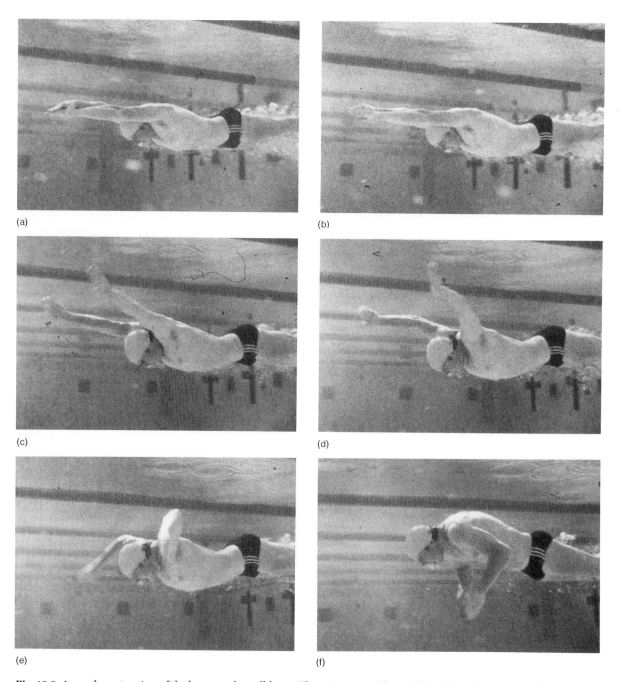

(a)

(b)

(c)

(d)

(e)

(f)

Fig. 10.5 An underwater view of the breaststroke pulldown. The swimmer is Glenn Mills (NCAA Champion in the 200 yards breaststroke).

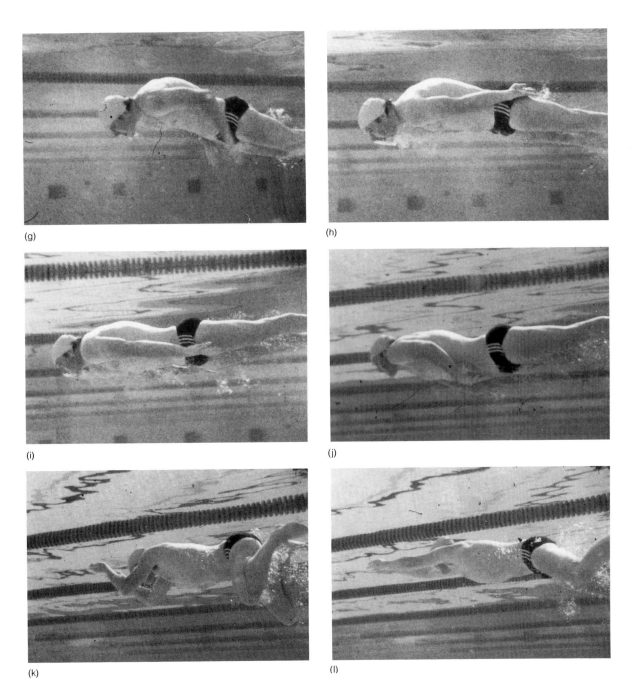

(g)

(h)

(i)

(j)

(k)

(l)

Fig. 10.5 (contd)

sideward with the palms of the hands. The movement should be made gently and with little effort.

The insweep

The insweep is shown in Fig. 10.5e and f. Once the catch has been made, the swimmer sculls the hands down and in under the body with a large semi-circular sweep, similar to the insweep of the butterfly. The insweep ends when the swimmer's hands come together under the chest (Fig. 10.5). This is made possible by continued flexion of the arms until they are bent nearly 90° when the hands come together under the body.

The swimmer rotates the palms of the hands inward throughout the insweep until they are pitched inward and upward when the movement is completed. The velocity of the hands increases moderately from the beginning to the end of the insweep. This is a very propulsive movement but not as propulsive as the upsweep that follows.

The upsweep

The upsweep can be seen in Fig. 10.5f−h. After completing the insweep, the swimmer sweeps the arms out, up and back until they are completely extended and just above the thighs.

The swimmer rotates the palms out during this movement and keeps the elbows flexed and palms facing back until the hands approach the front of the thighs. This part of the upsweep is very much like the corresponding movement in the butterfly. The techniques change once the hands reach the thighs, however. From that point the swimmer extends the arms up and out at the elbows to throw the water up and away from the thighs.

The upsweep ends with the arms completely extended above the thighs and with the hands facing away from the body. The velocity of the hands decelerates during the transition from insweep to upsweep, followed by a rapid acceleration to maximum speed at the end of the movement.

The second glide

Once the upsweep is completed, the swimmer turns the palms inward and places them against the thighs

to aid in streamlining the body during the glide that follows. The swimmer then glides in a streamlined position for a short time (Fig. 10.5i). Then, the arms recover forward and the swimmer kicks to the surface.

Arm recovery and kick to the surface

This phase of the underwater armstroke is shown in Fig. 10.5j−l. Swimmers should begin recovering the arms forward when they feel the speed of the underwater armstroke decreasing. This will occur quickly, therefore they will glide for only a short time.

The swimmer in Fig. 10.5 can be seen to slide the hands forward underneath the body by flexing them at the elbows. The upper arms and elbows are held close to the sides and the forearms and hands are underneath the body and very close to the skin. The swimmer's palms are facing upward with one hand lying over the other so that they can slip forward, on edge, with a minimum of resistance (Fig. 10.5).

The swimmer begins to extend the arms forward when they pass the head (Fig. 10.5k). They extend forward with elbows close and hands facing one another, forming the shape of an arrowhead. The arms continue extending until they are nearly straight. Then, they should begin the outsweep without hesitation. The swimmer's palms should face downward. These arm recovery movements should be made gently to minimize resistive drag.

The swimmer begins recovering the legs forward when the arms are midway through the recovery (Fig. 10.5). The leg recovery should also be gentle to keep drag to a minimum. The movement is primarily accomplished by flexing the legs at the knees and pulling the heels up toward the buttocks. The knees stay reasonably close together during the recovery so that the legs are within the confines of the body, thereby reducing drag.

The leg recovery is the period during the swimmer's movement toward the surface when speed will decelerate most. Consequently, the swimmer should move through this stage as quickly as possible and the timing should be such that the succeeding kick brings the swimmer to the surface.

The swimmer extends the arms forward and up toward the surface while recovering the legs. The swimmer then executes the propulsive phase of the kick which should bring the swimmer to the surface just before it is completed. The swimmer begins sweeping the arms out during the final stages of the kick in order to be ready to catch and sweep them in with no delay when the body breaks through the surface. The swimmer should *not* glide to the surface unless necessary to prevent disqualification. The speed will drop off quickly after finishing the kick so the swimmer must start the armstroke immediately. At the same time, the swimmer must comply with the rules for this stroke by making sure the head surfaces just before the arm makes the catch. The rule states that the swimmer's head must break through the surface of the water before the arms reach the widest point in the next armstroke. Swimmers should try to reach the end of the outsweep at the same time that the head breaks the surface. This technique requires precise timing and is worth learning due to the time it can save. Studies have shown that pulling up and through the surface will increase the speed by approximately 0.3 s as compared to gliding to the surface. This means almost a full second improvement in 100- and 200-m events. It can improve swimmers' times by over 2 s in 200-m events.

The swimmer takes a breath at the normal point in the armstroke once the head reaches the surface, that is, during the arm recovery. Swimmers should *not* breathe before starting the outsweep nor during the time the arms are traveling outwards.

Recommended reading

Belokovsky, V. & Ivanchenko, E. (1975) A hydrokinetic apparatus for the study and improvement of leg move-ments in the breaststroke. In Lewillie, L. & Clarys, J.P. (eds) *Swimming II*. Baltimore, Maryland: University Park Press, pp. 64–69.

Bergen, P. (1978) Breaststroke. In Ousley, R.M. (ed.) *1977 ASCA World Clinic Yearbook*. Fort Lauderdale, Florida: American Swimming Coaches Association, pp. 99–106.

Bober, T. & Czabanski, B. (1975) Changes in breaststroke technique under different speed conditions. In Lewillie, L. & Clarys, J.P. (eds) *Swimming II*. Baltimore, Maryland: University Park Press, pp. 188–193.

Craig, A.B. Jr., Boomer, W.L. & Skehan, P.L. (1988) Patterns of velocity in breaststroke swimming. In Ungerechts, B., Wilke, K. & Reischle, K. (eds) *Swimming Science V*. Champaign, Illinois: Human Kinetics, pp. 73–77.

Czabanski, B. (1975) Asymmetry of the lower limbs in breaststroke swimming. In Lewillie, L. & Clarys, J.P.

(eds) *Swimming II*. Baltimore, Maryland: University Park Press, pp. 207–213.

Czabanski, B. & Koszyczyc, T. (1979) Relationship between stroke asymmetry and speed of breaststroke swimming. In Terauds, J. & Bedingfield, E.W. (eds) *Swimming III*. Baltimore, Maryland: University Park Press, pp. 148–152.

Daly, D., Persyn, U., Van Tilborgh, L. & Riemaker, D. (1988) Estimation of sprint performances in the breaststroke from body characteristics. In Ungerechts, B., Wilkie, K. & Reischle, K. (eds) *Swimming Science V*. Champaign, Illinois: Human Kinetics, pp. 101–107.

Firby, H. (1975) *Howard Firby on Swimming*. London: Pelham Books.

Haljand, R. (1984) A new scientific approach to analyzing swimming technique. In Cramer, J.L. (ed.) *How to Develop Olympic Level Swimmers: Scientific and Practical Foundations*. Helsinki: International Sports Media, pp. 72–105.

Huellhorst, U., Ungerechts, B.E. & Willimczik, K. (1988) Displacement and speed characteristics of the breaststroke turn—a cinematographic analysis. In Ungerechts, B.E., Wilke, K. & Reischle, K. (eds) *Swimming Science V*. Champaign, Illinois: Human Kinetics, pp. 93–98.

Mason, B.R., Patton, S.G. & Newton, A.P. (1989) Propulsion in breaststroke swimming. In: Morrison W.E. (ed.) *Proceedings of the VII International Symposium on Biomechanics in Sports*. Melbourne, Australia: Footscray Institute of Technology, pp. 257–267.

Nagy, J. (1989) From a technical angle: breaking down the technical elements of the wave-action breaststroke. *Swim. Tech.* **26**:16–19.

Nimz, R., Rader, U., Wilkie, K. & Skipka, W. (1988) The relationship of anthropometric measures to different types of breaststroke kicks. In Ungerechts, B., Wilkie, K. & Reischle, K. (eds) *Swimming Science V*. Champaign Illinois: Human Kinetics, pp. 115–119.

Pai, Y-C. (1986) A hydrodynamic study of the oscillation motion in swimming. In Hay, J.G. (ed.) *Starting, Stroking and Turning*. Iowa City, Iowa: Biomechanics Laboratory, University of Iowa, pp. 145–150.

Persyn, U., De Maeyer, J. & Vervaecke, H. (1975) Investi-gation of hydrodynamic determinants of competitive swimming strokes. In Lewillie, L. & Clarys, J.P. (eds) *Swimming II*. Baltimore, Maryland: University Park Press, pp. 214–222.

Schleihauf, R.E. Jr (1976) A hydrodynamic analysis of breaststroke pulling efficiency. *Swim. Tech.* **12**:100–105.

Schleihauf, R.E., Higgins, J.R., Hinrichs, R. *et al.* (1988) Propulsive techniques: front crawl stroke, butterfly, back-stroke and breaststroke. In Ungerechts, B., Wilke, K. & Reischle, K. (eds) *Swimming Science V*. Champaign, Illinois: Human Kinetics, pp. 53–60.

Thayer, A., Schleihauf, R.E., Higgins, R.E. *et al.* (1986) A hydrodynamic analysis of breaststroke swimmers. In

Hay, J.G. (ed.) *Starting, Stroking and Turning*. Iowa City, Iowa: Biomechanics Laboratory, University of Iowa, pp. 131–143.

Van Tilborgh, L., Willens, E.J. & Persyn, U. (1988) Evaluation of breaststroke propulsion and resistance — resultant impulses from film analysis. In Ungerechts, B., Wilke, K. & Reischle, K. (eds) *Swimming Science V*. Champaign, Illinois: Human Kinetics, pp. 67–71.

Vervaecke, H.U.B. & Persyn, U.J.J. (1979) Effectiveness of the breaststroke leg movement in relation to selected time-space, anthropometric, flexibility, and force data. In Terauds, J. & Bedingfield, E.W. (eds) *Swimming III*. Baltimore, Maryland: University Park Press, pp. 320–328.

Chapter 11

Starts and turns

The various starts and turns that competitive swimmers use are described here under the following six headings.

1 The grab start.
2 The track start.
3 The backstroke start.
4 The freestyle flip turn.
5 The backstroke turn.
6 The open turn used by butterfly and breaststroke swimmers.

The grab start

This start was introduced by Hanauer in 1967 and has rapidly gained in popularity since that time. The difference between it and earlier popular starts is that swimmers grip the front edge of the block while waiting for the starting signal. They pull the body forward off the starting platform when it sounds.

Several research studies have certified the grab start as faster than other methods. The grab start is superior because swimmers can get their body moving toward the water faster by pulling against the starting platform with their hands than by swinging the arms backward. They decelerate more quickly with the grab start once they enter the water because the arms do not generate the amount of force that can be produced by a circular backswing. However, the ability to get the body moving quickly apparently outweighs the loss of momentum that occurs after entry. Times, therefore, are faster to selected points in the pool where swimmers usually surface. For example, Thorsen (1975) found that horizontal and vertical velocities were greater with the circular backswing start, yet the grab start was faster by 0.1 s to the point of entry.

Another important change in starting technique is known as the *pike* or *scoop dive*. In this style, swimmers travel through the air in a high arc, often piking (bending) at the waist, so they can enter the water at a very steep angle. Before this style, was introduced, swimmers were advised to dive almost straight out and to enter the water at a very slight angle. The differences between the two dives are illustrated in Fig. 11.1.

The major advantage of the pike dive seems to be that

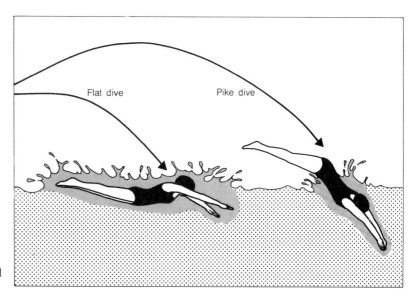

Flat dive   Pike dive

Fig. 11.1 A comparison of the pike and flat dives.

swimmers encounter less drag when they enter the water, consequently they travel faster during the glide under water. Another advantage is that swimmers who use the pike dive generally travel a greater distance through the air before entering the water.

As you can see in Fig. 11.1, the body of the swimmer using a flat dive hits the water at several places at once. This will cause the body to decelerate quite rapidly during the glide. With the pike dive, the swimmer's entire body enters the water at nearly the same point. The body slips underwater with less turbulence, which should allow a faster underwater glide.

A word of caution is in order regarding the pike dive. It is very dangerous when used in shallow pools. The angle of entry causes a swimmer to travel deeper with this dive than with other methods. Several accidents have been reported where swimmers have hit their face and head on the bottom while attempting this dive in less than 1.5 m of water. A small number have suffered serious neck injuries, leaving them paralyzed. This dive should *not* be attempted in pools that are *less than 1.8 m (6 ft)* deep. The depth swimmers reached with the pike dive varied from 1.0 to 1.7 m (3–5 ft) in a study by Counsilman and associates (1988).

Important phases of the grab start are shown in Fig. 11.2. For descriptive purposes, it has been divided into:

1 the preparatory position;
2 the pull;
3 the drive from the block;
4 the flight;
5 the entry;
6 the glide;
7 the pull-out.

The preparatory position

Swimmers should stand at the rear of the starting platform until the starter gives them permission to assume the preparatory position by saying; "take your marks." The position they should take after that command is shown in Fig. 11.2a. The toes of both the swimmers's feet grip the front edge of the starting platform. The feet are approximately shoulder-width apart. The swimmers grasps the front edge of the starting platform with the first and second joints of the

fingers. The hands may be either inside or outside the feet. It is not known, at the present time, whether one of these methods is superior to the other. The knees are flexed approximately 30–40° and the elbows are also flexed slightly. The head is down and the swimmer is looking at the water just beyond the starting platform.

While in the preparatory position, swimmers should lean forward and tense the leg muscles so they can get in motion faster once the starting signal sounds. They should maintain balance with the hands.

The pull

This phase is shown in Fig. 11.2b. At the sound of the starting signal, the swimmer pulls up against the starting platform. This pulls the hips and, consequently, the center of gravity down and forward beyond the front edge of the starting platform as the swimmer begins falling toward the water. The swimmer flexes the legs at the knees and hips as he falls forward. This prepares the swimmer to thrust the body off the platform once in position to do so.

There is no need for swimmers to use a long or powerful arm pull to get the body in motion. This will not add speed or force to the dive. All he needs to do is get the body moving forward; gravity takes over after that. No amount of additional pulling will increase the speed at which the center of gravity moves forward past the front edge of the starting platform.

The drive from the block

This phase of the start is shown in Fig. 11.2c–e. The swimmer releases the front of the starting platform immediately after the body starts moving forward. He falls downward and forward until the knees are flexed approximately 80°. At that point, the legs are extended to drive the body off the starting platform. The leg drive is executed by a powerful extension at the hip and knee joints followed by extension of the feet at the ankles.

After the hands release the block, the arms are extended forward in a semi-circular path until they are pointing at the area where the swimmer wishes to enter the water. The arms bend rapidly during the first half of the movement as they come up under the chin. Then they are extended forward and down as the swimmer leaves the platform. The head follows the movements of the arms, looking down as the arms are extended down when leaving the starting platform. This point is very important. Swimmers' *heads* must start down for the water before the *feet* leave the starting platform. If the swimmer keeps the head up as he leaves the platform, he will not be able to execute the pike in time to make a clean entry.

The angle of take-off, formed by the top of the starting platform and the swimmer's legs, should be approximately 40−50° (Fig. 11.2e). This angle will give swimmers the arc-like trajectory they need for a clean entry.

The flight

This phase of the grab start is shown in Fig. 11.2f and g. After leaving the starting platform, the swimmer travels through the air with the trunk in an extended position. He pikes at the waist as the body passes the peak of the flight (Fig. 11.2g). After piking, the legs are lifted up in line with the trunk for a streamlined entry.

The entry

The entire body should try to enter the water through the hole that is made with the hands. The entry is shown in Fig. 11.2h and i. The swimmer's body enters the water in a streamlined position with the arms fully extended and together. The head is down between the arms. The legs are fully extended and together with feet extended back (toes pointed).

The angle of entry should be approximately 30−40° from the surface of the water (Beritzhoff, 1974). This steep angle will cause swimmers to plunge deep beneath the surface unless they make some adjustments to change the direction the body is traveling. The directional change is accomplished by snapping the legs down in a dolphin kicking motion while at the same time lifting the hands toward the surface. The timing of these actions will vary according to how quickly swimmers wish to reach the surface. They should begin as the body enters the water in shorter races. They can wait until after the body is submerged in longer races. Of course, the technique should not be used in breaststroke races because these swimmers want to stay under the water longer.

The glide

After the entry, swimmers should glide in a stream-lined position for a short time. There should be no arch to the back nor pike at the waist. The position should be held until they are approaching the velocity of the race. Obviously, swimmers will not glide very long in short races; on the other hand, they will glide for a somewhat longer time in middle-distance and distance races. Swimmers should never continue to glide until they fall below race velocity simply to gain additional distance from the dive. They will lose time and waste muscular effort accelerating the body back to race speed.

The pull-out

Swimmers should begin kicking just before reaching race speed in butterfly and freestyle races . Two dolphin kicks or 2−4 flutter kicks should bring them close enough to the surface so that one underwater armstroke will complete the job. The upper body should remain streamlined during these kicks. The first armstroke should be powerful, bringing them up through the surface traveling forward at race speed. The underwater armstroke for breaststroke swimmers was covered in Chapter 10.

Swimmers in all three other strokes should concentrate on moving forward during the pull-out. They should not pull the body up to the surface at a steep angle. They should pull and kick themselves up diagonally so they reach the surface traveling forward much more than they are moving upward.

Once on the surface, athletes should not delay in attaining the proper stroke rhythm for the race they are swimming. Breathing and looking around are two of the most common causes for such delays. For that reason, it is best for the swimmer, in all events except breaststroke, to delay breathing until the end of the first stroke, or even until the second stroke after surfacing. Sprinters should certainly delay taking the first breath until they are a much greater distance down the pool.

The track start

This form of starting is a recent adaptation of the grab start, particularly where preventing injuries is

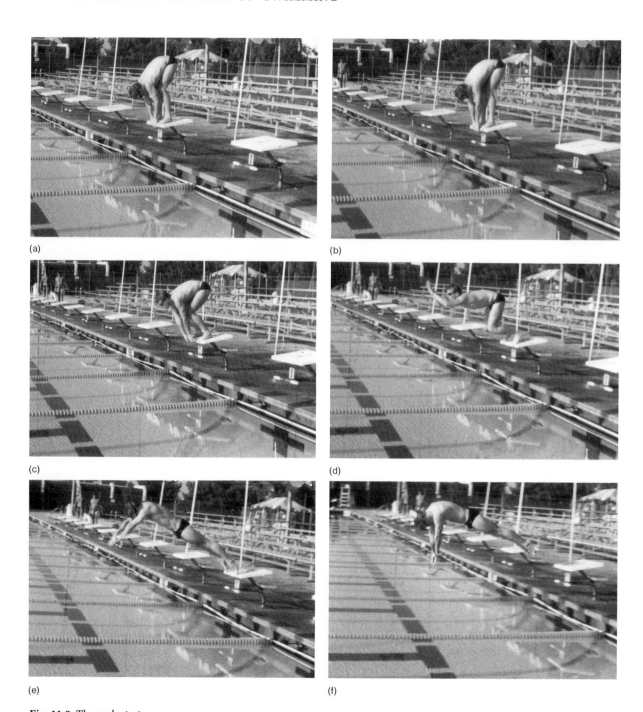

(a)

(b)

(c)

(d)

(e)

(f)

Fig. 11.2 The grab start.

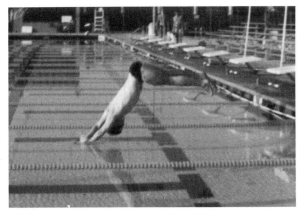

(g)

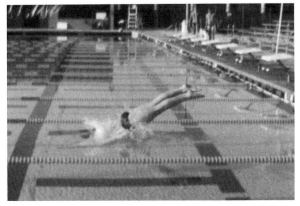

(h)

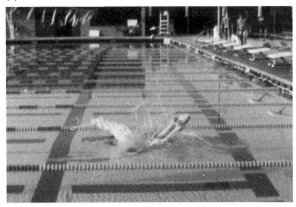

(i)

Fig. 11.2 (contd)

concerned. It has been used by several swimmers on the international level. The major difference between it and the traditional grab start is in the preparatory position on the starting platform. The swimmer in Fig. 11.3 is shown in the preparatory position for the track start. She has one foot back. Two major advantages have been proposed for this style.

First, swimmers can get into the water faster. This may be because their center of gravity travels almost straight forward beyond the starting platform until they reach the point where it begins falling toward the water. With the pike dive, the center of gravity travels up a greater distance after leaving the block, increasing the time it takes to reach the entry position.

Second, the swimmer's legs can deliver a greater forward thrust when they have two impulses rather than one. With the track start, swimmers push first with the rear leg and then with the front leg.

To date there have been three studies comparing the track start to other styles of starting. In one, there was no difference between the two styles in the time to reach 5, 10 and 12 m. In another, the track start was significantly slower and in a third, the track start was faster for a distance of 12.5 yards.

Apparently, the jury is still out on the track start. Swimmers who use the style seem to get off the block faster but they enter the water at a somewhat flatter angle and lose time during the glide. On the other hand, swimmers who use the conventional starting position (both feet at the front edge of the block) are slower leaving the block but enter the water at an angle that permits a faster glide. The mechanics of the track start have been described in the same phases used for the grab start. A swimmer is shown performing the start in Fig. 11.3.

The preparatory position

The swimmer has the toes of one foot over the front edge with the other foot back, pressing against the incline of the starting platform. The ball of the rear foot should be near the rear edge of the starting block. The head is down and she is gripping the front edge of the block with both hands. The swimmer is learning back so the weight is on the rear foot (Fig. 11.3a).

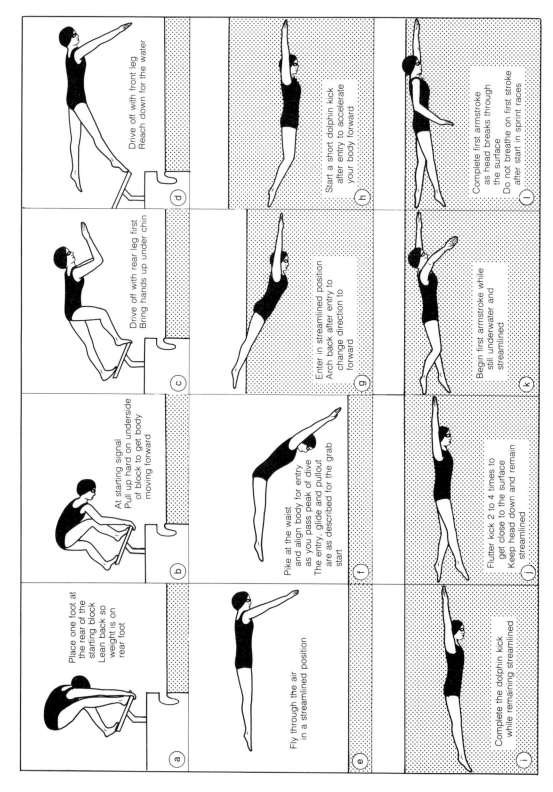

Fig. 11.3 The track start.

The pull and drive from the starting platform

When the starting signal sounds, the body is pulled downward and forward with the hands and arms. The swimmer then drives off the block, first by extending the rear leg, followed immediately by an extension of the front leg (Fig. 11.3b). Simultaneously, the arms should extend forward in a semi-circular path until they are pointing to the place where the swimmer plans to enter the water. Swimmers should try for the steepest angle of take-off that is compatible with the low position at the start.

The flight

Figure 11.3e−g shows the flight phase of the track start. After leaving the starting platform, the swimmer flies through the air in an arc that is somewhat flatter than the arc of the pike dive. This will make it almost impossible for the swimmer to enter the water in one spot. Nevertheless, the swimmer should try for the cleanest, most streamlined entry possible by piking slightly at the waist during the flight so she can achieve a better angle of entry.

In addition to the preparatory position, the biggest difference between the track and grab starts is in the angle of take-off. The track-start swimmer does not drive off the block at a large angle. To do so would cause the center of gravity to rise too high during the flight through the air, which in turn would negate one of the advantages of the track start.

After entering the water, the glide and pull-out should be performed in the same manner as described for the grab start; the only exception might be that track-start swimmers will not glide quite so long. As mentioned, they generally lose speed faster because they do not enter the water as cleanly.

The backstroke start

Short- and long-course rules have now been standardized so that, in the preparatory position, swimmers must have the feet entirely underwater in all backstroke races. A swimmer is shown doing a backstroke start in Fig. 11.4. The mechanics of this start have been described as:
1 the preparatory position;
2 the drive from the wall;
3 the flight ;
4 the entry;
5 the glide and kick;
6 the pull-out.

The preparatory position

While waiting for the command, "take your marks," swimmers should be in the water facing the wall and gripping the backstroke bar with both hands. The feet should be entirely underwater and in contact with the end wall. The balls of the feet and toes should be against the wall; the heels should be away from the wall. The leg should be bent and the hips in the water.

When commanded to take your marks, the swimmer in Fig. 11.4a has pulled the body into a crouched position. The head is down, the arms flexed at the elbows. The hips are in the water with the buttocks close to the heels.

Some swimmers have the feet together on the wall while others prefer to use a staggered position with one foot slightly below the other. Research has not identified the superior method, so the best advice is to try both methods and select the one which seems best.

The drive from the wall

This phase of the start can be seen in Fig. 11.4b−e. When the starting signal sounds, the swimmer throws the head up and back, looking for the opposite end of the pool. Almost immediately thereafter, he thrusts the body up and back by pushing down and in against the bar with the hands. Once the arms are extended, the swimmer releases the bar and brings the arms over the head as quickly as possible. In the meantime, the body is driven up and away from the wall by extending the legs at the knees and the feet at the ankles.

There are at least two reasons for recommending that backstrokers swing the arms overhead rather than around to the side in the traditional manner. First, this technique will get the arms overhead faster so the body can be aligned for the entry. Second, an overhead arm swing should encourage a higher arc and more arch during the flight which will, in turn, provide for a more streamlined entry.

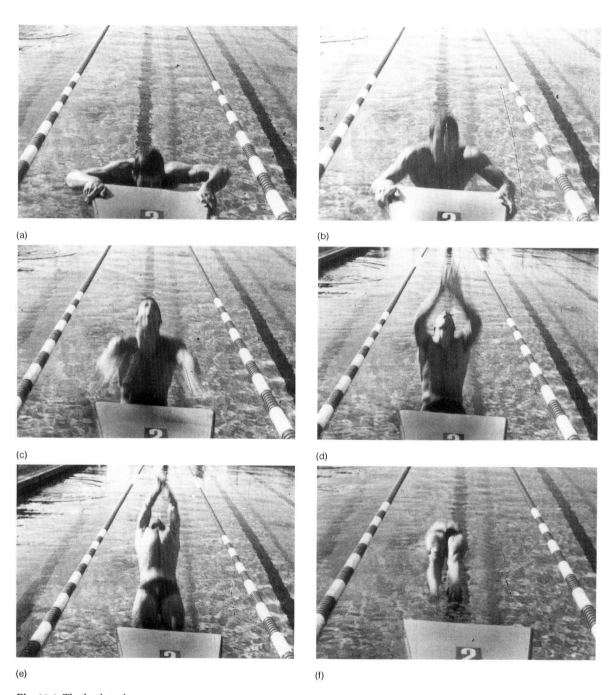

(a)

(b)

(c)

(d)

(e)

(f)

Fig. 11.4 The backstroke start.

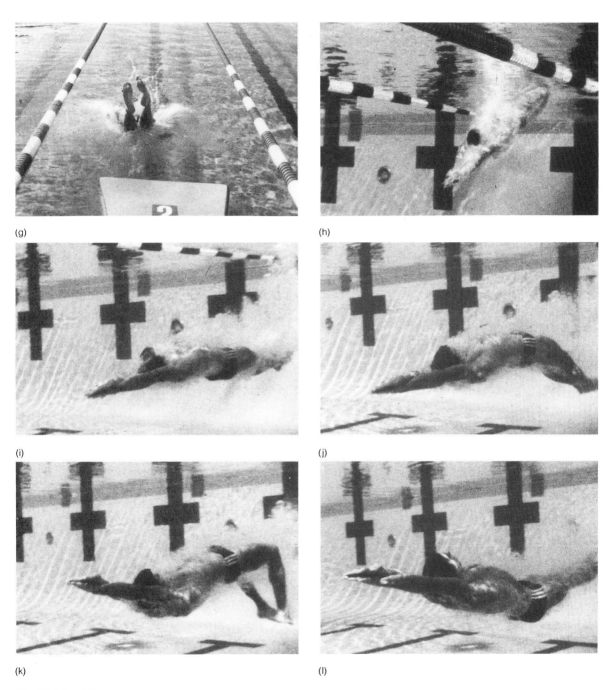

(g) (h)

(i) (j)

(k) (l)

Fig. 11.4 (contd)

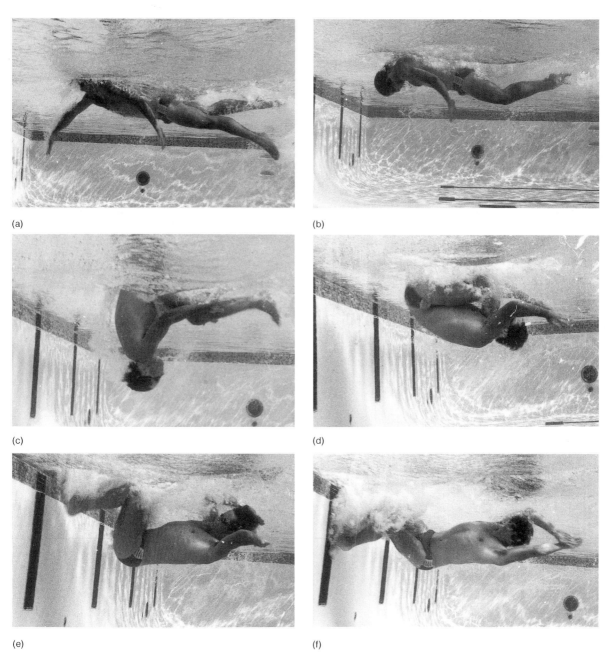

(a)

(b)

(c)

(d)

(e)

(f)

Fig. 11.5 The freestyle flip turn.

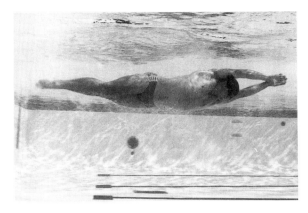

(g)

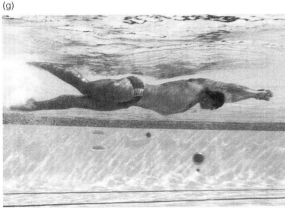

(h)

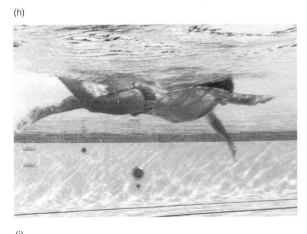

(i)

Fig. 11.5 (contd)

The flight

This phase of the backstroke start is shown in Fig. 11.4f. The swimmer's body travels through the air in an arc. The head is back and the arms are extended overhead. The legs and feet are also extended.

Swimmers should endeavor to get the entire body out of the water during the flight. This will be difficult because the feet will tend to drag through the water after pushing off the end wall. Nevertheless, if they get a reasonably high angle of take-off and arch the back sufficiently during the glide, they should be able to keep the lower legs and feet out of the water during most of the flight.

The entry

Figure 11.4h shows the entry position. It should be made in a streamlined position, with arms extended and together. The head is down between the arms. The legs and feet remain in extended positions. Swimmers should make every effort to enter the body through the same "hole" in the water opened by the hands and head. This is difficult to accomplish because the body is so near the water during the flight through the air. Consequently, the hips will usually enter the water slightly behind the point where the head entered. Swimmers can keep the legs from dragging through the water by lifting them to a slightly piked position during the entry.

The glide and kick

After entering the water, the swimmer should lift the arms slightly and bring the legs downward sharply to change the direction of the body from down to forward. The swimmer should glide in a streamlined position until approaching race speed. He should begin kicking at that point.

A recent innovation has been for backstroke swimmers to dolphin-kick underwater before surfacing. A large number of swimmers have found this technique is faster than swimming on the surface. International rules only permit swimmers to use the dolphin-kick for 15 m after each turn. There are, however, presently not restrictions on the distance backstroke swimmers can kick under the surface.

Swimmers who have good dolphin kicks should

probably use this technique to achieve the maximum allowable or tolerable distance. They should train so they can stay underwater for at least 3−6 kicks after every turn. Swimmers who are not good dolphin-kickers are probably better advised to flutter-kick 2−4 times after a short glide, before pulling the body through the surface.

The pull-out

The pull-out should be timed so swimmers reach the surface just as the pull-out motion has been completed. They can then recover that arm over the water and get into the normal swimming rhythm with no delay. They should not lift the head from a streamlined position until they reach the surface. Once on the surface, they should establish the stroking frequency for the race as quickly as possible.

Turns

The flip turn is the most popular method for freestyle races. Swimmers in breaststroke and butterfly races favor a similar open turn.

The freestyle flip turn

Underwater views of a swimmer performing a flip turn can be seen in Fig. 11.5. The flip turn is a forward somersault with a one-eighth twist followed by a push-off from the wall. Swimmers rotate the remaining seven-eighths to a prone position during the drive from the wall and the following glide. For explanatory purposes, the parts of the trun that will be described are:

1 the approach;
2 the turn;
3 the push-off;
4 the glide;
5 the pull-out.

The approach

The swimmer in Fig. 11.5a is approaching the wall. He should have sighted the wall several strokes out in order to make modifications in the approach that will allow him to swim into the turn with no loss of speed.

Most swimmers begin that final armstroke 1.7−2.0 m

(5.5−6.5 ft) from the wall (Chow *et al.*, 1984). Sprinters will tend to start the turn sooner because they are traveling into the wall faster. It is very important to maintain race speed as swimmers approach the turn. The majority slow down to anticipate the turn, which costs them precious seconds over the course of a race.

The turn

The mechanics of the turn are shown in Fig. 11.5b−e. The swimmer has left the opposite arm in the water back at the hip when he began the final armstroke. He ducks his head underwater and begins to somersault over while completing the second half of the final underwater armstroke. The action is one of following the hand back and up toward the surface with the head.

The swimmer tucks the legs tight into the stomach and somersaults almost straight over in a tucked position (Fig. 11.5d). Notice that he executes a small dolphin kick during the final armstroke to assist in pushing the hips up.

Once the final armstroke has been completed, the swimmer leaves both arms back at the hips. When the somersault is half completed, he turns the palms of both hands down and pulls them toward the head to help bring it toward the surface.

The head comes up between the arms as the feet reach the wall so the body is aligned and ready for the push-off at the instant the feet make contact (Fig. 11.5e). The hands are also overhead with elbows flexed for the same reason.

The swimmer executes a slight twist to the side as the feet come into the wall so they can be planted with toes facing out and up in the same direction in which the body is turned. The twist is accomplished by turning the head to the side in the second half of the somersault. Most swimmers will turn the head away from the arm that was used to stroke into the turn.

The speed of the somersault is really controlled by the swimmer's head movements. As quickly as possible, the swimmer drives the head down, back and then up toward the surface to an aligned position between the arms.

The push-off

This phase of the turn is shown in Fig. 11.5f and g. When the feet reach the wall, they are planted at a depth of approximately 30–40 cm (12–15 in). The swimmer begins extending the legs immediately when the feet make contact with the wall.

The push-off is executed while the swimmer is on his back (except for the slight rotation to the side, as mentioned earlier). The swimmer rotates toward a prone position while extending the legs so that he is on his side by the time the feet leave the wall. He completes the turn to a prone position during the glide that follows. This rotation is assisted by the movements of the legs. The swimmer comes off the wall with the top leg crossed over the bottom and helps the body rotate to a prone position by uncrossing and bringing the top leg down during the glide.

The drive off the wall should be powerful. The swimmer in Fig. 11.5 extends the arms and legs simultaneously to add impetus to the push-off. The push-off should be made horizontally: it should *not* be angled upward.

The glide

After pushing off, the swimmer glides until he approaches race speed. At that time, the swimmer takes 2–4 flutter kicks and pulls the head up through the surface with the first armstroke. The glide should be streamlined, with the arms extended overhead and the head down between the arms. This position can be seen in Fig. 11.5h. The back is straight and the legs and feet are extended and together.

The pull-out

The swimmer begins the pull-out when he feels that one underwater armstroke will bring the head up through the surface. That armstroke should be timed so the head breaks through the surface when he is midway through the armstroke. The swimmer should remain streamlined with the head down until it breaks through the surface. After that, the head can be carried in a normal swimming position.

Swimmers should never breathe during the armstroke that carries them into the turn. This will delay the beginning of the somersault.

The issue of when to take the first breath after the turn is controversial. At present, the most popular technique is to delay that breath at least until the second armstroke. Swimmers have been taught to take the first stroke out of the turn with the arm that is opposite the breathing side in order to delay breathing until the second stroke is underway. The wisdom behind this technique is that many swimmers delay getting into their race rhythm when they breathe on the first stroke out of the turn. Unfortunately, this technique has spawned a generation of swimmers who lose time by breathing as they stroke into the turn so they can delay breathing coming out of the turn. I believe they lose more time when they delay the somersault than would be lost by breathing on the first stroke after the turn. This will be particularly true if they concentrate on establishing the stroke rhythm as they breathe coming off the wall.

Delaying the breath out of the turn may be a good technique to use in sprint races, provided swimmers do not breathe going into the turn. However, they may be better advised to breathe on the first stroke out of the turn in races of 400 m and longer so they will not be encouraged to breathe as they begin the somersault.

The backstroke turn

In January 1991, FINA (the international governing body for competitive swimming) adopted new rules for the backstroke turn and for the distance over which the dolphin kick could be used, following the start and each turn in backstroke races. Swimmers are no longer required to touch the wall with their hand at the turn and the distance they can dolphin kick underwater was lengthened from 10 to 15 m.

The turn

The new FINA rule on turns goes as follows:

"Upon completion of each length, some part of the swimmer must touch the wall. During the turn the shoulders may turn past the vertical toward the breast. If the swimmer turns past the vertical, such motion must be part of a continuous turning action and the swimmer must return to a position on the back before the feet leave the wall."

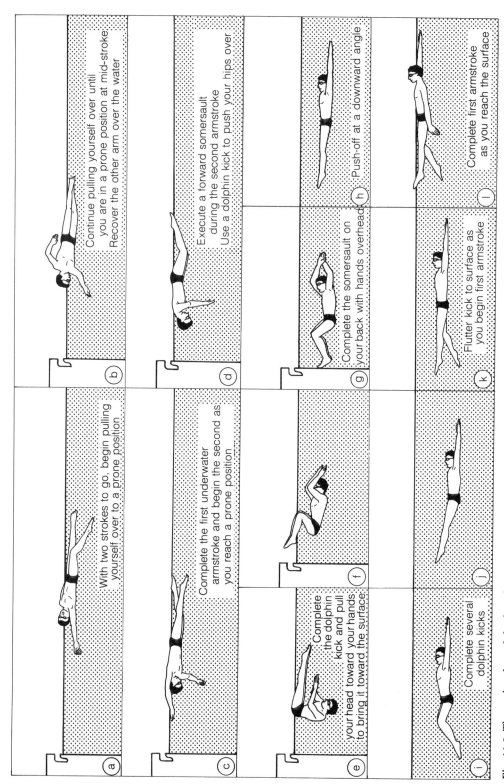

Fig. 11.6 The no-hand touch backstroke turn.

(a) With two strokes to go, begin pulling yourself over to a prone position.

(b) Continue pulling yourself over until you are in a prone position at mid-stroke. Recover the other arm over the water.

(c) Complete the first underwater armstroke and begin the second as you reach a prone position.

(d) Execute a forward somersault during the second armstroke. Use a dolphin kick to push your hips over.

(e) Complete the dolphin kick and pull your head toward your hands to bring it toward the surface.

(f) [figure only]

(g) Complete the somersault on your back with hands overhead.

(h) Push-off at a downward angle.

(i) Complete several dolphin kicks.

(j) [figure only]

(k) Flutter kick to surface as you begin first armstroke.

(l) Complete first armstroke as you reach the surface.

The present interpretation of this rule is that swimmers can leave the position on their backs after they begin their second to last stroke of each length. They may then take one stroke while in a prone position as they somersault into the turn, *provided* the turn is executed as one continuous motion.

The dolphin kick

The new ruling for dolphin kicking states in part that:

"... it is permissible for the swimmer to be completely submerged during the turn and for a distance of not more than 15 meters (16.4 yards) after the start and each turn. By that point, the head must have broken the surface of the water."

United States Swimming and NISCA (the National Interscholastic Swimming Coaches Association) have adopted the "no hand-touch" backstroke turn for competition in the USA and the NCAA will undoubtedly follow suit for intercollegiate competition.

All swimmers should take advantage of the no-hand touch backstroke turn. It allows them to start turning earlier during each length of the pool and it also permits them to somersault over more quickly.

Swimmers should also take advantage of the opportunity to kick underwater for a greater distance. There seems little doubt that they can move faster underwater using a dolphin kick than they can when swimming backstroke on the surface. Consequently, they should use the dolphin kick for as much of the allowable 15 m as possible. Of course, this advice applies only to swimmers who have good dolphin kicks. Poor kickers will probably find it faster to surface and swim backstroke after the turn.

Although some may consider it potentially more fatiguing to dolphin kick underwater for 15 m, the history of swimming has demonstrated that swimmers who were willing to test their limits were capable of much more than had initially been imagined.

Description of the backstroke turn

The no-hand touch backstroke turn has only been used in competition for 3 months at the time of this writing. It will be sometime longer before innovative and intuitive swimmers demonstrate the best technique or techniques to us. This, together with the fact that rule

interpretations may change as the turn is used in more major competitions, could mean that the following description may not stand the test of time. These facts, notwithstanding, this author believes that the turn illustrated in Fig. 11.6 is the fastest method within the present interpretation of the new rule.

The prerequisite for a good backstroke turn is for swimmers to judge their distance from the wall with a minimum of *looking around*. They should use the backstroke flags to determine when they are approaching the turn, and then count the number of strokes needed before they begin rotating to a prone position.

Ideally, it is best to swim into the turn without looking for the wall beforehand. The new rule makes this much easier for all swimmers to do. Since they can begin the turn two armstrokes from the wall, they can turn on their stomach earlier and thus see the wall, meaning they no longer need to worry about hitting their arm or head. Also, should they misjudge the turn slightly, they can make adjustments during the last armstroke that will take them into the wall properly after they have rotated to a prone position.

The turn should begin two armstrokes from the wall. The underwater portion of the first of those armstrokes should begin with the swimmer on his back (Fig. 11.6a). He should begin rotating toward the pulling arm, to a prone position, once that armstroke is underway. In the meantime, the other arm should recover over the water in a manner similar to the high-elbow recovery used in the front crawl stroke (Fig. 11.6b). The swimmer should be in a completely prone position as the stroking arm comes under his chest. The other arm should be entering the water at this time (Fig. 11.6c). The in and up sculling motion of the stroking arm should be used to assist the rotation from a supine to a prone position.

Once a prone position is reached, the turn is executed like a freestyle flip except, of course, that the swimmer stays on his back after the push-off. The swimmer makes a strong upsweep with the stroking arm and then leaves it at his side. He should sight the wall at this time to assist in making any adjustments that may be required to bring his feet to the wall quickly. A full underwater stroke is then completed with the other arm which is left back at the hip. The head should be tucked into the chest and the swimmer should execute a dolphin kick to assist in getting his hips over the water (Fig. 11.6d).

Once both hands are back at his sides, the swimmer should turn his palms toward the bottom and use them to pull his head up and his feet over (Fig. 11.6e−f). Both hands should meet overhead before the swimmer's feet reach the wall. His head should be back between his arms and he should have his upper body and arms aligned so he can push-off with no delay once his feet make contact with the wall (Fig. 11.6g). His feet should be planted on the wall several inches below the surface so he can make a deep push-off that will facilitate use of the dolphin kick.

His arms and legs should extend simultaneously as he drives off the wall on his back. He should push-off in a slightly downward direction to glide under the surface turbulence and to keep his body deeper during the dolphin kick (Fig. 11.6h). His body should be streamlined from head to toes during the glide.

After gliding a short distance, the swimmer should begin dolphin kicking, if this is his preference, or he should take 2−4 flutter kicks and begin his pull-out. As mentioned earlier, swimmers with "good legs" are advised to take several dolphin kicks after the push-off, traveling as much of the allowable distance as possible in this manner (Fig. 11.6l−j).

The swimmer should begin flutter kicking shortly before he starts pulling himself toward the surface (Fig. 11.6k). He should begin an underwater armstroke after 2−4 flutter kicks. His head should be brought up through the surface with a normal stroke (Fig. 11.6l). His head should remain streamlined, in line with the other arm, until it reaches the surface. There should be no delay establishing the proper stroke frequency for the race once he reaches the surface.

Many swimmers make the mistake of gliding to the surface before they begin stroking; this means that they decelerate markedly. Another common mistake they make is to begin the pull-out before they have kicked their bodies close to the surface. Consequently, they complete the underwater portion of the arm-stroke too early and must glide until they reach the surface before they can recover the arm and start the next stroke.

The butterfly and breaststroke turns

The turns that swimmers use in butterfly and breast-stroke are almost identical from the time they touch the wall until they are gliding. The following phases

have been used to described the turn:

1 The approach.
2 The turn.
3 The push-off.
4 The glide and pull-out.

The turn is shown from underneath in Fig. 11.7.

The approach

Swimmers in both strokes should focus on the wall as they approach so they can adjust the strokes to reach it just as they extend the arms forward during the recovery. The final kick should be made powerfully so they hit the wall with as much momentum as possible. That momentum will help them get the upper body moving in the opposite direction by providing a rebound-like action off the wall. Ideally they want to make contact with the wall just as the propulsive phase of that kick is ending. Swimmers will decelerate and increase the time into the wall when they glide. If they must glide to the wall, they should begin drawing the legs under them during the glide so the turn is underway when contact has been made.

They must touch the wall with both hands simul-taneously with the shoulders level. The swimmer in Fig. 11.7a is touching the wall properly.

The turn

Once the touch is made, the legs are pulled under the body by tucking them tightly into the stomach. As mentioned earlier, the swimmer may begin pulling the legs up before the touch is made if gliding into the wall. Simultaneously, one shoulder is lifted in the direction the swimmer plans to turn the body (the left shoulder if turning to the left and vice versa). That hand is quickly removed from the wall and brought back to the ribs by flexing the elbow. It is then extended back in the direction from which the swimmer just came.

In the meantime, the swimmer has grasped the gutter (if one is available) with the other hand and pulls the hips and legs forward into the wall. This is done by flexing the arm. This sequence of events is pictured in Fig. 11.7b−e.

When the legs are halfway to the wall, the swimmer pushes the body away by extending the arm. Then, the arm is brought over the water to meet the other hand. There will be no part of the swimmer's body in contact with the wall during this phase of the turn. Nevertheless, the momentum the swimmer developed when the trunk was pushed away will also drive the feet into the wall.

In the meantime, the other arm is used to help bring the head down into the water. The swimmer does this by turning the palm of that hand up and pushing it toward the surface.

The push-off

This phase of the turn can be seen in Fig. 11.7f and g. Swimmers should try to have both hands overhead and the body aligned when the feet reach the wall. Then they should push off immediately. The feet are planted on the wall with toes pointing to the side. The push-off is made by extending the arms and legs simultaneously and it is made on the side. The swimmer rotates toward a prone position while the legs are extending. That rotation is completed during the glide that follows. It is assisted by bringing the top leg down over the bottom leg after the feet leave the wall.

Although swimmers should attempt to have both arms overhead and the body aligned, it is not possible to be perfectly aligned before the feet reach the wall. Generally, one arm will be extending down into the water when the feet reach the wall. Swimmers should not wait until body is aligned before pushing off: they can always complete the alignment during the push-off. This may affect the streamlining of the push-off somewhat, but the time they save getting off the wall will more than compensate for this loss and the speed of the entire turn will be faster. Swimmers should be able to get in a streamlined position while they are pushing off, even if they start before the body is perfectly aligned.

The glide and pull-out

Figure 11.7h shows the swimmer gliding after the push-off. The swimmer glides in a streamlined position until approaching race speed. At that time, butterfly swimmers should execute two dolphin kicks and begin an armstroke that will bring them up through the surface. In sprint events, the swimmer should wait at least until the second stroke before taking a breath. In 200 m races they may take a breath at the end of that first underwater armstroke.

Breaststroke swimmers should execute an underwater armstroke and kick to the surface (see Chapter 10).

Swimmers should take a breath as they are falling back into the water. They should train themselves to take only one breath, no matter how tired they are. Hanging on the wall to get an extra breath will add unwanted time to races.

There are several key coaching points that can help swimmers learn to turn faster. It is important that they stay on the side throughout the turn. The legs should be brought up directly underneath the body in a tucked position so that they travel the minimum distance possible into the wall.

The arm should be brought over the water with a high elbow and slipped into the water, fingertips first, behind the swimmer's head. This technique will help swimmers remain in the vertical plane during the turn. It wastes time to spin the body around to the side.

They should not turn the face down until after they enter the water. They will tend to spin around if they look down while the face is traveling over the water.

The mechanics of the turn will change only slightly if there is no gutter available. Swimmers simply place the palms of both hands flat against the wall at the surface. Then they should pull one arm back as described in this section. In the meantime, they let the body ride into the wall by flexing the other arm. The legs should be tucked tightly into the stomach while this is taking place. Once the legs are passing underneath, they should push the head up and away from the wall by extending that arm vigorously. After that, the turn is completed in the same manner as described earlier in this section.

There is important difference between the open turns used in butterfly and breaststroke races. The turns are similar in every respect except the angle of the push-off. Butterfly swimmers should push off horizontally. On the other hand, breaststrokers should angle the push-off down so they can glide deeper, where the underwater pull-down and glide can be executed more effectively. This position was shown in Fig. 10.1.

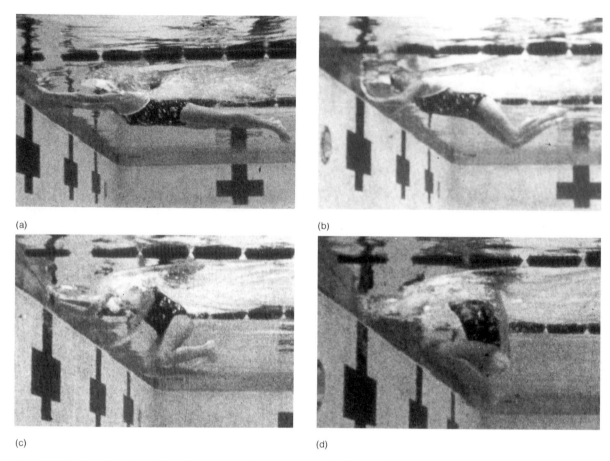

(a)

(b)

(c)

(d)

Fig. 11.7 Underwater views of a swimmer executing an open turn in breaststroke.

Recommended reading

Ayalon, A., Van Gheluwe, B. & Kanitz, M. (1975) A comparison of four styles of racing start in swimming. In Lewillie, L. & Clarys, J.P. (eds) *Swimming II*. Baltimore, Maryland: University Park Press, pp. 233–240.

Beritzhoff, S.T. (1974) *The relative effectiveness of two breaststroke starting techniques among selected intercollegiate swimmers*. Master's thesis, California State University, Chico, California.

Bowers, J.E. & Cavanaugh P.R. (1975) A biomechanical comparison of the grab and conventional sprint starts in competitive swimming. In Lewillie, L. & Clarys, J.P. (eds) *Swimming II*. Baltimore, Maryland: University Park Press, pp. 225–232.

Cavanaugh, P.R., Palmgren, J.V. & Kerr, B.A. (1975) A device to measure forces at the hand during the grab start in swimming. In Lewillie, L. & Clarys, J.P. (eds) *Swimming II*. Baltimore, Maryland: University Park Press, pp. 43–50.

Chow, J.W-C., Hay, J.G., Wilson, B.D. & Imel, C. (1984) Turning techniques of elite swimmers. *J. Sports Sci.* **2**:241–255.

Counsilman, J.E., Counsilman, B.E., Nomura, T. & Endo, M. (1988) Three types of grab starts for competitive swimming. In Ungerechts, B.E., Wilke, K. & Reischle, K. (eds) *Swimming Science V*. Champaign, Illinois: Human Kinetics, pp. 81–91.

Disch, J.G., Hosler, W.W. & Bloom, J.A. (1979) Effects of weight, height, and reach on the performance of the conventional and grab starts in swimming. In Terauds, J. & Bedingfield, E.W. (eds) *Swimming III*. Baltimore, Maryland: University Park Press, pp. 215–221.

Fitzgerald, J. (1973) The track start in swimming. *Swim. Tech.* **10**:89–94.

Gibson, G. & Holt, L.E. (1976) A cinema-computer analysis of selected starting techniques. *Swim. Tech.* **13**:75–76, 79.

Groves, R. & Roberts, J.A. (1972) A further investigation of the optimum angle of projection for the racing start in

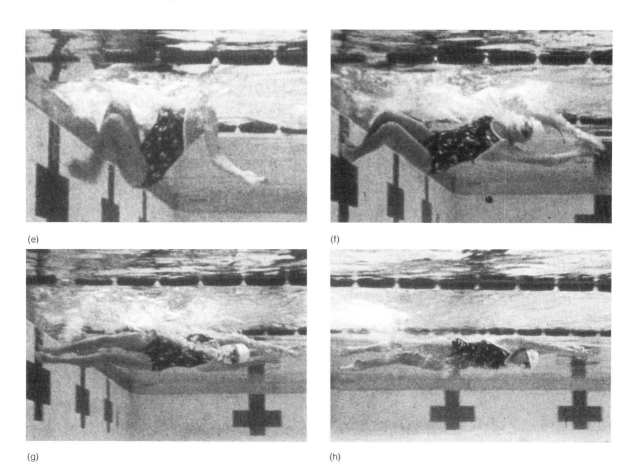

(e) (f)

(g) (h)

Fig. 11.7 (contd)

swimming. *Res. Q.* **43**:167–174.

Guimares, A.C.S. & Hay, J.G. (1985) A mechanical analysis of the grab starting technique in swimming. *Int. J. Sports Biomech.* **1**:25–35.

Hanauer, E. (1967) The grab start. *Swim. World* **8**:5, 42.

Hanauer, E.S. (1972) Grab start faster than conventional start. *Swim. World* **13**:8–9, 54–55.

Hay, J.G. (1986) The status of research on the biomechanics of swimming. In Hay, J.G. (ed.) *Starting, Stroking and Turning.* Iowa City, Iowa: Biomechanics Laboratory, University of Iowa, pp. 53–76.

Hobbie, P. (1980) Analysis of the flat vs. the hole entry. *Swim. Tech.* **16**:112–117.

Huellhorst, U., Ungerechts, B.E. & Willimczik, K, (1988) Displacement and speed characteristics of the breaststroke turn—a cinematographic analysis. In Ungerechts, B.E, Wilke, K. & Reischle, K. (eds) *Swimming Science V.* Champaign, Illinois: Human Kinetics, pp. 93–98.

Jorgenson, L.W. (1971) *A cinematographical and descriptive*

comparison of three selected freestyle racing starts in competitive swimming. Doctoral dissertation, Louisiana State University, Baton Rouge, Louisiana.

LaRue, R.J. (1983) A biomechanical comparison of the grab start and the track start in competitive swimming. *Abstr. Res. Papers* **1**:20.

Lewis, S. (1980) Comparison of five swimming start techniques. *Swim. Tech.* **16**:124–128.

Lowell, J.C. (1975). Analysis of the grab start and the conventional start. *Swim. Tech.* **12**:66–69, 76.

Michaels, R.A. (1973) A time distance comparison of the conventional and the grab start. *Swim. Tech.* **10**:16–17.

Michaels, R.A. (1974) Is the underwater pushoff faster? *Swim. Tech.* **11**:12.

Miller, J.A., Hay, J.G. & Wilson, B.D. (1984) Starting techniques of elite swimmers. *J. Sports Sci.* **2**:213–223.

Parker, S. (1974) Taking the flip one step further. *Swim. Tech.* **11**:75.

Pelchat, C. (1971) *A biomechanical analysis of selected*

racing starts in swimming. Unpublished Master's thesis, Pennsylvania State University, University Park, Pennsylvania.

Ransom, G.G. (1973) The no breathe flip turn. *Swim. Tech.* **10**:70−82.

Roffer, B.J. & Nelson, R.C. (1972) The grab start is faster. *Swim. Tech.* **8**:101−102.

Stratten, G. (1970) A comparison of three backstroke starts. *Swim. Tech.* **7**:55−60.

Thayer, A.L. & Hay, J.G. (1984) Motivating start and turn improvement. *Swim. Tech.* **20**:17−20.

Thorsen, E.A. (1975) Comparison of the conventional and grab start in swimming. *Tidsofkr. fur Legensp.* **39**:130−138.

Turner, J.C. (1974) The mechanical advantages of the grab start speak for themselves. *Swim. Tech.* **10**:111−112.

Van Slooten, P.H. (1973) An analysis of two forward swim starts using cinematography. *Swim. Tech.* **10**:85−88.

Wilson, D.S. & Mariano, G.W. (1983) Kinematic analysis of three starts. *Swim. Tech.* **19**:30−34.

Winters, C.N. (1968) *A comparison of the grip start in competitive swimming.* Master's thesis, Southeast Missouri State College, Cape Girardeau, Missouri.

Zatsiorsky, V.M., Bulgakova, N. Zh. & Chaplinsky, N.M. (1979) Biomechanical analysis of starting techniques in swimming. In Terauds, J. & Bedingfield, E.W. (eds) *Swimming III.* Baltimore, Maryland: University Park Press, pp. 199−206.

Section 3

Training

Chapter 12

Adaptations to swimming training

Repeated days and weeks of training can be considered as a positive form of stress because training improves the body's capacities for energy production, tolerance to physical stress, and swimming performance. The major physical changes occur within the first 6–10 weeks of training. The magnitude of these adaptations is generally considered to be controlled by the volume of exercise performed during training, leading many coaches and athletes to believe that the swimmer who does the most training will be the best performer. As a result, we often consider the quantity and quality of training to be synonymous. That is to say, we rate the value of a workout in terms of meters swum, rather than the speed at which it is performed. This philosophy has resulted in programs that are nonspecific to the demands of competitive swimming and often impose unrealistic demands on the swimmer. It must be realized that the rate of adaptation to training is limited and cannot be forced beyond the body's capacity for development. Too much training may result in only small improvements, and, in some cases, a breakdown in the processes of adaptation (i.e., overtraining and chronic fatigue). The key concept to remember is that muscle will adapt optimally to exercise which moderately exceeds its capacity, requiring a gradual progression in the training load to maximize performance. There is a limit to the physiological and anatomical development that can be achieved with training—a factor that is probably determined by genetics. Swimmers are not all created with the same ability to tolerate training. Consequently, improvements with training differ from individual to individual, which explains why swimmers who exercise under the same regimen frequently exhibit different levels of improvement.

The improvements in endurance that occur with daily aerobic training appear to be the result of changes in both central and peripheral circulation (e.g., cardiac output, muscle blood flow) and muscle metabolism (e.g., muscle respiratory capacity). Training changes within the muscles range from an improvement in blood flow around the fibers to dramatic changes in the muscle's energy-producing systems.

One of the most important changes that occurs during training is an increase in the number of capillaries surrounding each muscle fiber (Fig. 12.1). Endurance-trained swimmers may have 50% more capillaries in their arm muscles than sedentary individuals. An increase in the number of capillaries allows greater exchange of gases, heat, and fuels between the blood and the working muscle fibers.

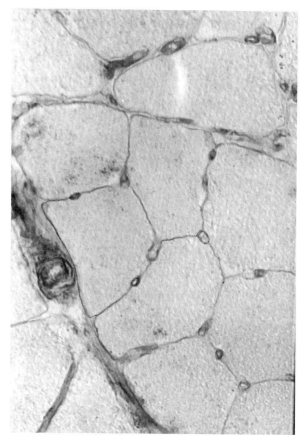

Fig. 12.1 Cross-sectional view of muscle showing the capillaries between the fibers. Note that there are approximately 3–4 capillaries around each fiber.

This increased exchange maintains an environment conducive to energy production and repeated muscle contractions. It appears that most of the increase in muscle capillary density occurs within the first few months of training; however, little research has been performed to determine what changes occur with longer periods of training.

Myoglobin, a compound similar to hemoglobin, acts as a storage compartment for oxygen within the muscle fibers, supporting aerobic metabolism when oxygen becomes limited during muscular effort. Aerobic training, such as short rest intervals and continuous swims of 400 m or more, can increase the myoglobin content of muscle, thereby enhancing its aerobic potential. In addition, endurance training also causes mitochondrial changes that improve the capacity of the muscle fibers to produce adenosine triphosphate (ATP). In the laboratory it is possible to measure the aerobic capacity of a specimen of muscle tissue obtained by needle biopsy. This procedure, termed the Q_{O_2} of muscle, determines the maximal oxygen uptake of a piece of muscle. In the untrained state muscles have a Q_{O_2} of 1500 $\mu l \cdot h^{-1} \cdot g^{-1}$. Swimmers who have been training 5000–12 000 m·day^{-1} have a Q_{O_2} in their shoulder muscles that is approximately twice as high as the untrained individual. Highly trained marathon runners, those who run more than 15 km·day^{-1}, have leg muscle Q_{O_2} values in excess of 4000 $\mu l \cdot h^{-1} \cdot g^{-1}$—a value nearly three times that of the untrained muscle.

Although it appears that the respiratory capacity of muscle increases with increasing training volume, swimming more than 30 km·week^{-1} does not increase the Q_{O_2}. The highest average values reported in human muscle (5174 $\mu l \cdot h^{-1} \cdot g^{-1}$) were in swimmers who had trained at only 5000 m·day^{-1}—higher (4756 $\mu l \cdot h^{-1} \cdot g^{-1}$) than when they trained at 10 000 m·day^{-1}. Thus, it appears that there is a limit to the muscle's capacity to adapt to aerobic training, with maximal improvements occurring at a training level of about 4000–6000 m·day^{-1}. This means that training in excess of these levels may do little to improve aerobic capacity.

The production of ATP depends on the action of special protein molecules called *enzymes*, which speed the chemical reactions of energy metabolism. As a result of aerobic training, the amount of these enzymes increases dramatically. Figure 12.2 illus-

trates the changes in the muscle's oxidative enzymes during 12 weeks of gradually increased training. It is interesting to note that these enzymes continue to rise throughout the period of training, but that little change in whole-body maximal oxygen uptake occurred during the final 6 weeks of training. It is also interesting to observe that during this same period the enzymes of glycolysis remained unchanged or tended to decline slightly.

The concentrations of muscle enzymes such as succinate dehydrogenase (SDH) and citrate synthase are dramatically influenced by endurance training. Even moderate amounts of daily activity will increase the muscle's aerobic capacity and the activity of these enzymes. For example, recreational swimming for as little as 20 min·day^{-1} has been shown to increase muscle SDH activity by more than 25% above the levels seen in sedentary individuals. Training more vigorously (60–90 min·day^{-1}), on the other hand, produces a two- to threefold increase in muscle SDH activity.

Adjustments in the action of the aerobic enzymes make it possible for the endurance-trained muscle to burn fat more effectively, thereby lessening the demands placed on its limited supply of glycogen. Samples of muscle taken from the thigh of men before and after cycle training have shown a 30% increase in their ability to burn free fatty acids. Other studies have reported that endurance training also increases the release of free fatty acids from the fat cells during exercise, thereby making them available for the muscle's use. Thus, improvements in the muscle's aerobic energy system result in a greater capacity to produce energy, and to shift toward a greater reliance on fat for ATP production.

Endurance training places repeated demands on the muscle's energy supplies of glycogen and fat. Muscle glycogen, in particular, may be drastically reduced with each training session. As a result, the mechanisms responsible for the replacement of glycogen stimulate greater stores when the swimmer has adequate rest and sufficient dietary carbohydrate. When distance swimmers, for example, stop training for several days and eat a diet rich in carbohydrates (400–550 g·day^{-1}) their muscle glycogen levels will increase to nearly twice the levels seen in sedentary individuals who follow the same regimen.

In addition to its greater glycogen stores, endurance-

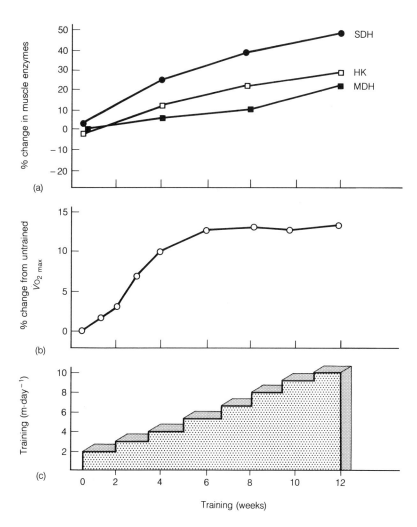

Fig. 12.2 (a) Changes in muscle oxidative enzyme activities and (b) percentage change in maximal oxygen uptake ($\dot{V}_{O_2 \, max}$) for a group of swimmers during (c) a progressive increase in training distance. Note that the swimmers' $\dot{V}_{O_2 \, max}$ improved only during the first 6 weeks of training when they were swimming 5000 m per day. Though they continued to increase their training volume, there was no additional improvement in aerobic capacity. SDH, Succinate dehydrogenase; HK, hexokinase; MDH, malic dehydrogenase.

trained muscle fibers have substantially more fat (i.e., triglyceride) than can be found in untrained fibers. Although there is only limited information regarding this improved fuel storage with endurance training, a 1.8-fold increase in muscle triglyceride content has been found to occur after only 8 weeks of endurance running. In general, the droplets of triglyceride are distributed throughout the muscle fiber, but are in close proximity to the mitochondria, making them readily available as a fuel source during exercise. In addition, many of the muscle enzymes (e.g., lipoprotein lipase, and carnitine palmityl transferase) responsible for the oxidation of fat are increased with endurance training.

As noted earlier, not all individuals have the same potential for adaptation to training. Men or women who perform a given training regimen will experience varied levels of muscular and circulatory improvements; some will show a large adjustment, while others may experience little or no change in their aerobic capacity. In addition, there seems to be an upper limit to the amount of adaptation that can be achieved with endurance training. Athletes who train with progressively greater workloads will eventually reach a maximal level of improvement; additional increments in the training volume will not improve their endurance. This point is illustrated in Fig. 12.3, which shows the responses of two groups of

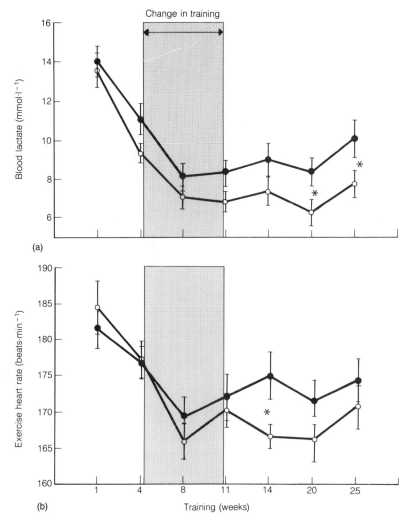

(a)

(b)

Fig. 12.3 Changes in (a) blood lactate and (b) heart rate during a standardized 365.8-m (400-yd) swim for swimmers who trained once per day (○) and those who trained twice per day (●). The latter group trained twice per day only during the 4th to 11th weeks (shaded area).

swimmers who trained either once or twice per day for 8 weeks. The swimmers' heart rates and blood lactate values decreased dramatically with the initiation of training, but showed no additional changes despite the twofold increase in training for those who trained twice per day.

Thus, it seems that there is an optimal amount of physical exercise that will produce maximal improvements in aerobic capacity and endurance performance. Although this optimal training load probably differs from one individual to another, observations with swimmers suggests that, on the average, the ideal training regimen may be equivalent to an energy expenditure of between 6000 and 10 000 kcal·week^{-1}, (25 200−42 000 kJ·week^{-1}) which translates to between 25 and 30 km·week^{-1} (4000−6000 m·day^{-1}). Of course, these are only estimates of the stimulus required for muscular conditioning, since some swimmers may show greater improvements with more training, while others may show the best results with substantially less training.

Aerobic training

Although the amount of work performed during training seems to be the most important determinant for developing aerobic endurance, peak performance also depends on the quality, or speed, of swimming training. The major fault with long-distance, low-intensity training is that it fails to develop the neurological patterns of muscle fiber recruitment, biomechanical skill, and the energy systems needed during swimming competitions. High-intensity speed training may include either intermittent exercise (intervals) or continuous exercise at near competition pace. Although interval training has been used for many years, most athletes consider this form of training to be highly anaerobic. While some interval training can be performed at speeds that produce a large amount of lactate, it is also possible to use this training format as a means to develop the aerobic system. Although long continuous swimming will develop the aerobic system, repeated bouts at a faster pace with brief rest intervals will achieve the same benefits. This form of *aerobic interval* training has become the foundation for swimming conditioning, involving repeated swims (50–200 m) at slightly slower than race pace, but with very brief (5–15 s) rest intervals.

It can be argued that a single continuous bout of exercise can give the same aerobic benefits as a set of aerobic intervals, but there are some swimmers who find continuous endurance swimming boring. When it comes to the aerobic aspects of training, personal preference may be the deciding factor. At present there is no direct evidence to show that aerobic interval training will produce greater muscular adaptation than continuous training bouts. Whether the training is performed as one long bout of continuous exercise or in a series of shorter intervals, the aerobic muscular benefits seem to be the same.

Anaerobic training

As mentioned earlier, a large part of the energy used during competitive swimming is derived from the anaerobic breakdown of muscle glycogen and the muscle's ATP and phosphocreatine (PCr) stores. In competitive events lasting only a few seconds, most of the energy demands are met by the breakdown of ATP and PCr. This anaerobic system is controlled by several enzymes, namely myokinase and creatine phosphokinase, though neither of these enzymes limits the rate of ATP resynthesis. Maximal sprint swimming lasting more than 4–5 s relies on the breakdown of glycogen to replace ATP and PCr. In

this energy system there are two key enzymes that limit the rate of ATP formation: phosphorylase and phosphofructokinase.

How does anaerobic sprint training improve performance? In addition to enhancing muscle strength, sprint training has been shown to improve the muscle's buffering capacity, that is, the ability to tolerate lactic acid produced within the muscle. Since the accumulation of lactate and free hydrogen ions within the muscle is considered to be responsible for fatigue during sprint exercise, an increase in muscle buffering capacity would delay the onset of fatigue during anaerobic exercise. It is interesting to note that the muscle's buffer capacity increased 12–50% as a result of 8 weeks of sprint training, but was not changed with endurance training. As with other muscular adaptations (e.g., enzymes) to training, changes in buffer capacity are specific to the intensity of exercise performed during training.

As a result of this increase in muscle buffer capacity, sprint-trained subjects accumulate more blood and muscle lactate during and following an all-out sprint test. It appears that with an enhanced buffer capacity the subjects' muscles can continue to generate energy for a longer period before critically high concentrations of lactate and hydrogen (H^+) develop, leading to an inhibition of the contractile process. It is interesting to note that under similar circumstances (i.e., sprinting to exhaustion), endurance-trained subjects do not accumulate as much muscle lactate or experience the unusually low pH values seen in sprint-trained men. Since aerobically trained muscles have significantly lower glycolytic enzymes, it may be that they have a lower capacity for anaerobic metabolism. More information is needed to explain the implications of the muscular changes that accompany both anaerobic and aerobic training.

As has been mentioned, both aerobic and anaerobic training produce remarkable adaptations in skeletal muscle. As noted earlier, improvements in capillary blood flow and the muscle's energy systems appear to be specific to the intensity and duration of the exercise performed during training. Anaerobic training, for example, will enhance muscular strength, buffering capacity, and glycolytic energy production, but may have little effect on the aerobic capacity of the muscle. Aerobic activities, on the other hand, increase the muscle's respiratory capacity and capillarization without altering its glycolytic potential or buffering capacity. Individuals who train solely for aerobic events may even show a decline in explosive muscular power. Little is known about the interaction between these two forms of training. Whether both systems can be trained to their full potential at the same time is unclear, although evidence suggests that it is possible to develop the aerobic and anaerobic benefits using various forms of intermittent and continuous exercise.

How much training is enough? The controversy

There is at present some debate concerning the amount of training required for swimmers to achieve maximal physical benefits. There are those who argue that swimmers can only reach their full potential if they swim more than $10\,000$ m·day^{-1} (i.e., 3–4 h·day^{-1}), whereas others contend that the same benefits can be obtained with as little as $4000-6000$ m·day^{-1} (i.e., 1.5–2 h·day^{-1}). This debate over how much physical training is needed for optimal performance is based on the contention that improvements in conditioning are related to the amount of exercise that can be performed in training (i.e., the number of meters swum per day). This leads to the assumption that the best swimmer is the one who does the most training.

In the early 1950s swimming training was typically limited to $1500-2000$ m·day^{-1}. Over the past 30–40 years swimming coaches have learned through trial and error that in order to produce the best results, swimmers must swim as many meters as possible each week. An obsession with daily training distance has become the foundation of the swimming coach's training plan. Any discussion of training immediately turns to how many meters the swimmers have been performing each day. The intent of the following discussion is not to prove or disprove the traditional theories of the need for large training volumes. Rather, we will attempt to take an objective view of why we train swimmers, what we hope to gain, and to illustrate the possible gains and pitfalls of long or short training volume.

First, we must remind ourselves that the purpose of training is to prepare the swimmer for the demands of competition. This must involve the physiological,

biomechanical, and psychological aspects of preparation. Though the physiological aspects of training have been extensively studied, there is only limited information concerning the psychological and biomechanical benefits of a heavy training regimen on performance. We must not ignore the potential advantage of hard training in building confidence among swimmers who believe they are better than their competitors because they have trained harder. Equally, the many hours of training will certainly add to the swimmers' skill and efficiency. Thus, there are some intangible aspects to training that may not be readily evident from the scientific literature.

With the exception of the 400-, 800-, and 1500-m events, the majority (approximately 70%) of swimming competitions are completed in less than 2 min, suggesting that a large part of the energy needed for these events is derived anaerobically, and that success depends on muscle strength and power. But training must improve more than the swimmer's energy supply and strength. It can be argued that swimming technique is by far the most important factor determining success in swimming. There are many swimmers with exceptional strength and endurance who fail to approach the élite level of competition because they lack the skill needed to use their talents. Thus, it is generally agreed that swimming training should:

1 maximize the swimmer's aerobic and anaerobic energy systems;
2 improve swimming strength and power; and
3 develop an efficient technique.

One rule of training to remember is that the adaptations to regular exercise are specific to the type of activity performed during training. When the body is stressed it attempts to compensate by developing a greater tolerance to handle future bouts of stress. If, for example, swimmers were asked to perform an easy 3000-m swim every day for 4 weeks, their bodies would develop the endurance to tolerate a 3000-m swim, but would gain little or no strength. In addition, they might develop a more efficient style that would enable them to swim the 3000 m with less effort. Thus, the benefits of such a training bout are specific to that event, but would have little value for performance in shorter sprints (e.g., 50 m).

In light of the brevity of most swimming events (i.e., less than 2 min) the specific gains desired from training are those of strength, aerobic and anaerobic endurance, and the mechanics for efficient sprint swimming. Based on the principle of *training specificity* we would expect the best possible gains from a training program that emphasizes these factors, namely short, repeated sprint swims. But the debate is not over the need for quality (i.e., sprint) training. Rather, the issue is whether the same benefits can be achieved with training loads of 5000 (one training session per day) and 10 000 m (two training sessions per day). Unfortunately, there are few studies to provide us with the empirical evidence to answer this question, though a recent study with collegiate male swimmers has shown similar performance results

from both levels of training.

As illustrated in Fig. 12.4, two matched groups of Division I collegiate swimmers were studied over a 24-week training period, which included a period of training in one group of more than 10 000 m·day^{-1}. The training for the swimmers in the other group did not exceed 5000 m·day^{-1}. Both groups experienced similar physiological adaptations and performance gains. Measurements made at rest and after endurance swimming suggested that the additional training performed by the men in the long-distance group did not significantly enhance their aerobic or anaerobic capacities above those attained by the short-distance group (Table 12.1).

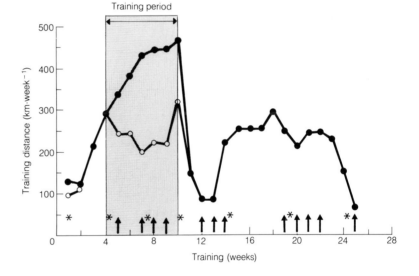

Fig. 12.4 The training plan used for the group of swimmers who trained twice per day (●) (noted by the shaded area) and those in the group who trained only once per day (○). ↑, Competition; *, testing. From Costill *et al.* (1990).

Table 12.1 Mean (± s.e.) muscle fiber composition (% type I fibers), phosphofructokinase (PFK), phosphorylase, and citrate synthase (CS) activities (μmol·min^{-1}·g^{-1}) before (pre) and after (post) 6 weeks of training in two groups of swimmers

Group	Type I fibers (%)	PFK Pre	PFK Post	Phosphorylase Pre	Phosphorylase Post	CS Pre	CS Post
Short-distance (n = 5)	65.5 (±8.9)	17.9 (±6.0)	16.8 (±4.5)	26.5 (±2.8)	24.8 (±1.8)	34.9 (±3.6)	38.9* (±5.8)
Long-distance (n = 4)	74.5 (±2.4)	20.4 (±4.0)	21.5 (±2.3)	22.8 (±2.0)	23.8 (±3.1)	33.4 (±1.7)	41.4* (±3.8)

* Significant difference (*p*<0.05) between pre and post values.

The major finding of this investigation was that the additional training imposed on the long-distance group (weeks 5−11) did not produce a greater improvement in performance. To the contrary, during this period of increased training these swimmers showed no improvement in swimming power and experienced a significant decline in sprinting ability (Fig. 12.5). This finding is in keeping with an earlier report that swimmers experience a decline in arm strength and power during periods of heavy training. Arm power was observed to be at its lowest level when the swimmers were training at approximately 9000 m·day^{-1}, and highest when the swimmers tapered their training to 2700 m·day^{-1} for a 3-week period. This finding in not confined to swimming training, since a similar decline in the ability to generate peak tension during distance-running training has been reported.

The cause for this decline in muscular force with heavy training is unknown, though it has been shown that during intense periods of training there is a decrease in single-fiber peak tension, suggesting that the decline in force may be specific to the fiber's contractile mechanism and independent of neural control. Whatever the cause, the loss of muscular strength with intense training appears to be temporary and is quickly recovered after a few days or weeks of reduced training, as is often the experience with tapering.

Although it is tempting to suggest that all swimmers should confine their training to one training session of 3000−5000 m·day^{-1}, it is possible that the swimmers used in this study may not represent the wide range of abilities and experience seen in more élite or less talented swimmers. Nor do they describe the training requirements needed by female and age-group (<16 years) swimmers. Nevertheless, the present data make it clear that the extra time and energy used in training twice per day did not improve performance to a greater degree than was achieved by the men who trained only once per day. In fact, increased training may reduce speed and power — factors essential for success in competitive swimming.

In light of this effect on swimming power, a group of collegiate swimmers reduced their training from an average of 8742 m·day^{-1} in 1983 to 4517 m·day^{-1} in 1985. Since these men had been tested every 3−4 weeks during training throughout this 3-year period, it was possible to assess the influence of this reduction in training on their physical conditioning and competitive performances. The mean time for 5−6 competitions for each swimmer was calculated for the 100-yd (91.4-m) and 200-yd (182.8-m) events in 1983, 1984, and 1985. As shown in Fig. 12.6, the mean times for these men were significantly faster in 1985 than in either of the preceding years. All of the swimmers achieved lifetime-best performances at the 1985 conference championship competition, which

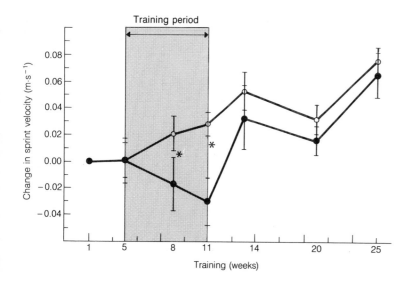

Fig. 12.5 Changes in sprint swimming velocity during 25 weeks of training. Note that the group who trained twice a day (●) tended to get slower during the period of heaviest training, whereas the group who trained only once per day (○), showed a steady improvement in sprinting throughout the training period. * $p<0.05$.

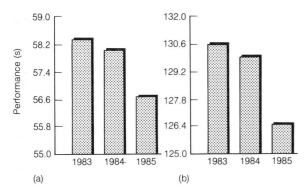

Fig. 12.6 Mean performances for (a) 100-yd and (b) 200-yd (91.4- and 182.9-m) swimming events during the 1983, 1984, and 1985 competitive collegiate season. Means include data from front crawl, backstroke, breaststroke and butterfly events. Note that the swimming times were fastest during 1985 when the swimmers only trained once per day at an average distance of $4000-6000$ m·day^{-1}.

followed a further taper in training to only 2240 m·day^{-1} for the final 2 weeks of the season. No significant differences were found in maximal oxygen uptake or the amount of blood lactate after the standard 182.8-m swim between the tests in 1984 and 1985. The men were, however, significantly more powerful in 1985 when tested on the swim bench and during a swimming power test. Thus, it appears that the men achieved the same endurance training effect in 1985 with roughly half the training load that had been employed in 1983 and 1984, yet remained stronger and performed better.

Although it is tempting to suggest that all swimmers will perform better if they confine their training to one training session of $4000-6000$ m·day^{-1}, it is possible that the swimmers used in this study may not represent the wide range of abilities seen in age-group males and females, or in more élite swimmers. In an effort to compare the improvements in performance for swimmers who train for more than 10 000 m·day^{-1} with those who swim approximately half that distance, the percentage of improvement in the 100-yd (91.4-m) front crawl from year to year was calculated for NCAA (National Collegiate Athletic Association) qualifiers (males) and the subjects [Ball State University (BSU) swimming team] used in the previously mentioned studies. The NCAA qualifiers were assumed to represent élite swimmers who generally train at more than 10 000 m·day^{-1}, whereas

the BSU swimmers trained an average of only $4000-5000$ m·day^{-1}. As shown in Fig. 12.7, the NCAA male swimmers experienced an average improvement of 0.8% per year (approximately 0.37 s·year^{-1}), which was identical to that observed for the BSU swimmers. Similar findings were also observed for competitors in other events (i.e., 200-, 500-, and 1650-yd front crawl). Thus, élite swimmers appear to show no greater improvement in performance than those training with only one session per day. These findings suggest that the data generated using the BSU swimmers are applicable for élite swimmers as well.

Our knowledge of the need for specificity in training might lead us to assume that several hours of daily training may not provide the adaptations needed for optimal sprint swimming performance. Since the majority of the competitive swimming events last less than 2 min, it is difficult to understand how training at speeds that are markedly slower than competitive pace for $3-4$ h·day^{-1} will prepare the swimmer for the supramaximal efforts of competition.

Although there may be some psychological advant-

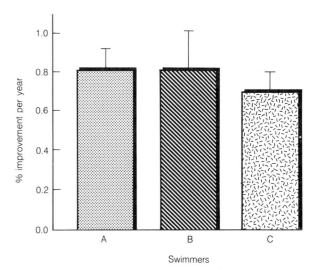

Fig. 12.7 Average improvements per year for élite (A: NCAA, $n=205$) and nonélite (B: BSU, $n=43$; C: MAC, $n=161$) collegiate swimmers. These data demonstrate that the élite and nonélite swimmers showed similar improvements from year to year despite the fact that the élite swimmers trained at nearly twice the volume of the nonélite swimmers. Training programs: NCAA, >10 000 m·day^{-1}; BSU, <5000 m·day^{-1}; MAC, $5000-10 000$ m·day^{-1}. MAC, mid-American Conference.

ages to hard training, there are also some negative factors to consider. Training for 3−4 h·day^{-1} may exceed the psychological and physical tolerance of some swimmers who possess the potential to reach the élite level. As a result, they may drop out of the sport before achieving their best performances. Thus, we are faced with the question: "how many good swimmers failed to become élite because they burned out before realizing their full potential?"

What then are the benefits of the *megameter* training programs? The fact that swimmers are able to tolerate the hours of intense training does not mean that they automatically become better swimmers. So long as the training program is progressive and does not overly tax the swimmers, they will adapt to the stress of training, making it possible to tolerate the training demands. Thus, it may be that long and multiple training sessions simply prepare the swimmer for long and multiple training sessions, which may or may not have any bearing on the swimmer's performance in a 1- or 2-min sprint event.

Unfortunately, this discussion will not finalize the debate over the issue of how much training is enough for maximal development, but it is clear that similar performance results can be achieved with less than 3−4 h of training each day. Although the training requirement may differ from swimmer to swimmer, there appears to be a greater risk of overtraining or chronically fatiguing swimmers than undertraining them. It appears that in mature élite-level swimmers, the physiological, biomechanical, and psychological development needed for peak performance can be achieved in 1.5−2 h of training per day. The traditional fear of underexercising the swimmer seems to be unwarranted, since shorter training sessions will simply enable the swimmer to train at better quality, thereby emphasizing training specificity.

Tapering

As noted earlier, periods of intense training reduce muscular strength, lessening the swimmer's sprinting performance. To produce their best performances, most swimmers reduce their training for 2−3 weeks or more before a major competition. Most coaches have learned from experience that this period does not cause the swimmer to lose conditioning, but results in a significant improvement in sprinting speed.

Tapering programs may differ dramatically but the general intent is to remove the stress of training for a period of 2 weeks or more. Some coaches prefer gradually to reduce the training volume over that period, whereas other may drop the training load in a single day to only 30% of the normal training volume. Although there is no clear advantage of either plan, it has been shown that individuals who are somewhat overtrained or chronically fatigued from training may benefit from the rapid drop in training, since it allows a longer period to recover. This plan also reduces the possibility of undertapering the swimmer.

Swimmers who reduce their training from an average of 10 000 to 3200 m·day^{-1} over a 15-day period show no loss in maximal oxygen uptake or endurance performance. Similar findings have been observed in swimmers who train at approximately 5000 m·day^{-1} and then reduce their training to 2000 m·day^{-1}. Surprisingly, measurements of blood lactate after a standard 200-m swim are generally higher after a period of tapering. Likewise, heart rates during swimming may be a few beats higher after the taper than during periods of heavy training. The causes for these changes in heart rate and blood lactate are not fully understood, though they appear to have little bearing on performance. Generally, swimming performance improves an average of 3.5% or more as a result of tapering. Such improvements are consistent across all the events (i.e., 50−1500 m).

The most notable change during the taper period is a marked increase in muscular strength. As a consequence of reduced training, swimmers demonstrated an increase in arm strength and power of from 17.7 to 24.6%. It is difficult to determine whether these improvements in muscle strength are the consequence of changes within the muscle's contractile mechanism or an improvement in muscle fiber recruitment. The underlying factors responsible for improved performance with tapering may be the focus of future studies, since it appears to play an important role in the fine-tuning of the swimmer's skills.

Body hair removal

The removal of body hair prior to major swimming competitions is an accepted practice which may contribute to the improvements in performance typically observed at championship meets. Although few studies have been conducted to explain the benefits of shaving-down, it has been suggested that hair removal may reduce skin resistance, thereby lessening the physiological demands of swimming at a given speed. A study by Sharp and Costill (1989) has shown that removing exposed body hair significantly decreases blood lactate, oxygen uptake, and heart rate during a standardized 400-yd (365.8-m) breaststroke swim. These findings, in combination with measurements of velocity decay after a maximal underwater leg push-off from the side of the pool, are taken as evidence that the mechanism for improvement in competitive swimming performance following a shave-down is related to a reduction of active drag. Thus, it is concluded that the use of this procedure before major competitions provides a measurable physiological advantage for the swimmer.

Recommended reading

Costill, D.L. (1977) Adaptations in skeletal muscle during training for sprint and endurance swimming. In Eriksson, B. & Furberg, B. (eds) *Swimming Medicine IV*. Baltimore, Maryland: University Park Press, pp. 233–248.

Costill, D.L. (1985) The 1985 C.H. McCloy research lecture: practical problems in exercise physiology research. *Res. Q.* **56**:378–384.

Costill, D.L., Coyle, E.F., Fink, W.F., Lesmes, G.R. & Witzmann, F.A. (1979) Adaptations in skeletal muscle following strength training. *J. Appl. Physiol. Resp. Environ. Exerc. Physiol.* **46**:96–99.

Costill, D.L., Fink, W.J., Hargreaves, M., King, D.S., Thomas, R. & Fielding, R. (1985) Metabolic characteristics of skeletal muscle during detraining from competitive swimming. *Med. Sci. Sports Exerc.* **17**:339–343.

Costill, D.L., Thomas, R., Robergs, R.A., Pascoe, D.D., Lambert, C.P. & Fink, W.J. (1991) Adaptations to swimming training: influence of training volume. *Med. Sci. Sports Exerc.* **23**:371–377.

Davies, C. & Knibbs, A. (1971) The training stimulus: the effects of intensity, duration and frequency of effort on maximum aerobic power output. *Int. Z. Angew. Physiol.* **29**:299–305.

Hermansen, L. (1971) Lactate production during exercise. In Pernow, B. & Saltin, B. (eds) *Muscle Metabolism During Exercise*. New York: Plenum Press.

Kirwan, J.P., Costill, D.L., Flynn, M.G. *et al.* (1988) Physiological responses to successive days of intense training in competitive swimmers. *Med. Sci. Sports Exerc.* **20**:255–259.

Lesmes, G.R., Costill, D.L., Coyle, E.F. & Fink, W.J. (1978) Muscle strength and power changes during maximal isokinetic training. *Med. Sci. Sports* **10**:266–269.

Saltin, B., Nazar, K., Costill, D.L. *et al.* (1976) The nature of the training response: peripheral and central adaptations to one-legged exercise. *Acta Physiol. Scand.* **96**:289–305.

Saltin, B. & Rowell, L.B. (1980) Functional adaptations to physical activity and inactivity. *Fed. Proc.* **39**:1506–1513.

Sharp, R.L. & Costill, D.L. (1989) Influence of body hair removal on physiological responses during breaststroke swimming. *Med. Sci. Sports Exerc.* **21**:576–580.

Sharp, R.L., Costill, D.L., Fink, W.J. & King, D.S. (1986) Effects of eight weeks of bicycle ergometer sprint training on human muscle buffer capacity. *Int. J. Sports Med.* **7**:13–17.

Chapter 13

Principles of training

The purpose of training programs is to produce metabolic, physiological and psychological adaptations that allow swimmers to perform better. The term *adaptation* refers to changes that occur in response to training. An example of the adaptation process follows. When training increases the demand for aerobic energy, the number and size of muscle mitochondria will increase so that these "chemical factories" where aerobic metabolism takes place become larger and more numerous. This will enable athletes to provide more energy from aerobic metabolism.

There are at least three steps in the adaptation process. Using the increase of muscle mitochondria as an example, the first step involves creating the need for more aerobic energy. Training must be sufficient in both duration and intensity to accomplish this. The second step is to provide the proper nutrients to build and repair mitochondrial tissue. In step three, the athletes must be given enough rest to build and repair that tissue.

Finally, it will be necessary to increase the duration and intensity of training to create further adaptations once plateaus occur. This brings us to the first two principles of training—overload and progression. Overload provides a method for producing adaptations while progression insures that a continued overload takes place. A third principle concerns the nature of adaptations. The human body adapt to the type of exercise being performed in a very specific, rather than general, manner. This, as the definition implies, is the principle of specificity.

The overload principle

The basic tenant of this principle is that adaptations will not occur unless the demands of training are greater than the usual demands made upon a particular physiological mechanism. This principle, although simple in definition, is quite complex in application. The complexity lies in the fact that, while the demands of training must be sufficient to stimulate adaptation, they cannot be too great or the training effect will be lost through injury or overtraining. If the amount of overload exceeds the tolerance of a particular physiological system, that system will break down.

The progression principle

A particular training load will only remain an overload until the swimmer adapts to it. At that point, the intensity and/or duration must be increased before any further adaptations will take place. The stepwise process of increasing overload is called *progression*.

Figure 13.1 illustrates the importance of overload and progression in the training process. It depicts changes in the blood lactic acid content of a man over a training period of approximately 50 days. Changes in aerobic capacity were examined in this study. A reduction in blood lactic acid content was used as a measure of improvement. As seen in Fig. 13.1, these reductions took place only when training speeds were progressively increased.

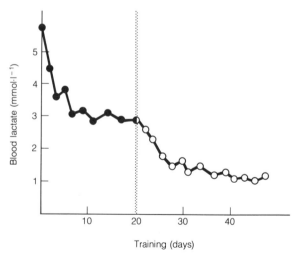

Fig. 13.1 The effect of overload and progression on aerobic endurance as measured by decreases in blood lactic acid. Training speeds: ●, 7 mph (27 km·h); ○, 8.5 mph (13.5 km·h^{-1}). Adapted from Åstrand & Rodahl (1977), with permission.

On day 1 the athlete portrayed in Fig. 13.1 began running at a speed of 7 mph. The lactic acid content of his blood decreased from slightly more than 5 mmol·l^{-1} to less than 3 mmol·l^{-1} after 10 days of training. Obviously, running at 7 mph was an overload during the first 10 days of training. Notice, however, that blood lactic acid did not decrease further over the next days of training at 7 mph (days 10–20). This was because the athlete's aerobic system had adapted to running at that speed and it no longer represented an overload.

After day 20, a new overload was applied by increasing the running speed to 8.5 mph. Another significant reduction of blood lactic acid took place during the first 10 days at the new speed (days 20–30). This improvement of aerobic capacity was followed by a plateau over the next 20 days (days 30–50) of running. The study was concluded after day 50.

Figure 13.1 clearly shows that athletes, including swimmers, cannot train at the same speeds week after week and expect to continue improving their aerobic capacities. This statement is equally true for other physiological capacities. For best results, they should gradually increase their training speeds throughout the season.

There are also other ways to increase training overloads progressively. In addition to training speeds, the other variables that can be manipulated to produce a progressive overload are *volume* and *density*. Volume refers to training mileage. That mileage can be expressed as the distances for repeat sets, as daily mileage, weekly mileage, and as mileage completed during any seasonal phase. Density concerns the amount of work accomplished in a certain time. The rest intervals between repeats are the usual expression of this variable.

Overload and progression can be applied by increasing one or more of these variables while maintaining the others at their usual level. For example, increasing swimming speed without reducing volume or density will provide for overload and progression. An increase of volume with no change in speed or density will do likewise. Finally, density can be increased when the rest interval between repeats is reduced while speed and volume remain unchanged.

Many programs do not include deliberate progression plans, yet some swimmers improve because they are highly motivated and train at progressively faster speeds as they become capable of doing so. There are many other swimmers who do not adapt well to this "hit-or-miss" approach, however. Some do not put forth sufficient effort while others injure themselves by trying to progress too fast. Coaches should program systems of progression into their training plans. Systemic increases in training intensity, duration and density will produce greater adaptations with less risk of injury.

The principle of specificity

The last principle of training that will be discussed is specificity. Like overload, the principle of specificity is straightforward in definition but complex in application. By definition, this principle states that the physiological processes most improved by training will be those that are stressed most. The problem in applying specificity to the training process happens when coaches translate this principle too narrowly. Some have misinterpreted it to mean that athletes should swim their training volume at under-distance competition speeds where the demands of training are identical to those of competition. While this is certainly one form of specific training, it is not the only nor the most important form. Truly specific training involves a much broader interpretation — one that includes all the various phases of the metabolic system that supply energy for adenosine triphosphate (ATP) replacement during races.

To review, the three energy systems are the ATP–PCr (phosphocreatine) or nonaerobic system, the anaerobic system and the aerobic system. Race-speed swimming will train these systems to provide energy in approximately the same proportions as during competition. Consequently, *only the dominant energy system will be stressed sufficiently to produce a maximum training effect.* The other energy systems may not be stressed optimally and will, therefore, not improve as much as they might with another form of training. This, in turn, will not allow them to make the contribution to the energy supply during races that they might otherwise make.

Too much emphasis on race-pace training will stress the anaerobic system most while the remaining two will be neglected. The anaerobic system will be stressed most by underdistance race-speed repeats simply because this system plays a limiting role at all race distances in competitive swimming. When repeats are swum at race speed, the fatigue created by anaerobic metabolism will limit the volume in all sets but those designed for races of 1500 m. Consequently, the aerobic system will not receive the stimulation it needs to adapt maximally.

Likewise, the nonaerobic system will not receive sufficient stimulation for maximum improvement by swimming at race speed. Training speeds need to be faster than those in competition to overload this system. There are three types of specificity that should be included in training.

1 training that is specific to race-pace;
2 training that is specific to muscle fibers;
3 training that is specific to energy systems.

There are a large number of studies that endorse the concept of training specificity according to energy systems and muscle fibers. Figure 13.2 illustrates the results of one such study. It depicts the effects of both sprint and endurance training programs on the three energy systems. Figure 13.2a shows the effects of these two programs on the ATP−PCr reaction. Notice that the sprint training program improved this reaction most, while endurance training improved it only slightly. The relative effect of sprint and endurance training on blood lactic acid content is shown in Fig. 13.2b. A reduction of this end-product of anaerobic metabolism was produced most by endurance training and least by sprint training. If you remember, a reduction in blood lactic acid accumulation reflects improved aerobic capacity. Figure 13.2c shows

the effects of sprint and endurance training on the maximum amount of lactic acid that can accumulate in the blood after exercise. An increase in this amount is a desirable anaerobic training effect because it shows that athletes can get more energy from glycolysis before becoming fatigued. This effect was produced only by sprint training. It is interesting that endurance training actually reduced lactic acid accumulation in the blood. This result indicates the possibility that an athlete's capacity for anaerobic metabolism may be reduced by endurance training.

The importance of training specific muscle fibers can be illustrated by contrasting the training effects on trained and untrained limbs. Two approaches have been taken in studies of this type. In the first, one leg or arm was trained while the opposite limb served as a control. A second approach was to train one set of limbs, either the arms or legs, while the other set was used as a control. The overwhelming result was that in the majority of these works, the trained limb or limbs improved in size, performance, anaerobic capacity, and aerobic capacity more than their untrained counterpart (Clausen *et al.*, 1971; Saltin *et al.*, 1976; Pate *et al.*, 1978, Hardman & Williams, 1983; Glina *et al.*, 1984; Loftin *et al.* 1988).

Figure 13.3 shows the results of one such study. Subjects were endurance-trained on a bicycle ergometer. They pedaled with only one leg, while the other remained inactive. Notice that the lactic acid concentration decreased markedly in the trained leg but only slightly in the untrained leg after training.

In another study of this type, arm exercise resulted in an 80% increase of work output for the upper limbs

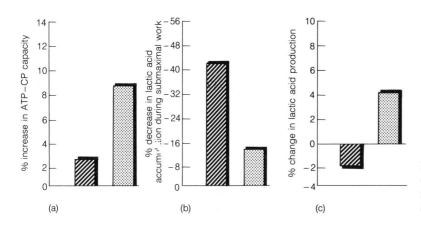

Fig. 13.2 Effects of sprint (▨) and endurance (▧) training on (a) the nonaerobic, (b) aerobic, and (c) anaerobic energy systems.

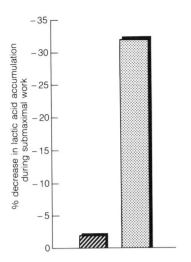

Fig. 13.3 Comparison of aerobic training effects on a trained (▨) and untrained (▨) limb. From Fox & Mathews (1981), with permission.

but only an 18% increase for the legs. In still another, the trained leg improved endurance performance by 340% and maximal oxygen uptake by 19.5%. Improvements in the untrained leg were 151% and 10.5% respectively.

In these studies, the improved performances of the untrained limbs probably resulted from increased circulatory and respiratory capacities. They made it possible for those systems to deliver more oxygen and nutrients to all the tissues in the body, including those that were not trained. This category of training effects is characterized as *central* because any type of exercise will improve their function and contribute to improved performances in other nonspecific types of exercise. Another category of training effects is referred to as *peripheral* because it concerns those changes taking place only in the muscle fibers exercised. Peripheral training effects are specific to the muscle fibers used and are only transferable to other activities where those same fibers do the work.

Studies where muscle biopsies have been used to assess differences of physiological capacity between trained and untrained muscle fibers have provided enlightening information about the importance of peripheral training effects. These studies have shown consistently that only the fibers used in training increase their: (i) mitochondrial size and number;

(ii) myoglobin content; (iii) glycogen, ATP and PCr storage; (iv) aerobic, nonaerobic, and anaerobic enzyme activity; (v) capillary density; (vi) buffering capacity; and (vii) protein content.

This brings us to the most important part of this discussion. Swimmers cannot depend on nonspecific training for top performances. They cannot hope to become conditioned for maximum performance unless they use the same muscle fibers in training that they will use in competition. Further, they must train the energy systems within these muscle fibers for maximum adaptations. This means that athletes cannot achieve maximum adaptations in swimming muscles by running or circuit training. These methods may be good supplements but they should never supplant swimming as the major training form. It also means that swimmers should not do all of their endurance training with the freestyle. They will not achieve maximum endurance in some of the different muscle fibers that are used in the butterfly, backstroke or breaststroke if they swim these strokes only during sprint training. For best results, they must swim both endurance and sprint repeats in the stroke or strokes they plan to use in competition on a regular basis.

Recommended reading

Åstrand, P.-O. & Rodahl, K. (1977) *Textbook of Work Physiology.* New York: McGraw-Hill.

Clausen, J.P., Klausen, K., Rasmussen, B. & Trap-Jensen, J. (1971) Effect of selective arm and leg training on cardiac output and regional blood flow. *Acta Physiol. Scand.* **82**:35–36a.

Fox, E.L. & Mathews, D.K. (1981) *The Physiological Basis of Physical Education and Athletics.* New York: Saunders College Publishing.

Gergley, T., McArdle, W., DeJesus, P., Toner, M., Jacobowitz, S. & Spina, P. (1984) Specificity of arm training on aerobic power during swimming and running. *Med. Sci. Sports Exerc.* **16(4)**:349–354.

Glina, J.C., Caiozzo, V.J., Bielen, R.J., Prietto, C.A., McMaster, W.C. (1984) Anaerobic threshold for leg cycling and arm cranking (abstract). *Med. Sci. Sports Exerc,* **16(2)**:109.

Hardman, A.E., & Williams, C. (1983) Single leg maximum oxygen uptake and endurance performance before and after short-term training. *Int. J. Sports Med.* **5** (Suppl.):122–123.

Houston, M.E. & Thomson, J.A. (1977) The response of endurance adapted adults to intense anaerobic training. *Eur. J. Appl. Physiol.* **36**:207–213.

Hutinger, P. (1970) *Comparison of isokinetic, isotonic, and isometric developed strength to speed in swimming the crawl stroke.* Doctoral dissertation, Indiana University.

Jacobs, I., Esbjornsson, M., Sylven, C., Holm, I. & Jansson, E. (1987) Sprint training effect on muscle myoglobin, enzymes, fiber types, and blood lactates. *Med. Sci. Sports Exerc.* **19(4)**:368−374.

Loftin, M., Boileau, R.A., Massey, B.H. & Lohman, T.G. (1988) Effect of arm training on central and peripheral circulatory function. *Med. Sci. Sports Exerc.* **20(2)**:136−141.

Nakamura, Y., Takei, Y., Mutoh, Y. & Miyashita, M. (1985) Specificity of exercise duration for anaerobic type training (abstract). *Med. Sci. Sports Exerc.* **17(2)**:268.

Pate, R.R., Hughes, R.D., Chandler, J.V. & Ratliffe, J.L. (1978) Effects of arm training on retention of training effects derived from leg training. *Med. Sci. Sports* **10**:71−74.

Saltin, B., Nazar, K., Costill, D.L. *et al.* (1976) The nature of the training response: peripheral and central adaptations to one-legged exercise. *Acta Physiol. Scand.* **96**:289−305.

Sharp, R.L. (1986) Muscle strength and power as related to competitive swimming *J. Swim. Res.* **2(2)**:5−10.

Sharp, R.L., Costill, D.L. & King, D.S. (1983) Power characteristics of swimmers at the 1982 US Senior National Long Course Swimming Championships. *J. Swim. Res.* **2(2)**:5−10.

Chapter 14

A training plan

Planning involves separating the training year into smaller and more manageable units. The principal reason for planning is to insure systematic adaptations that will bring swimmers to a peak at the time of their most important meets. The yearly plan should be constructed first; then, the seasonal plan and finally weekly and daily training plans should be constructed.

Planning the training year involves first deciding how many times swimmers will shave and taper for important meets. This will establish the number of seasons in each year. Next, each season should be divided into phases that emphasize different methods of training. Finally, each of these season phases should be subdivided into shorter subphases that provide for systematic progressions in training distance and intensity.

Yearly planning

The majority of coaches divide the training year into two or three seasons depending on the number of times they wish to shave and taper for important meets.

A two-season yearly plan

In this plan, the year is usually separated into short- and long-course seasons. The short-course or winter season culminates in a major national or international competition some time in March or April. The long-course or summer season ends with a meet of equal or greater importance in August. The swimmers are usually given 1 or 2 weeks for rest and recuperation between seasons.

A three-season yearly plan

Coaches who use this approach do so because they shave and taper for an important meet in December or January. In this case the first or fall season runs from September to January. The second or winter season is from January to April and the third or summer season goes from May to August.

Each season should include a minimum of 20 weeks for best results. This does not mean swimmers should do the same mileage at the same intensity for 20 weeks. The emphasis of training should change at 6–12-week intervals.

Season planning

Once the year has been divided into seasons, the next step is to separate each season into phases or macrocycles. Each macrocycle should have a different set of goals concerning the adaptations sought and the kinds of training used to produce them. The typical plan is to separate the season into four macrocycles.
1   The general endurance period.
2   The specific endurance period.
3   The competition period.
4   The taper period.

The general endurance period

The purposes of this training phase are to build a base of endurance, strength, flexibility, and psychological endurance and to improve techniques. It is a preparation period for the more intense training that will follow. It should be 6–10 weeks in length when conditions permit. Most of the training should be in the form of stroke drills, pulling and kicking, all at basic endurance speeds. The amounts of fast endurance and sprint training should gradually increase throughout this phase but they are not emphasized. Approximately 60% of the weekly mileage should be at the basic endurance level with 20% in the form of intense endurance swimming. Some sprint training should be included. The remainder of the weekly mileage should be devoted to warming up and swimming down. Athletes should swim all strokes and repeat distances in training. Their specialties should not be emphasized during this phase. This is also true of sprinters, although they should not be expected to do as much mileage as the middle-distance and distance swimmers.

A considerable amount of time—perhaps 3—4 h·week^{-1}—should be spent on dry land training for the purpose of increasing the size and strength of all of the major muscle groups. Distance swimmers may, if they wish, forego dry land training in favor of swimming additional mileage each week. They may also substitute stroke-specific circuit training on land aimed at improving muscular endurance for their 400—500-m events.

Stretching exercises should be conducted daily, stressing the joints of the ankles, lower back and shoulders. This is the time for instructions on technique and for diagnosing the strokes of swimmers with video tape. Various forms of psychological training can also be conducted, such as visualization and relaxation drills.

The specific endurance period

The emphasis remains on improving endurance in this phase. This phase should be between 8 and 12 weeks long when time permits.

The major differences between this phase and the general endurance phase are that more endurance training is done at an intense level, and that a great deal of the training is done in the swimmer's specialty stroke or strokes. Aerobic training mileage should reach its highest level during this phase. The amount of intense endurance training should increase by approximately 15—20%.

Stretching exercises should continue to be used. The emphasis on dry-land resistance training should shift to fast repetitions designed to produce muscular power. During the last portion of this phase, most of the dry-land training should consist of stroke-simulated exercises, at competition turnover rates. Some of this training can also be done in the water against resistance. In water, sprint-assisted training can also be introduced at this time, although the main emphasis on this form of training should be saved until the next phase.

The amount of sprint training should also double during this phase. Psychological training can continue although the emphasis should shift toward discussion of personal conflicts that may interfere with training and performance. The swimmers should be per-

forming visualization and relaxation drills on their own.

Sprinters should train with less mileage and greater average intensity than swimmers in other events. They should also move into the next macrocycle, the competition phase, 2 or 3 weeks before athletes who swim longer events. Distance swimmers should discontinue dry-land training in favor of swimming more mileage per week.

The competition period

This is the period of the season when most of the important competitions should be scheduled. It is also the time when the emphasis of training shifts from endurance to sprinting. The stress should be on race-specific training, anaerobic training and power training with enough endurance mileage to maintain the improvements that were made during the previous two phases.

Research studies on the optimum duration for training anaerobic capacity and muscular power are sparse and contradictory, although coaches generally agree that 4—8 weeks is optimum for these purposes (Paulsson, 1984; Wilke & Madsen, 1986). Accordingly, the competitive period is generally scheduled for the final 4—8 weeks prior to the beginning of the taper.

Weekly mileage should be reduced, perhaps by 25%, to allow for longer rest intervals and faster swims. The amount of basic and intense endurance training should each be reduced by approximately 10% while the percentages of anaerobic and sprint training should be increased by about 10%.

Sprinters should be using sprint-assisted training, race-pace swimming, and power training to a greater extent than other swimmers. Middle-distance and distance swimmers should be using more short-rest repeats designed to improve both aerobic and anaerobic capacities in their race-specific training.

Flexibility training should continue although the amount can be reduced to a maintenance level. Dry-land training should consist of stroke-simulated circuit training exercises that are designed to increase muscular power. They can be done on land or in the water.

No further changes in stroke mechanics should be suggested except for those swimmers who are making very serious mistakes. Athletes want to feel they are swimming at maximum effort without having to decrease that effort to stroke in a certain way. The only exception to this suggestion is that they should continue to concentrate on swimming as economically as possible, using the combination of stroke length and rate that puts them on pace with the least expenditure of energy.

The taper period

The final phase of each season is the taper. It is a period of reduced volume and intensity that should last 2–5 weeks. The taper was covered in more detail in Chapter 12.

Weekly and daily planning

Once the task of planning the season has been completed the real work begins—the planning of weekly and daily training programs. The best results will be achieved when they are planned meticulously. The purpose of this section is to provide some suggestions for planning effectively. Weekly planning will be discussed first.

The following categories of training will be included in each weekly session:

1 *Basic endurance training*. This refers to short-rest repeats at a moderate rate. They can include stroke drills, kicking and pulling. The purpose is to improve aerobic capacity without depleting muscle glycogen.
2 *Intense endurance training*. These are long sets of short-rest repeats. They should be swum at the fastest possible average speed. The purpose is to improve aerobic capacity at the fastest possible rate.
3 *Race-specific training*. These are sets of under-distance repeats that are swum at or near race speed. The rest intervals can be medium or short. The purpose is to improve the aerobic and anaerobic capacity of distance swimmers. Middle-distance and sprint swimmers will find that these repeats will have their most significant effect on anaerobic capacity.
4 *Sprint training*. These are sets of repeats that are swum at very fast speeds. The repeat distances can vary from 12.5 to 200 m. The purpose is to improve anaerobic capacity and muscular power. These sets should not be as long or as difficult to perform as the race-specific swims.

Planning weekly programs

The important considerations are to include enough of each type of training to induce maximum adaptation. At the same time, athletes must be provided with enough rest to replace the energy used. There are two general guidelines for the strategic placement of the various types of training.

1 At least three major sets of intense endurance training should be included each week. An equal number of sprint sets should also be scheduled.
2 Never swim more than two sets of intense endurance training in a row without providing at least 24 h of reduced intensity or mileage.

The literature clearly shows that a particular form of training is most effective when performed between 3 and 5 days per week. Consequently, it seems reasonable that each type of training should be used at least that frequently.

The literature also demonstrates that the glycogen in muscles will be nearly depleted after 1 or 2 h of intense training. As you now know, 24–48 h of recovery time is needed for replacement of the muscle glycogen used in training. Intense endurance training and long sets of race-pace swimming cause the greatest depletion. Consequently, the placement of these kinds of training should be given first consideration when constructing weekly plans.

While it is true that the rate of glycogen use is greater during sprint training, the sets are shorter, so the amount of depletion will be less. Therefore, small amounts of sprint training can be scheduled during days when glycogen repletion is needed. The amount of glycogen used during sprint sets will be more than offset by the amount repleted so the net result will be an increased storage of that substance.

Basic endurance training can be used in training sessions when glycogen repletion is desired. The swimming speeds should be slow enough to allow stored fat to supply a large percentage of the energy. In this way, the rate of glycogen use on those days will, once again, be less than its rate of repletion.

A suggested weekly plan that includes two training sessions per day

A typical training week includes two sessions per day Monday through Friday and one session on Saturday.

There are at least two general methods for placing the various kinds of training throughout the week that will provide adequate time to replace muscle glycogen. One method can be termed *alternating*: one intense endurance or long anaerobic set should be performed every 24−36 h. In the other method, swimmers can perform two of these sets in a row before allowing 36−48 h for recovery. That method of placement has been termed *combined*.

An alternating method for cycling through the week is shown in Table 14.1. Intense endurance training and anaerobic training should be placed first because, as mentioned, they require greater amounts of muscle glycogen than other types of swimming repeats. The intense endurance sets have been scheduled for Monday afternoon, Wednesday morning and Thursday afternoon. One long anaerobic set was placed on Saturday morning. Another was scheduled for Friday afternoon since the swimmers would be getting $1\frac{1}{2}$ days off after Saturday morning. These placements permit at least 36 h for muscle glycogen repletion.

Short sets of sprints, stroke drills and basic endurance training have been filled in during the remaining sessions. Four sprint sets are placed at times when muscle glycogen should be partially replaced and the athletes can swim very fast. In this case they are scheduled for Monday and Friday mornings, and Tuesday and Wednesday afternoons. They could also have been placed in any of several other sessions since they are not stressful and will not

use a significant amount of muscle glycogen.

Placing the main sets in this manner does not preclude the use of short sprint sets (100−300 m) or medium-sized basic endurance sets during other sessions. Specialty sprint drills such as sprint-assisted and sprint-resisted training can also be fitted into this plan during two or three sessions per week.

A combined method for cycling training through the week

One combined method for cycling the various types of training through the week is shown in Table 14.2. In this case, the intense endurance and race-specific sets are arranged so they fall on two successive training sessions. After that, the swimmers are provided with 36−48 h for replacing muscle glycogen.

Intense endurance and race-specific sets have been placed on Monday morning and afternoon sessions, on Wednesday afternoon and Thursday morning, and on Friday afternoon and Saturday morning. Sprint training has been placed in the sessions on Tuesday, Thursday and Friday afternoons. Basic endurance training has been scheduled for Tuesday morning and afternoon, Wednesday and Friday mornings and Thursday afternoon.

These are two of literally hundreds of ways in which training can be cycled throughout the week. It should not be difficult to develop many other weekly plans using the two rules given earlier in this chapter.

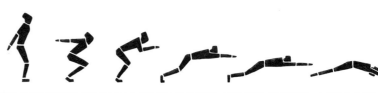

Table 14.1 An alternate method for weekly planning when two training sessions per day are used

	Monday	Tuesday	Wednesday	Thursday	Friday	Saturday
a.m.	Basic endurance Sprint	Basic endurance	Intense endurance	Basic endurance	Basic endurance Sprint	Race-specific
p.m.	Intense endurance	Basic endurance Sprint	Basic endurance Sprint	Intense endurance	Basic endurance Race-specific	

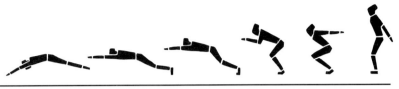

Table 14.2 A combined method for weekly planning when two training sessions per day are used

	Monday	Tuesday	Wednesday	Thursday	Friday	Saturday
a.m.	Intense endurance	Basic endurance	Basic endurance	Race-specific	Basic endurance	Race-specific
p.m.	Intense endurance	Basic endurance Sprint	Intense endurance	Basic endurance Sprint	Sprint Intense endurance	

Planning for one training session per day

Swimmers who are training once per day are not as likely to become glycogen-depleted because they will be having 24 h of complete rest between each session. Nevertheless, it is probably a good idea to use either an alternating or combined schedule in case their diets are low in carbohydrates.

An alternating arrangement for once-a-day training

Table 14.3 illustrates an alternating method for swimmers who are training 5 days per week and swimming a meet on Saturday afternoon. The intense endurance and race-specific sets are scheduled for Monday, Wednesday and Friday. The meet can be used as another race-specific training session. Sprint training and basic endurance sets form the bulk of training mileage on Tuesday and Thursday. A third sprint training set is also placed on Monday. Some basic endurance swimming should also be included on Monday, Wednesday and Friday, although it should not be the main set.

A combined arrangement for once-a-day training

This way of placing the various levels is shown in Table 14.4. The intense endurance and race-specific sets have been scheduled for Monday, Tuesday and Friday afternoons and Saturday morning. One additional race-specific set was placed on Tuesday afternoon. This spot was selected because the swimmers will have 2 recovery days immediately after. The training sessions on Wednesday and Thursday are made up primarily of basic endurance and sprint training. One additional sprint training set was scheduled for Friday since the swimmers would only be training once on Saturday or they might be competing.

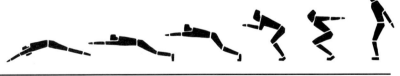

Table 14.3 An alternating method for weekly planning when swimmers are training once per day

	Monday	Tuesday	Wednesday	Thursday	Friday	Saturday
p.m.	Sprint Intense endurance	Basic endurance Sprint	Race-specific	Basic endurance Sprint	Intense endurance	Race-specific

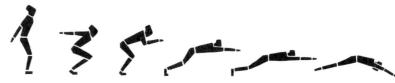

Table 14.4 A combined method for weekly planning when swimmers are training once per day

	Monday	Tuesday	Wednesday	Thursday	Friday	Saturday
p.m.	Intense endurance	Intense endurance Race-specific	Basic endurance Sprint	Basic endurance Sprint	Sprint Intense endurance	Race-specific

Daily planning

Daily training sessions should be planned to encourage athletes to swim each set of repeats at the most effective intensity. Some general guidelines for such planning are given below.

1   Short sprint sets should usually be placed early in the session before the swimmers are too fatigued to swim fast. It is far more common to place them at the end so swimmers leave the pool feeling exhilarated. There is no reason to discontinue this practice during sessions where the intensity is low. However, when major sprint sets are scheduled on the same day with intense endurance and race-specific repeats, it would be better to complete them early in the session.

2   Major sets of intense endurance and race-specific training should be placed late in the daily session. As stated earlier, these sets cause substantial depletions of muscle glycogen. Once that happens, athletes will tend to swim the remaining sets at recovery speeds where the training effects will be minimal. For this reason, it is far better for them to swim their basic endurance sets early in the session so they will be completed at a moderate pace. The same statement is true of sprint sets and short sets of race-specific repeats except, of course, that they should be swum at fast speeds.

A sample daily training structure is shown in Table 14.5. It is designed primarily to improve aerobic capacity with some anaerobic and sprint training included. Following are the reasons for the placing of each segment.

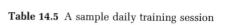

Table 14.5 A sample daily training session

1   *Warm-up*
Swim 300 m
Pull 300 m
Swim 4 × 50 m on 1 min
Descend

800 m

2   *Sprint training*
Swim 6 × 50 m on 3 min
Swim 150 m between each 50

300 m sprint training
750 m recovery swimming

3   *Basic endurance*
Pull 6 × 200 m on 2.30 min

1200 m

4   *Basic endurance*
Kick 150, 100, 50
Descend each and repeat 4 times
Rests 3, 2, and 1 min

1200 m

5   *Intense endurance*
Swim 4 × 500 m on 7 min

2000 m

6   *Recovery set*
Swim 8 × 100 on 1.45 min
Start at basic endurance speed and swim each repeat slower until recovered

800 m

Total = 7050 m

The session begins with a warm-up of 800 m. Swimming speed should progress to a basic endurance level during the 300-m repeats, so the warm-up serves a training purpose as well. This is followed by 4 × 50-m swims on a 1-min interval. The time for each swim should get faster until the athletes are swimming reasonably fast on the last repeat. A sprint set of 6 × 50-m swims is placed next so the swimmers can sprint before they become too fatigued. This is followed by pulling and kicking sets in the form of stroke drills. These serve the double purpose of improving endurance and stroke techniques.

The main set is next: 4 × 500-m swims on a short rest. These swims should be completed at the fastest possible average speed. However, the last swim should be the fastest one in the set to insure that the athletes overload aerobic metabolism before they become fatigued. The final segment of the training session is 800 m of easy swimming to aid recovery.

Recommended reading

Paulsson, L.-E (1984) Developing sprint champions through strength training and other tricks. In Cramer, J.L. (ed.) *How to Develop Olympic Level Swimmers: Scientific and Practical Foundations*. Helsinki, Finland: International Sports Media, pp. 138–159.

Wilke, K. & Madsen, O. (1986) *Coaching the Young Swimmer*. London: Pelham Books.

Chapter 15

Training for specific events

Thus far, the information presented on training has been of a general nature. The purposes of this chapter are twofold: to make some specific suggestions for training athletes in strokes other than freestyle and to suggest some modifications of the general plan for sprinters and middle-distance swimmers.

Training for sprint and distance events

Training the sprinter

Sprinters are defined as swimmers who specialize in the 50- and 100-m events. Muscular power and anaerobic endurance are musts for these swimmers. There are, however, several reasons why sprinters need aerobic endurance: a good aerobic base will allow them to train more intensely later in the season, and aerobic training will increase the quantity of muscle glycogen and provide greater use of fats during endurance training. Both of these changes will reduce muscle glycogen use during training so that more and longer sprint sets can be completed without the swimmer becoming exhausted. A third reason is that endurance training will shorten the recovery time between swims in competition and between training sessions.

The difficult task to accomplish when training sprinters, is to maintain a proper balance between endurance and sprint training. "How much endurance mileage is too much?" is a question that cannot be answered at this time. Even if it could, the answer would probably be somewhat different for each athlete.

The first step in achieving this balance is to reduce the quantity of endurance training as compared to the amounts completed by middle-distance and distance swimmers. We can only speculate as to how great that

reduction should be. The opinions of successful coaches range from reductions of one-third to one-half of the usual weekly mileage.

The second step is to alter the proportions of the two types of endurance training to include more basic mileage and less intense endurance swimming. A suggestion would be to plan two additional race-specific sets and two additional spring sets into their weekly programs.

The final step is to include additional amounts of sprint training in their programs. It is particularly important to include additional amounts of sprint training in the general and specific preparation periods to guard against significant loss of speed during these periods of increased endurance mileage.

Sprinters will have lower anaerobic thresholds than swimmers in other events even though they may be ranked higher in their events. Their muscle physiology is well constructed genetically for events requiring power and speed and they tend to rely more on anaerobic metabolism at slower speeds. You should expect sprinters to repeat between 3 and 5 s slower per 100 m on endurance sets than middle-distance swimmers of similar relative ability. By the same token, expect them to swim those repeats at lower heart rates, perhaps 150–170 beats·min^{-1}, and at lower percentage of maximum effort, in the range of 70–80%.

While their lack of aerobic capacity causes them to have difficulty swimming endurance repeats, their power and speed should allow them to shine when they do sprint training. Sprinters can be expected to swim sprint 50s 6–8 s faster than they swim repeats of that same distance in endurance sets. Times in fast 100-m repeats may be 10–12 s faster than endurance training speeds.

Sprinters should spend more time on resistance training both on land and in the water. On land, it can take the form of weight training, circuit training and/or swim bench training. Regardless of the form of training, the emphasis should be on improving muscular power and anaerobic endurance. Therefore, the combinations of repetitions and sets should vary. Some exercises should incorporate a small number of maximum efforts, executed at fast speeds for several sets. Three to six sets of 4–12 repetitions are suggested. In other exercises, the emphasis should be on training for approximately 20–40 s at a time, for

3−5 sets, with exercise rates that are similar to, or faster than, the stroke rates swimmers use in races.

Stroke rates and stroke lengths should be monitored carefully during sprint sets. The swimmers should be conscious of trying to maintain competition stroke rates, and maintaining the greatest possible stroke length without reducing that rate.

Sprinters can train twice per day without becoming overtrained. By the same token, they can probably train once per day without undertraining. Their training balance and the systems of overload and progression they use are much more important considerations than the number of training sessions per week.

Training the distance swimmer

Where training balance is concerned, the problems of distance swimmers are the converse of those of sprinters. Distance swimmers must maximize aerobic capacity even if this means that muscular power and anaerobic capacity are compromised. This is not to say that they should avoid sprint training. Quite the contrary, anaerobic capacity is important to success in the 1500/1650 m, although not to the same extent that aerobic capacity determines performance.

Distance swimmers should, of course, swim more mileage per week than swimmers in shorter events. Most of the additional mileage should be in the form of basic and intense endurance training. Part of this increase can be accomplished by swimming race-specific repeats. Those repeats should stress aerobic metabolism for swimmers in distance events. In other words, instead of swimming medium-length sets of 100 repeats at 200-m speed, distance swimmers should be swimming longer sets of that same distance at 1500-m speed. Their sprint training should emphasize anaerobic capacity more than power. They will swim fewer 25s and more 50s and 100s.

Distance swimmers will have higher anaerobic thresholds than swimmers in other events. Accordingly, they will be able to swim much faster during endurance sets than swimmers in shorter events with the same relative ability. Expect distance swimmers to train at somewhat higher heart rates and percentage efforts than other swimmers during endurance sets.

Distance swimmers will not be able to improve on their endurance repeat times very much during sprint sets. Their muscle physiology allows them to swim endurance sets much closer to their maximum speeds than other swimmers. They may only be able to swim sprint 50s 3−5 s faster than their pace for intense endurance sets. Times for high-speed 100 m repeats may only be 6−8 s faster than endurance paces.

The value of heavy-resistance land training is questionable for distance swimmers. Their events do not require great power. In the absence of research, the decision to include dry-land weight or circuit training in the programs for distance swimmers must remain a matter of individual preference. These programs should never be included at the expense of adequate training mileage, however.

Training for events other than freestyle

It was stated earlier that the major training effects which produce improvements in performance take place in each of the individual fibers within large groups of muscles. Although certain fibers are probably used when swimming all of the competitive strokes, there are undoubtedly some that are used only when athletes swim a particular stroke. The only way to insure that those muscle fibers adapt is to swim that stroke in training. Further, the stroke or strokes of preference must be swum during both endurance and sprint training. For these reasons, backstroke breaststroke and butterfly swimmers should not swim freestyle in all or even most of their endurance sets. Freestyle training can be emphasized for all swimmers during the general preparation period. After that, however, swimmers with other specialties should be sure to spend at least 4−6 weeks stressing endurance training in their specialties. They should also spend an additional 4−6 weeks stressing sprint training in that same stroke or strokes.

Freestyle swimming can be done in most, but not all, basic endurance sets. Athletes should swim their specialties during some, perhaps even the majority, of their intense endurance sets, however. It has been suggested that more than half of swimmers' training mileage should be swum in their specialties during the specific preparation and competitive periods of each season. Much of their kicking mileage should also be in their specialties during those periods.

Training for backstroke

Large teams and crowded training conditions have discouraged many athletes from swimming backstroke in training. This is unfortunate and should be remedied. Coaches should encouraged backstroke swimmers to swim their stroke in all forms of training. Backstroke flags should be up at every training session to encourage them to do so.

The kick is much more important to success in backstroke swimming than it is for the freestyle swimmer. It probably contributes more to propulsion in this stroke because the swimmer's supine position allows for a longer propulsive upbeat of the legs. Backstroke swimmers should spend more time in kicking drills than front crawl swimmers. The principal emphasis should be on improving the aerobic endurance of the leg muscles. Backstrokers will tend to relax their legs when swimming endurance sets and the aerobic capacities of their leg muscles may suffer. Some freestylers use their legs so little in races of 100 and 200 m that they can train with reduced kicking and not have it affect their potential performances. The same thing cannot be said for backstrokers. The vast majority will be using a six-beat kick in these races. They cannot afford to have that kick create an inordinate demand for anaerobic energy because the aerobic capacity of their leg muscles is poorly developed.

The stress of sprint swimming will require a stronger kick and therefore should be sufficient for improving the anaerobic energy systems in their leg muscles, without the need for special kicking drills. Backstroke swimmers should be encouraged to use their legs in sprint sets. They should not be allowed to use a reduced-effort or broken-tempo kick to save energy. By the same token, they should be encouraged to use a six-beat kick in all endurance sets. It does not have to be a strong six-beat kick since vigorous kicking would reduce their ability to swim the set without becoming unusually fatigued. Nevertheless, they should not be allowed to use two- or four-beat rhythms.

The mechanics of the kick should also be stressed. Coaches should make sure that backstroke swimmers are kicking correctly and that they have sufficient ankle extension (plantar flexing) ability to do so. If not, they should use flexibility exercises designed to improve ankle extension ability until it is adequate.

Training for butterfly

All remarks about the kick in the previous section apply equally, if not more so, to butterfly swimming. Butterflyers must have good aerobic endurance in their leg muscles, excellent ankle extension ability and good kicking mechanics.

Many coaches and swimmers harbor the misconception that they should not swim butterfly for long distances in training. Nothing could be further from the truth. Butterflyers need aerobic endurance in the muscle fibers they use. As mentioned earlier, there is no guarantee that freestyle swimming will provide this. Muscle fiber involvement, although similar, is probably not identical in both strokes.

The advice just given must be tempered by the fact that swimming butterfly in long repeats is more difficult than swimming freestyle. Consequently, it is more stressful and swimmers' stroke mechanics tend to deteriorate more. Large amounts of endurance swimming using the butterfly stroke may upset the balance between aerobic and anaerobic training and increase the probability of swimmers in this stroke becoming overtrained.

For these reasons, butterfly swimmers should not do as much endurance mileage in their specialty as was suggested for backstrokers. Fortunately, the mechanics of the front crawl and butterfly strokes are more alike than those of any other two competitive strokes. Therefore, a greater amount of the butterfly swimmers' training can be done using freestyle. Swimmers on high-mileage programs should probably swim only 20–30% of their training volume using butterfly.

Training for breaststroke

All remarks about the importance of kicking in backstroke and butterfly swimmers go double or triple for athletes in this stroke. What has been noted about athletes' swimming endurance and sprint repeats in their specialties also applies. The mechanical difference between breaststroke and other competitive styles is greater than between any other two competitive styles. It stands to reason, therefore that the overlap in muscle fiber use will be less for breaststroke swimming and other styles than for any other combination of competitive strokes.

Breaststrokers should kick as much as their knees will stand because the kick plays such a dominant role in this stroke. This does not mean they should do more kicking than swimmers in other strokes, however. The potential for knee problems and the serious ramifications of those problems make it necessary to administer kicking repeats with the dual considerations of improving leg endurance and preventing sore knees.

When prescribing training, coaches should keep in mind that breaststrokers, unlike swimmers in other strokes, rely on their kicks as much or more so as their armstrokes during endurance sets. Consequently, full-stroke swimming will improve the aerobic and anaerobic capacities of their leg muscles but they may tend to do less work with their arms than swimmers in other strokes. For this reason, full-stroke breaststroke swimming will reduce the amount of kicking needed for improving any energy system. So, when the potential for sore knees forces a choice between kicking or swimming breaststroke, swimmers should make the latter choice.

The dominance of the kick in breaststroke swimming suggests that breaststrokers should include a substantial amount of pulling in their training programs. The practice of pulling with a dolphin kick should be discouraged. It is a good stroke drill but not very effective for improving endurance or anaerobic power in the arms. It is easy to compensate for a weak pull by emphasizing the dolphin kick so that the training stimulus on the arm muscles remains too low for optimum adaptations to take place. If you suspect that certain breaststrokers are not using their arms

fully, it would be a good idea to include more pulling in their weekly schedules.

Surprisingly, the energy demands of breaststroke swimming are even greater than those of the butterfly. Their minimum and maximum velocities generally fluctuate more than 1 m·s^{-1} during each stroke cycle. Swimmers in other strokes seldom fluctuate more than 1 m·s^{-1} at any point in their cycles. Breaststroke swimmers expend more energy accelerating their bodies with each stroke than swimmers do with any other competitive style. For this reason, they, like butterflyers, will need more anaerobic energy at slower speeds. So, in endurance sets, it should be expected that the relative speed of breaststrokers will not be as fast as swimmers in other strokes.

Unlike butterflyers, breaststrokers should not swim a smaller percentage of their endurance or sprint mileage in their specialties. They need adequate specific mileage at all levels of training to produce the aerobic and anaerobic adaptations required in their muscles.

When sore knees make it impossible to swim breaststroke, a sizeable amount of the full-stroke swimming can be replaced by breaststroke pulling and butterfly swimming. The similarity between the butterfly and breaststroke armstrokes is greater than between breaststroke and either of the two remaining competitive styles. The similarity is so great, in fact, that breaststroke swimmers with weak armstrokes would be well advised to swim a lot of butterfly in training. It is unfortunate that many breaststrokers are not well skilled in butterfly. It is an excellent supplement for their training.

Chapter 16

Training for strength and power

We have witnessed a complete turnaround in thinking about resistance training during the past three decades. Athletes in our sport were told they should not lift weights in the 1950s. The belief was that weight training would build bulky muscles and decrease flexibility. Attitudes toward resistance training have changed so much that we now believe swimmers must engage in resistance training if they wish to be successful. One of the most controversial areas in sport concerns the procedures for performing this training.

Experts disagree about the physiological mechanisms responsible for strength improvements. Do muscles become stronger, or do athletes simply learn to release neural inhibitions so they can use the strength they already possess? Research and testimonials from those who have performed unusual feats of strength under stress indicate that an untapped reserve resides in human muscles. Do increases of strength necessarily lead to improvements in performance? A long-standing belief about the relationship between weight training and athletic performance is that any form of exercise which increases muscular strength will allow athletes to exert greater force in other types of work. However, research has demonstrated that strength gains are specific to the method used in training. People improve their strength most on tests using the same equipment, exercises, and rates of motion that they used in training. Improvements are considerably more modest when the tests of strength are dissimilar.

What are the implications of these controversies for swim training? Should swimmers perform all of their resistance training with bands and swim benches to enhance the learning effect or should they do standard, nonspecific weight-training exercises to increase muscle size and strength?

Some experts have tried to resolve this issue with the following theory. Early increases of strength are due to learning effects. The brain learns to use the strength in the muscles to perform a particular movement. Changes of this nature take place rapidly and are responsible for the improvements seen during the first 6 weeks, before a significant increase of muscle size is noticed. Later increases of strength are due to muscles growing larger (*hypertrophy*). Some experts believe that once this hypertrophy takes place, athletes can train their muscles to apply their newly developed strength in the execution of sports skills. This theory provides a sensible basis for the practices that coaches and athletes feel have been successful, until these controversies are resolved through research.

Swimmers should spend the first one-third to one-half of their seasons doing nonspecific resistance training to increase muscle size and strength. Then, they should spend the next third doing stroke-simulating exercises against resistance both on land and in the water. Doing their training in this order will allow them to take the raw material they developed earlier and train their nervous systems to use more of it later in the season.

Is it necessary to increase muscle size to improve strength, especially when we already have more potential strength in our muscles than we will ever use? In other words, should swimmers simply dispense with nonspecific training and do only stroke-simulated training against resistance? That is another question which is unanswerable, at present.

One question that can be answered concerns the effect of resistance training on bulking-up. Neither women nor men need be concerned about increasing muscle size so much that they become bulky. Most do not possess the genetic predisposition to gain large amounts of muscle tissue. Those few who do can concentrate more on stroke-simulating exercises and spend less time with nonspecific heavy-resistance training so they can improve strength without inordinately large increases of muscle tissue.

The focus of this discussion has been on improving strength, and has oversimplified a very complex issue. Increasing strength is only the first step. It is the effect of that increase on power and muscular endurance that finally determines how fast athletes will swim. Those relationships will be discussed below.

Strength, power, and muscular endurance

To comprehend fully the link between strength training and swimming, we must first understand the relationships between strength and power and between strength and muscular endurance. *Strength* can be defined as the *amount of force* a person can apply *for one maximum effort*. This definition says nothing about the *speed* of applying force. *Power* refers to the *rate of force application*. That rate is a necessary aspect of strength expression in most sports, and swimming is no exception. Swimmers must have a reasonable turnover rate in races to be competitive, in addition to an ability to apply force with their strokes. Where swimming fast is concerned, both the forces applied and their rates of application are important to success.

Muscular endurance pertains to the fatiguability of muscles. This measure involves the length of time that certain levels of power output can be maintained. Swimmers rarely exert one powerful effort except on the start and on turns. In all other parts of their races they use some portion of their maximum power in a repetitive manner, stroke after stroke, until the race is completed. In this case, swimmers who can maintain the highest average power output have a great advantage over their competitors.

The relationship between strength, power, and swimming speed

While most of us believe that powerful swimmers are faster, the relationship between power and swimming speed has not been easy to prove. A study by Sharp *et al.* (1982) reported a high relationship between power generated during one maximal pull on a swim bench and swimming speed for 25 yd (22.75 m). That study had a great influence on the swimming community and is often cited as a justification for strength training. However, in another study Sharp *et al.* (1983) were unable to find a strong relationship between power measured on a swim bench and speed in a group of national-level swimmers. The national-level swimmers constituted a much more homogeneous group, consisting of athletes who were closer in age and performance. This result might lead us to believe that power is not an important feature of fast swimming, at least among mature athletes. A more

reasonable assumption, however, would be that that power measured on land does not accurately reflect power in the water.

This hypothesis was tested by adapting the conrol mechanism from a biokinetic swim bench to record stroking power in the water (see Chapter 17). Swimmers attached one end of the cable to their waist by means of a harness. Then they sprinted 25 yd (22.75 m) several times, against the resistance supplied by the various settings on the control mechanism. When power was tested in this way, a very high relationship with swimming speed was found to exist, even among homogeneous groups of athletes. The correlation between swimming power and sprinting time for 22.75 m was 0.82. A slightly higher relationship of 0.84 was also reported between swimming speed and the peak force athletes generated during the power swim. On the other hand, dry-land tests of stroking power on the swim bench yielded a nonsignificant correlation with swimming speed of 0.62 for these same athletes.

These results suggest that the force and power athletes can generate during 22.75 m of sprint swimming is very important to success in sprinting. They further suggest that the amount of force swimmers can apply with each stroke also has a very close connection with speed. It seems wise, then, to engage in activities that will improve muscular power, at least for events from 50 to 400 m.

Muscular endurance

Although the relationship with speed is high, swimmers never exert maximum amounts of power in any aspect of racing. Even races as short as 50 m require a minimum of 18–20 strokes with each arm. This is analogous to performing 18–20 repetitions of a weight-training exercise. Anyone with a passing knowledge of weight training knows that maximum force cannot be exerted when the number of repetitions is that great. Accordingly, swimmers intuitively choose to exert a portion of their force at some optimal turnover rate until the race has been completed. In short races, that portion will be very close to maximum, while in longer races it will be considerably less.

Regardless of the race distance, swimmers who can maintain a higher percentage of their maximum force should obviously have an advantage. Miyashita and Kanehisa (1983) reported a significant relationship between improvements in muscular power and swimming speed for events as short as 50 m. What caused this improvement? Was it a high level of power, improved aerobic capacity, or an increase of muscle-buffering capacities? All three of these physiological mechanisms were probably involved. Accordingly, a combination of swim training that includes aerobic and anaerobic elements, and resistance training that improves strength and power, should improve muscular endurance adequately. Athletes should not need special land training to help in improving this capacity.

Improving muscular strength and power

All strength training is based on the principles of overload and progression. As strength increases the resistance must also increase to continue overloading the muscles so strength will increase even more. The most obvious way for modern-day athletes to apply the progressive-resistance principle is to add more weight each time it is determined they are capable of doing so. Sets and repetitions are used to make these determinations.

Sets and repetitions

The majority of studies have shown that 4−8 repetitions for 3 or more sets are optimum for improving muscular strength, although programs that include up to 12 repetitions have also been very effective. Eight to 12 repetitions are usually recommended for training the legs. No differences in strength gains were found between programs including as few as 3 sets of 10 repetitions and as many as 15 sets of 10 repetitions.

Resistance

The most important factor in any resistance program designed to increase muscular strength is the amount of force athletes apply to move a particular amount of weight. The number of repetitions and sets they perform is secondary to using resistance that creates an overload on muscles. For developing muscular strength, the resistance should be 70−90% of the

maximum resistance they can lift for one repetition. Power will be improved most with resistance in the range of 30−80% of maximum.

Frequency

Most experts agree that training 3 days per week is optimum, although both 2 and 5 days per week have been used effectively (Braith *et al.*, 1989). The program should require 30−45 min and include 6−12 exercises.

Exercise selection

The exercises that should be performed are those that work the major muscle groups swimmers use to propel themselves through the water. In addition, they should mimic swimming movements as much as possible. The major muscle groups used include those that bring swimmers' arms from a position overhead to their hips. They are the pectoralis major muscles of the chest, the latissimus dorsi muscles of the back, the rhomboids, the trapezius, and the frontal (anterior) deltoids. The inward sweeps of their arms are accomplished by the biceps, brachialis, brachioradialis, and supinator muscles of the upper arm and forearm. The teres major and minor of the upper back are also used. The muscles that sweep the arm out and up from under the body are the middle and posterior deltoids. The triceps and anconeus are the primary muscles involved in extending the arms at their elbows.

The downbeats of flutter and dolphin kicks, the upbeat of the backstroke and knee extension in the breaststroke are accomplished by the knee extensors and the hip flexors. The knee extensors are the quadriceps (rectus femoris, vastus intermedius, vastus medialis, and vastus lateralis). The hip flexors are the psoas major, iliacus, and pectineus. The upbeat of the kick is made possible by contraction of the hamstrings (biceps femoris, semitendinosus, and semimembranosus) and gluteus maximus. These muscles also extend the legs in breaststroke and during hip extension when they are starting and turning. Breaststrokers also require strength in the adductor muscles that are responsible for squeezing their legs together during the propulsive phase of their kick. These muscles are the adductor brevis, adductor longus, adductor magnus, and gracilis. In addition to the muscles involved in hip and knee extension, starts and turns require powerful extensions of the ankles which are made possible by the gastrocnemius, soleus and plantaris muscles.

The abdominal muscles, the rectus femoris, stabilize the trunk during stroking and kicking. The internal and external obliques on the sides of the abdominal area, and the erector spinae muscles of the middle and lower back assist them.

Some of the best resistance exercises for these muscles are listed in Table 16.1.

Military presses, dips and push-ups are not recommended. They can cause friction between the head of the humerus and the tendons of the shoulders which may exacerbate current cases of tendonitis or, perhaps, precipitate the condition.

To establish a resistance-training program, athletes should select 6–12 exercises which work all of the major muscle groups of the arms, trunk and legs.

Table 16.1 Resistance-training exercises

Joints or body parts involved	Exercises
Shoulder	
For downsweep and upsweep	Lat machine pulldowns to the front and behind the neck; upright rows, bent-over rowing, seated rows, straight-arm pullovers, bent-arm pullovers, bench press, chins, incline bench press, decline bench press; pulleys, shoulder shrugs, swim bench
For insweep	Lying lateral raises; side pulleys
Upper arm	Curls, triceps extensions
Forearm	Forearm curls, wrist curls
Lower back	Back hyperextensions, dead lifts
Abdomen	Sit-ups, side-twists
Hip and knee	Leg curls, leg extensions, leg presses; half-squats
Ankle	Calf raises
Adductor	Adductors with pulleys, adductor machine, ball squeezes

Increasing power

Obviously, muscular force (strength) plays an important role in the production of power. Speed of movement plays an equally important role, however. Recent studies have shown a high degree of specificity between strength and its speed of application. So, once strength has been increased, the emphasis should switch to increasing power (Moffroid & Whipple, 1970; Miyashita & Kanehisa, 1983).

One of the important items to consider in any program for improving swimming power is that the exercises should approximate stroking speeds. Unfortunately, that is an almost impossible task. The hand velocity patterns for competitive swimmers showed that they do not move their arms through the water at constant rates of speed (Maglischo *et al.*, 1986). Their underwater armstrokes consisted of pulses of speed with the hands decelerating and then accelerating with every major change of direction. In certain parts of their underwater armstrokes, swimmers' hands were traveling as fast as 6 m·s^{-1} (20 ft·s^{-1}), and at other times they were only moving at 1.5 m·s^{-1} (5 ft·s^{-1}). The average velocity of their hands was generally in the neighborhood of 3 m·s^{-1}, yet they were seldom moving at that speed.

If athletes are able to complete, for example, 10 repetitions in 5 s they they will be working in the range of maximum hand velocities. One repetition per second equals average hand velocities. A combination of the two repetition speeds should be used in power training.

The swim bench

Swim benches and minigyms can be used effectively to train strength and power. Strength training should be conducted at slow speed settings for 3 sets of 10–15 repetitions. This will provide enough time to produce a large amount of muscular force. Training at competition rates should accompany the slow-speed training for development of power. At least two different speed settings should be used for this purpose. One speed should simulate maximum speeds of hand movement, and the other should correspond to average hand speeds. Stroke rates for maximum hand velocities should be in the neighborhood of $4-6$ m·s^{-1}. Rates of $2-3$ m·s^{-1} will suffice for average hand velocities.

An example of an event-specific program for a swimmer with a goal time of 22 s in the 50-m freestyle would be to work for 22 s while trying to generate the highest score. Four to six sets should be performed. Half of those sets should be done at very fast speed settings and the remaining sets should be performed at slower speeds. The rest periods between sets should be in the neighborhood of $3-5$ min so the athletes can recover sufficiently to make another near-maximum effort.

Another method to achieve this same goal of 22 s for 50 m is to use multiple sets that are $10-15$ s in length. These allow athletes to exert more force and could possibly provide a better overload. Four to six sets are recommended.

Flexibility training

It has been suggested that increased joint flexibility enables the swimmer to perform better because of the following reasons.

1 An increased range of motion in certain joints should allow propulsive force to be applied over a longer period of time.

2 A greater range of motion in certain joints should permit recovery and kicking movements that do not disturb horizontal and lateral body alignment.

3 An increased range of motion may diminish the energy cost and increase the speed of swimming by reducing intramuscular resistance to motion.

The joints where a large range of motion could be advantageous to swimmers are the ankles, shoulders and lower back. Breaststroke swimmers may also profit from improving flexibility in the adductor muscles of the groin, the outward rotators of the knees and the knee extensors of the upper leg.

Freestyle, butterfly and backstroke swimmers should be able to maintain their feet in position to displace water back for a longer time during the downbeats of their kicks if they possess more-than-average ability to extend (*plantar flex*) their ankles. Swimmers in these strokes also need to be able to turn the soles of their feet in (*inversion*). This will improve their ability to position the feet to displace water back during the downbeats of the flutter and dolphin kicks and the upbeats of the back crawl flutter kick.

We are all aware of the importance of shoulder flexibility where the arm recoveries for the freestyle, butterfly and backstroke are concerned. A high-elbow recovery in freestyle will reduce the potential for the arm to pull the swimmer's body out of lateral alignment as it swings over the water. Butterfly swimmers need flexibility in the shoulders so they will not drag their arms through the water during the recovery. The ability to hyperflex the arms overhead is needed by backstrokers to insure a recovery that does not disrupt later alignment.

The dolphin motion of breaststroke and butterfly swimmers is assisted by their ability to hyperextend the lower back. Breaststrokers who use a dolphin motion in their strokes are in a similar position as they execute their arm and leg recoveries.

Propulsion during the breaststroke kick depends on a good range of motion at the ankles in a flexing motion (*dorsiflexion*), rather than extension. Breaststroke swimmers who can flex their ankles should be able to get their feet facing back earlier during the outsweep of their kick, so that they will be able to catch sooner and lengthen the propulsive phase. Breaststrokers should also be able to turn the soles of their feet in and out with ease (*eversion* and *inversion*). The outward motion will help them get a good angle of attack during the outsweep while an ability to rotate the feet in will provide a more propulsive position during the insweep.

Stretching exercises increase the range of motion in joints by lengthening their connective tissue. Muscles are not lengthened. Connective tissue is made up of a tough, fibrous protein material called *collagen*. It is resistant to stretch but it can be lengthened.

Stretching can be dangerous

A joint's resistance to stretch provides a protective mechanism that reduces the chances of it becoming overextended. Sprains, strains and tears are types of injuries that can result from muscles and connective tissue being forced beyond their present state of extensibility. Flexibility exercises should be aimed at stretching the connective tissue within muscles, but not the tendons and ligaments. Tears and dislocations are more likely to happen if they become weak or overextended.

It is good advice to administer stretching exercises

with special care by convincing swimmers to stretch only to the point where resistance is felt. They should improve their ranges of motion slowly and carefully without the usual attempts at super-overload they use in other aspects of training. There are also stretching exercises which, although they may be beneficial, are probably best eliminated from programs. These are exercises that stretch the arms backward from shoulder height and those that stretch the arms up and forward from behind the back. Both of these exercises, and others like them, force the head of the long bone in the arms (the *humerus*) forward against the tendons and ligaments that surround the shoulder joint. These are the same tendons and ligaments that become chronically inflamed when swimmers develop tendonitis. Consequently, it would be best to avoid any exercises that could precipitate or exacerbate this condition.

The other joints where stretching exercises should be avoided are the knees and hips. Although flexibility in these joints is a decided advantage in breaststroke, the potential for long-term damage is too great to recommend any special exercises for them.

Modes of flexibility training

Several types of stretching exercises have been used over the years. The five most popular methods are listed below.

1 *Ballistic stretching* involves moving joints rapidly and powerfully from one end of their range of motion to the other.

2 *Held-stretching* is the opposite of this method. Joints are moved gently and slowly to the limit of their range and then held there for 5–60 s.

3 *Partner-assisted methods* are static stretches with the pressure supplied by another person. The force supplied by the partner permits a greater degree of stretch than could be achieved without their help.

4 *Slow-dynamic stretching* is a reduced-speed version of ballistic methods. The joint is moved slowly, rather than quickly, through a range of motion. It can be combined with static stretching by holding for 5 or more seconds at the extended end of the range.

5 The *contract–relax method* is an outgrowth of proprioceptive neuromuscular facilitation techniques. It is based on the belief that when muscles are contracted first, they will relax more completely and

permit a greater range of motion.

Although each of these methods has its advocates, research has not shown one to be consistently superior to others (Beaulieu, 1980). All will increase the range of motion in joints. It seems that any exercise that stretches a joint will increase its range of motion. The degree of stretch plays a more important role than the mode of training. Two of these stretching methods are potentially more dangerous than the others and should be avoided, however.

Ballistic methods are considered most dangerous because it is difficult to control a fast-moving limb, so the potential for overstretching is greater. Partner-assisted stretching is the other dangerous method. There is always the danger than an enthusiastic athlete who is much stronger may stretch his or her partner's muscles and tendons beyond the breaking point.

Although it may seem contradictory to the statements just made, partner-stretching is recommended for improving ankle flexibility. There is little danger of exceeding their range of motion and the method is very effective.

Training procedures

As with other forms of training, the overload and progressive resistance principles should be applied to stretching exercises. As mentioned, they must be applied without pain. Although the stretch should always be terminated before pain is felt, the range of motion for particular exercises should be increased progressively throughout the season.

Stretching exercises should be performed daily for 10–20 min before training begins. In this way, athletes will have greater ranges of motion when they swim and may be able to use better techniques. Three to six sets of 10–15 repetitions have been recommended by experts (Beaulieu, 1980; Harre, 1982; Bompa, 1983).

Duration of held-stretch and contract–relax stretches

Recommendations have ranged from 6 to 60 s. Long stretches are probably a waste of time (Jerome, 1987). The training effect probably takes place in the first few seconds after the limits of the joint's range of motion are reached.

Recommended reading

Beaulieu, J.E. (1980) *Stretching for all Sports*. Pasadena, California: Athletic Press.

Bompa, T. (1983) *Theory and Methodology of Training*. Dubuque, Iowa: Kendall/Hunt.

Braith, R.W., Graves, J.E., Pollock, M.L., Leggett, S.L., Carpenter, D.M. & Colvin, A.B. (1989) Comparison of 2 vs. 3 days/week of variable resistance training during 10- and 18-week programs. *Int. J. Sports Med.* **6**:450−454.

Costill, D.L., King, D.S., Holdren, A. & Hargreaves, M. (1983) Swimmming speed vs. swimming power. *Swim. Tech.* **20**:20−22.

Harre, D. (1982) *Principles of Sports Training*. Berlin: Sportverlag.

Jerome, J. (1987) *Staying Supple: The Bountiful Pleasures of Stretching*. New York: Bantam Books.

Maglischo, C.W., Maglischo, E.W., Higgins, J. *et al.* (1986) A biomechanical analysis of the 1984 US Olympic swimming team: the distance freestylers. *J. Swim. Res.* **2**:12−16.

Miyashita, M. & Kanehisa, H. (1983) Effects of isokinetic, isotonic, and swim training on swimming performance. In Hollander, A.P., Huijing, P.A. & deGroot, G. (eds) *Biomechanics and Medicine in Swimming: International Series on Sport Sciences*, vol. 14. Champaign, Illinois: Human Kinetics, pp. 329−334.

Moffroid, M.T. & Whipple, R.H. (1970) Specificity of speed to exercise. *Phys. Therapy* **50**:1692−1700.

Sharp, R.L., Costill, D.L. & King, D.S. (1983) Power characteristics of swimmers at the 1982 US senior national long course swimming championships. *J. Swim. Res.* **2(2)**:5−10.

Sharp, R.L., Troup, J.P. & Costill, D.L. (1982) Relationship between power and sprint freestyle swimming. *Med. Sci. Sports Exerc.* **14**:53−56.

Section 4

Testing and

Medical Aspects

of Swimming

Chapter 17

Physiological evaluation

Although the stopwatch provides the best method of assessing the swimmer's adaptation to training, it offers few insights regarding the changes in the swimmer's physiology. As a result there have been numerous attempts to use physiological tests to gauge objectively the swimmer's improvements and to assist in planning the training program. Such tests include measurements of blood lactate, heart rates, and the rating of perceived exertion (RPE). Although the validity and sensitivity of these tests as indices of one's adaptation to training are open to some debate, it is generally agreed that they do correlate well with the swimmer's performance improvements during the early stages of training. There is, however, no evidence to support the concept that these tests provide sufficient information on which to base the swimmer's training regimen.

Measurement of blood lactate

The lactate threshold has been defined as that point in an exercise of increasing intensity at which the blood starts to accumulate lactate. It has been suggested that the lactate threshold is an indicator of the anaerobic processes of energy production within the muscle. This is not the case. Rather, the measurements of blood lactate accumulation simply provide a means of gauging the severity of the exercise relative to the subject's physiological limits. During easy swimming lactate remains only slightly above the resting level, showing a significant rise only when the muscles produce more lactate than is being removed by other body tissues. At that level of effort, lactate begins to accumulate in the blood; this may be referred to as the *lactate threshold*. An illustration of the lactate response at various swimming speeds is shown in Fig. 17.1. The lactate threshold can be expressed in terms

of the maximal oxygen uptake, $\% \dot{V}_{O_2 max}$, at which it occurs. An individual with a lactate threshold that occurred at 60% $\dot{V}_{O_2 max}$, for example, would have a greater endurance and performance potential than someone with a lactate threshold at 45% $\dot{V}_{O_2 max}$. The higher percentage indicates that the individual can exercise at relatively higher levels of effort before experiencing the physiological stresses associated with the onset of fatigue and ultimately exhaustion.

It should be pointed out that the accumulation of lactate in the blood is the combined result of:
1 lactate production in the muscles;
2 lactate diffusion from the muscles into the blood; and
3 the rate of oxidation and removal of lactate from the blood.

Thus, the amount of lactate measured in a blood sample may reflect both production and removal of lactate, while telling us little about the energetics of swimming. *The results of blood lactate values must be viewed cautiously*, since there are many potential interpretations and few valid applications of such data to our understanding of training and performance.

Nevertheless, when the swimmer is required to perform a standard swim at a relatively high intensity (approximately 80–100% $\dot{V}_{O_2 max}$), blood lactate is a reasonable indicator of swimming stress and can be used as one index of a swimmer's adjustment to

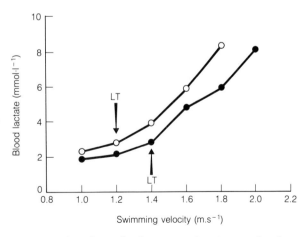

Fig. 17.1 The relationship between swimming speed and blood lactate accumulation for two swimmers. The arrow notes the lactate threshold (LT) for each swimmer. •, Trained swimmer; ○, untrained swimmer.

training. When required to perform a standardized 200- or 400-m swim at a set speed, swimmers show a dramatic decline in postexercise blood lactate during the first 6–10 weeks of training. Then, as with $\dot{V}_{O_2 max}$, there is little additional improvement, despite additional weeks and months of intense training. Thus, such testing is most useful during the early periods of adjustment to training.

Lactate-testing procedures

In most studies of lactate, blood is drawn from the arm, ear, or fingertip within 1–3 min after the standardized swim. Although venous forearm blood better represents the lactate production in the forearm muscles, samples taken with a needle and syringe are often perceived by the swimmers as being more traumatic. Capillary blood samples can be obtained from a puncture wound to the fingertip or earlobe. However, the size of the sample is usually small (approximately 25 μl), and is often more difficult to obtain if the wound fails to bleed sufficiently. Application of a vasodilator to the skin of the earlobe will increase blood flow to that area, making easier to collect a blood sample. For that reason the earlobe is the preferred site for sampling approximately 75 μl of blood.

Once the blood sample has been obtained, there are several methods for determining its lactate concentration. The standard enzymatic method for this analysis is detailed in Appendix A. Although this technique requires a modestly equipped biochemistry laboratory, it offers the advantage of accuracy and less cost. As an alternative method, automatic analyzers have been developed which make lactate determinations fast, easy, and reasonably accurate. The primary advantage of these analyzers is that they can be used at the pool, and the results are available for the coach within minutes after the trials.

In order to determine the swimmer's lactate threshold it is necessary to have him or her perform a series of 3 or 4 200- or 400-m swims at increasing speeds. An example of this testing sequence is shown in Fig. 17.2. If attempts are made to do all of the swims on the same day, at least 30 min should separate the swims to allow blood lactate to return to resting levels before starting the next swim. However, at the higher velocities, where more lactate is produced, even 30 min will not be sufficient time to normalize blood lactate. For that reason, some investigators recommend that the lactate swims be performed on separate days which, unfortunately, takes additional time away from training and reduces the sensitivity of the test.

The swimmer's adaptation to training can also be gauged with a single, standardized swim performed at about 95% of his or her best time for 200 or 400 m. This intensity is sufficient to produce a relatively high blood lactate when the swimmer is poorly trained, and reflects the gains in conditioning during subsequent tests. Such testing can be performed at 3–4-week intervals, using the same swimming velocity. A series of computer-controlled lights can be placed along the bottom of the swimming pool or a pace clock should be used to help the swimmer gauge the correct pace for each swim. As shown in Fig. 17.3, the results from these tests can be drawn up as a graph to illustrate the swimmer's adaptation to training. Lower blood lactate levels after this standardized swim suggest that the swimmer has become more

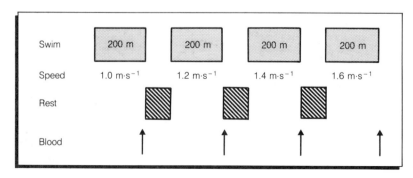

Fig. 17.2 Protocol for testing the lactate threshold. Arrows represent the time of blood sampling.

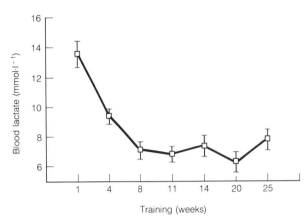

Fig. 17.3 Changes in blood lactate after a standardized 200-m front crawl swim during 24 weeks of training. (Distance, 400 m; speed, 1.45 m·s^{-1} (4:35); % max. speed, 95% at week 1.)

efficient, has improved aerobic capacity ($\dot{V}o_{2\,max}$), produces less lactate, and is able to remove lactate faster.

Heart rate measurements

Like blood lactate, exercise and postexercise heart rates increase in proportion to exercise intensity, and are lower if the swimmer improves endurance. If heart rates are recorded during or within the first 10 s following a swimming test, they provide a good indication of swimming effort and physical conditioning. There are, however, some limitations associated with the palpatated measurement of heart rate after exercise. First, pulse rates taken at the neck (carotid artery) or wrist (radial artery) are not easy to locate, and may lead to underestimates of the swimmer's heart rate during exercise. It is also hard to count the rate when the heart is beating at 2–3 times per second. In addition, counting the pulse for only 10 s induces a sizeable error when the rate is calculated as beats per minute (i.e., counts·10 s^{-1} × 6 = beats·min^{-1}). Finally, heart rates taken after the swim may underestimate the swimmer's heart rate during the exercise since the rate begins to decline within the first 10–20 s after the effort. Consequently, any delay in beginning the pulse count will result in a slower rate than that during exercise.

Therefore, heart rates provide the best indicator of stress when they are recorded during the activity. Current technology offers a simple, moderately inexpensive method for recording heart rates during swimming using radiotelemetry. A typical system is shown in Fig. 17.4. It has been our experience that the heart rate monitor transmitting unit must be securely taped to the chest in order to insure good contact and to prevent the water from displacing the unit during swimming. The receiving unit calculates and stores the heart rates at 5- or 15-s intervals throughout the

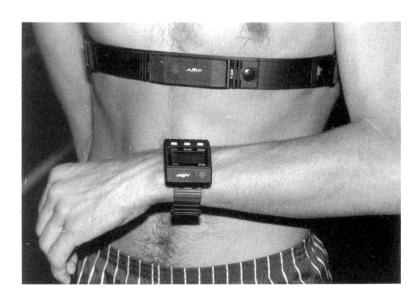

Fig. 17.4 Heart rate sending and receiving units.

test. An example of the graphic output from this system is shown in Fig. 17.5. Such measurements of heart rate provide an accurate indication of cardio-vascular stress during swimming, but it must be realized that heart rates during water exercise will be $8-10$ beats·min^{-1} lower than during similar levels of effort (% $\dot{V}_{O_2 max}$) on land.

Oxygen uptake tests

Energy expenditure during swimming is dependent on the velocity, body drag, and mechanical efficiency of the swimmer. The measurement of oxygen uptake during and immediately after swimming offers an indirect method to approximate the energy cost of swimming. As in other forms of exercise, oxygen uptake is linearly related to the intensity of the effort when the swimmer is performing in steady state and at less than $95-100\%$ $\dot{V}_{O_2 max}$. This means that estimates of energy expenditure during swimming apply only to swimming speeds that are considerably slower than those used in competition, which demand energy at levels that are between 150 and 200% $\dot{V}_{O_2 max}$. It is possible that a swimmer may appear quite economical while swimming at the slow, submaximal speeds required for oxygen uptake measurements, but may be quite inefficient during near maximal efforts. Thus, there is some doubt that measurements of oxygen uptake during swimming have any relevance to economy during competition.

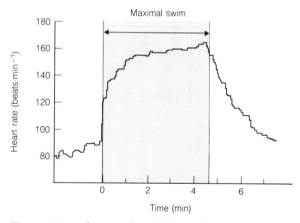

Fig. 17.5 A graphic recording for heart rate during warm-up, a 400-m swim, and recovery. $\dot{V}_{O_2} = 4.16$ l·min^{-1}; lactate = 9.5 mmol.

Nevertheless, these estimates of energy expenditure during swimming provide a useful tool to gauge improvements in swimming technique, and to assess the swimmer's aerobic capacity ($\dot{V}_{O_2 max}$).

Although oxygen uptake during swimming was first studied by Dubois-Reynolds in 1905, the most comprehensive studies were conducted by Holmer in 1974. Earlier studies had attempted to measure oxygen uptake during lake swimming, in swimming pools, and after brief periods (i.e., $1-2$ min) of breath-hold swimming. The development of a swimming flume has made it possible to reproduce the swim-mer's speed and eliminated a number of the technical problems associated with the earlier efforts to measure swimming energy expenditure.

Three separate techniques have been used in the measurement of oxygen uptake during swimming. These procedures include:

1 direct measurement during swimming in a pool or flume;

2 direct collection of expired air during tethered swimming; and

3 expired air collection immediately after a $300-400$-m swim.

Figure 17.6 illustrates each of the methods used for these tests. Tethered swimming requires the swimmer to exert sufficient effort to suspend a given weight and to remain stationary in the water. Consequently, this method does not lend itself to the measurements of free-swimming economy.

One of the major limitations to collecting expired gas samples during free-pool and flume swimming is that the instrumentation used (i.e., breathing valve and hoses) will add drag and alter one's body position during the test, thereby increasing the cost of swimming. To overcome this problem and to enable the swimmer to perform without restrictions, oxygen uptake values measured during recovery have been used to extrapolate backward to determine the $\dot{V}_{O_2}$ during swimming. This method of determining peak $\dot{V}_{O_2}$ and $\dot{V}_{O_2 max}$ during swimming has been shown to be both valid ($r = 0.99$) and reliable ($r = 0.92$), offering a less cumbersome means of assessing the energetics of swimming than by conventional methods. Each swimmer performs 2 or 3 400-m swims (front crawl, backstroke, or breaststroke) at an even, submaximal pace (approximately $0.8-1.4$ m·s^{-1}). The swimmers are instructed to take a breath approximately one

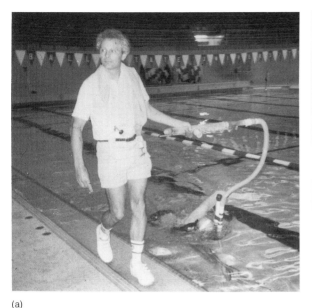

(a)

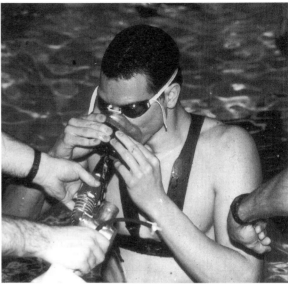

(b)

Fig. 17.6 (a) The apparatus used to measure oxygen uptake during testing in the pool. (b) The system used to estimate oxygen uptake using postexercise expired air collections. (c) The tethered system for measuring oxygen uptake.

(c)

stroke before the finish of the 400-m swim and to exhale the breath into the breathing mask as soon as it is sealed over the face, which takes about 1 s after the finish. Expired air is continuously collected in a Douglas bag for the first 20 or 40 s after the swim. Analysis of oxygen and carbon dioxide in the collected gas sample is subsequently used to calculate the $\dot{V}_{O_2}$ during the recovery period (Appendix B), and to estimate the $\dot{V}_{O_2}$ during the 400-m swim by the following equations.

1 *20-s gas collection*:

$$Y = 0.916X + 0.426$$

where X is the $\dot{V}_{O_2}$ during the first 20 s of recovery and

Y is the predicted $\dot{V}_{O_2}$ during the 400-m swim.

2 *40-s gas collection*:

$$Y = 0.910X + 0.710$$

where X is the $\dot{V}_{O_2}$ during the first 40 s of recovery.

Swimming economy, whether measured during the swim or by the postswim extrapolation of oxygen uptake, requires that the swimmer reach a steady-state pace lasting at least 4 min. Troup and Daniels (1986) have proposed that the swimmer perform 3 400-m front crawl swims at even pace, usually 1.0, 1.2, and 1.4 m·s^{-1}, but the pace selected for these tests will depend on the swimmer's ability. During the last 100 m of each 400-m swim, the expired air of the swimmer is collected, using a Douglas bag and specially designed breathing apparatus (Fig. 17.7). Expired gas samples are subsequently analyzed for oxygen and carbon dioxide by electronic or chemical methods. Calculations of oxygen uptake are performed using the equations listed in Appendix B. The graphic relationship of oxygen uptake and swimming velocity illustrates the increasing demand for oxygen with faster velocities, and the difference in economy for swimmers of varied abilities (Fig. 17.8).

Energy expended during swimming is used to pay the cost to maintain the body on the surface of the water and to generate the force required to overcome the water's resistance to motion. Though body weight in the water accounts for much of the cost of floating, lean body weight provides a better representation of the drag created by the movement of the body through the water. This may explain why the swimmer's energy cost to swim a given distance (ml of oxygen per m swum) correlates reasonably well ($r = 0.60$) with lean body weight.

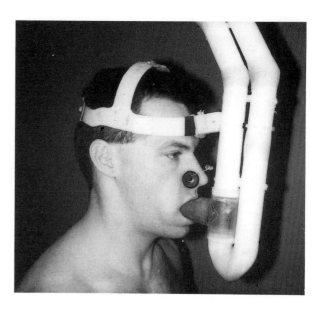

Fig. 17.7 Daniel's valve arrangement for measuring oxygen uptake.

Maximal oxygen uptake ($\dot{V}_{O_2\,max}$) during swimming

Although $\dot{V}_{O_2\,max}$ is often regarded as the best single measurement of one's physiological endurance capacity, it is not a consistently good predictor of success in competitive swimming. The winner of a 200-m front crawl race, for example, cannot be predicted from the swimmer's laboratory measurement of $\dot{V}_{O_2\,max}$. Élite male and female swimmers have often been reported to have $\dot{V}_{O_2\,max}$ values of

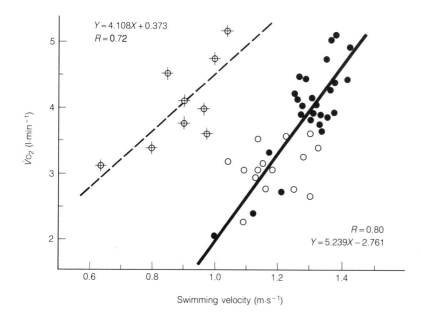

Fig. 17.8 The relationship between oxygen uptake ($\dot{V}_{O_2}$) and swimming velocity. ⊕, triathletes; ○, male competitive swimmers; ●, female competitive swimmers.

less than 60 ml·kg^{-1}·min^{-1}, well below that observed in élite endurance performers in other sports. Although it is well documented that $\dot{V}_{O2\,max}$ increases during the first 2 or 3 months of training, it will usually remain unchanged in subsequent months of high-intensity training. This suggests that there may be an individual limit to the amount of improvement in $\dot{V}_{O2\,max}$ that each swimmer can achieve during a given training season. This should *not* be interpreted to mean that one's aerobic capacity is unimportant in competitive swimming. To the contrary, aerobic energy production provides a large part of the energy during most swimming events and is highly responsive to the stress of training. Nevertheless, it appears that swimmers continue to improve their aerobic endurance, despite no measurable change in aerobic capacity.

Both tethered and free swimming bouts can be used for the determination of the swimmer's $\dot{V}_{O2\,max}$, though it is important that the swimmer should reach a level of exhaustion at the end of 5−7 min (tethered) or 400−600 m free swimming. This can be accomplished by asking the swimmer to perform a 400−600-m time trial that is evenly paced, though of maximal effort. To insure that an accurate value of oxygen uptake is obtained it is suggested that the test be performed at least twice with at least 30 min rest between trials.

Since $\dot{V}_{O2\,max}$ values are closely related to body size and weight, it not surprising to find that performance in a 400-m swim is best correlated with the $\dot{V}_{O2\,max}$ expressed per kg body weight in the water ($r = 0.74$). The swimmer's weight during submersion is explained in the section on body fat measurements, below.

Estimates of anaerobic capacity

Since a large portion of the energy used during sprint swimming is derived from anaerobic metabolism, a test to assess this capacity should prove helpful in determining the swimmer's potential for success in events from 50 to 400 m. Unlike the aerobic capacity ($\dot{V}_{O2\,max}$), there are no direct methods to measure one's anaerobic capacity. Several estimates have been developed for this purpose, though they are time-consuming and generally provide little more information than we might obtain from the stopwatch

during an all-out swim test or a set of maximal sprint intervals. Nevertheless, the following discussion is offered as an alternate method for estimating anaerobic capacity, using measurements of oxygen uptake and test of interval sets.

One method used to estimate the anaerobic capacity is to calculate the difference between one's estimated oxygen demand during all-out exercise and the $\dot{V}_{O2\,max}$. When the swimmer's oxygen uptake is determined at three or four different submaximal swimming speeds, it is possible to extrapolate a line to estimate the oxygen uptake at other swimming speeds above and below the $\dot{V}_{O2\,max}$. As shown in Fig. 17.9, the oxygen required above the $\dot{V}_{O2\,max}$ is referred to as the oxygen deficit and is assumed to represent the anaerobic capacity during a maximal-sprint swim. It is assumed, but not proven, that the swimmers with the greatest anaerobic capacity will have the largest oxygen deficit.

From the information shown in Fig. 17.9 it is possible to calculate the swimmer's oxygen deficit or anaerobic capacity for the 100-m swim by the following equations:

$$O_2 \text{ deficit} = [(100\text{-m time}) \times (\text{estimated } \dot{V}_{O2})] - [(100\text{-m time}) \times (\dot{V}_{O2\,max})].$$

$$\text{(Example)} = [(0.92 \text{ min}) \times (78 \text{ ml·kg}^{-1}\text{·min}^{-1})] - [(0.92 \text{ min}) \times (58 \text{ ml·kg}^{-1}\text{·min}^{-1})]$$
$$= [71.8 \text{ ml·kg}^{-1}] - [53.4 \text{ ml·kg}^{-1}]$$
$$= 18.4 \text{ ml·kg}^{-1} = O_2 \text{ deficit}.$$

A second but less complex index of the swimmer's capacity for anaerobic effort can be obtained from a series of short repeated sprints with a reasonably long rest interval between bouts. Examples of such anaerobic test sets are as follows:

10 × 50 m with 1 min 30 s rest

or

5 × 100 m with 3 min rest

The average times for these maximal swims can be used as an index of the swimmer's tolerance for anaerobic sprint effort. Unlike the aerobic capacity, however, the swimmer's maximal oxygen deficit and changes in the anaerobic test sets show only small improvements with training. Figure 17.10 illustrates the changes in $\dot{V}_{O2\,max}$, maximal oxygen deficit, and average times for an anaerobic test set during 24 weeks

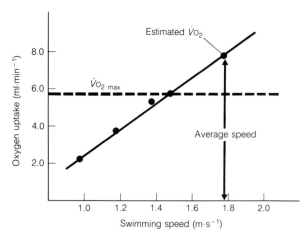

Fig. 17.9 Use of submaximal oxygen uptake to estimate the swimmer's oxygen uptake during a 100-m swim. Note that the estimated oxygen uptake ($ml \cdot kg^{-1} \cdot min^{-1}$) is above the swimmer's $\dot{V}_{O_2 max}$.

of training. It is interesting to note that most of the adaptations occurred during the first 8 weeks of training—a surprising finding, since the swimmers generally continue to show improvements in performance throughout the final 16 weeks of training. This would suggest that either the tests for anaerobic and aerobic fitness are not sensitive to performance changes or that the improvements in performance are related to factors such as swimming skill.

Stroke distance and velocity

As pointed out by Craig and Pendergast (1979), "Swimming, like most other methods of locomotion, involves the intermittent application of force which results in movement. In all of the stroke patterns used in swimming the mean velocity (V) is the product of the stroke rate (SR = strokes·min^{-1}) and distance moved through the water with each complete stroke (DS = distance·$stroke^{-1}$)."

$$V = SR \times DS.$$

As illustrated in Fig. 17.11, swimmers increase their swimming speed by a combination of taking more strokes and decreasing the distance per stroke. This ability to adjust stroke rate and distance per stroke seems to be learned as part of training. In an effort to gauge the swimmer's stroke economy, a stroke index (SI) can be calculated by multiplying the swimming velocity (V) by the distance per stroke (DS). This index assumes that at a given velocity, the swimmer who moves the greatest distance per stroke has the most effective swimming technique. This does not imply that the swimmer with the longest stroke expends the least energy, though there is some evidence to demonstrate that distance per stroke is a major determinant of success in middle-distance (i.e., 200–400-m) front crawl events.

Although there are more accurate methods of recording the swimmer's stroke rate and distance per

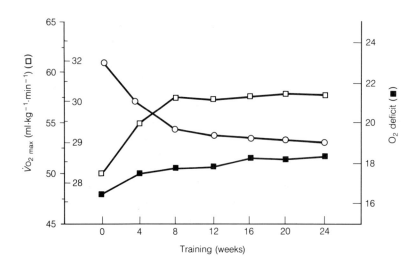

Fig. 17.10 Changes in maximal oxygen uptake ($\dot{V}_{O_2 max}$; □) O_2 deficit, (■), and performance time (○) during an interval set (10 × 50 m with 2-min rest).

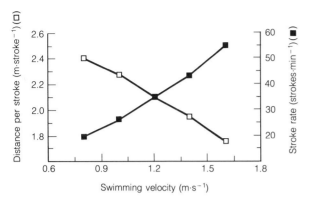

Fig. 17.11 The relationship between swimming velocity and the swimmer's distance per stroke (□) and stroke rate (■).

stroke, the simplest technique is to record the number of strokes taken (STK) per 50 m and the swimmer's time for 50 m (T, in s). This information can be used to calculate the stroke rate and distance moved with each stroke from the following equations:

$$V = 50 \text{ m}/T = \text{m·s}^{-1}$$
$$SR = (STK/T) \times 60 = STK\text{·min}^{-1}$$
$$DS = 50 \text{ m·STK}^{-1} = \text{m·stroke}^{-1}.$$

Example: If a swimmer swims 50 m in 30 s and takes 25 strokes, then his V, SR, and DS would be as follows:

$$V = 50 \text{ m·30 s}^{-1} = 1.66 \text{ m·s}^{-1}$$
$$SR = (25 \text{ strokes·30 s}^{-1}) \times 60 = 50 \text{ strokes·min}^{-1}$$
$$DS = 50 \text{ m·25 strokes}^{-1} = 2 \text{ m·strokes}^{-1}.$$

These simple calculations can be made for all four competitive strokes, and can be used by the coach as a method of assessing the swimmer's stroke economy.

Subjective ratings of effort

Sometimes the simplest tests of exercise stress are the best. This appears to be the case when we use the rating of perceived exertion (RPE) scale. By simply asking the swimmers to rate their sensations of effort we can gain as much overall information as can be obtained with other laboratory tests. About 20 years ago Gunnar Borg introduced a perceptual scale for use in exercise prescription for healthy and clinically limited individuals. The overall perceived exertion rating integrates various data, including

Table 17.1 The graded rating of perceived exertion (RPE) scale for rating the swimmer's perception of effort

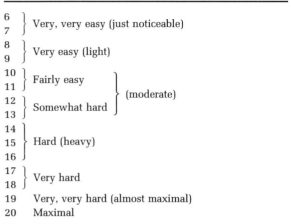

the signals elicited from the peripheral exercising muscles and joints, from the central cardiovascular and respiratory systems, and from the central nervous system. All these signals, perceptions, and experiences are integrated into a composite sensation of effort. The revised RPE scale developed by Borg is shown in Table 17.1.

The swimmer's RPE for a given swim has been shown to correlate highly with exercising heart rate, oxygen uptake, and blood lactate ($r = 0.8-0.9$). The scale values range from 6 to 20 and can be used to denote heart rates ranging from 60 to 200 beats·min^{-1}. This was intended to make the scale easier to use because a certain value on the scale, e.g., 13, would match approximately a heart rate of 130 beats·min^{-1}. However, this close relationship is not meant to be taken too literally because the meaning of a certain heart rate value as an indicator of exercise stress depends on the age of the athlete, type of exercise, anxiety and other factors. Nevertheless, the RPE is a simple, inexpensive way for the coach to gauge the stress experienced by the swimmer during training and identify conditions of chronic fatigue. In light of the strong relationship with the physiological indices of physical stress (i.e., heart rate, lactate, and oxygen uptake), the ease of administration, the immediate evaluation of training effort, and the cost-free nature of this test, it is surprising that it is not more widely used by coaches to assist in planning their swimmers' training program.

Strength and power testing

In male swimmers, a close relationship has been found between upper body strength and performance in sprint swimming ($r = 0.93$). Early studies attempted to use isometric and free-weight measurements in an effort to assess upper-body strength in competitive swimmers. Unfortunately, these methods were not specific to the requirements of swimming and, therefore, did not correlate highly with swimming performance. Recent technological advancements in strength-testing equipment, however, have enabled us to test the maximal force production in the arm muscles during activities that closely simulate the actions used in swimming. Although there are several isokinetic pieces of equipment capable of testing muscular strength, the Biokinetic™ swim bench produced by Isokinetics (Richmond, California) provides an opportunity to mimic the arm pull during butterfly and front crawl swimming (Fig. 17.12). Though it cannot duplicate the arm and hand actions used in the water, it does allow the swimmer to incorporate in one motion most of the muscle groups and the mechanics required during sprint swimming.

Although swim-bench tests of strength among age-group swimmers (swimmer less than 16 years old) correlates highly with sprint time for 25 m, this test does not discriminate between levels of sprint ability in élite competitors. This suggests that success in sprint swimming among older and élite swimmers may be determined primarily by technique rather than strength. Developments of a computer-based system to measure force and power during front crawl swimming (Costill *et al.*, 1986) has been shown to provide a sensitive and reliable method of determining muscular power in a manner that is closely related to sprint swimming performance in all groups of swimmers (Fig. 17.13).

The control mechanism from a Biokinetic™ system can be adapted using 20−30 m of stainless steel cable (approximately 65 kg), which is connected to the system's recoil wheel and to a harness belt. The recoil springs in the apparatus which normally cause the hand paddles to retrieve the wire must be disengaged and a variable speed motor attached to the coiling shaft. This enables the operator to engage a motor to rewind the cable after each test. During the test, the harness at the distal end of the cable is attached to the swimmer's waist. With the system set to release the

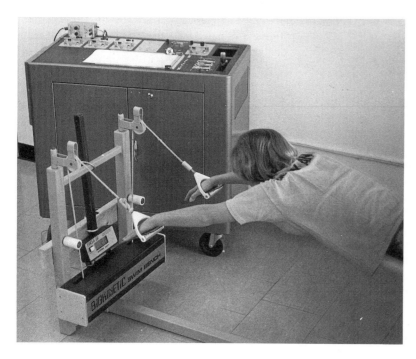

Fig. 17.12 The Biokinetic™ swim bench, used to measure upper-body strength and power, simulating a swimming arm pull.

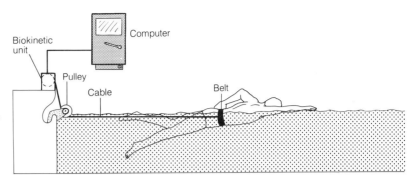

Fig. 17.13 The apparatus and computer system used to measure velocity, force, and power during tethered swimming. Courtesy of the Ball State University Human Performance Laboratory.

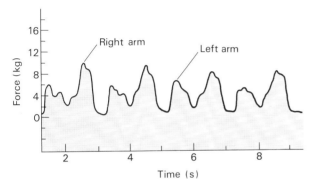

Fig. 17.14 A graphic recording of the force curve during front crawl swimming. Note the difference in height of the front crawl for this swimmer's right and left arm pulls. Mean power = 34.2 W.

cable at a given velocity 0.8 m·s^{-1}, females; 1.0 m·s^{-1}, males), the swimmers attempt to swim away from the apparatus with maximal effort for a distance of 12–15 m. The force generated against the cable by the swimmer is sensed by a force transducer in the Biokinetic™ system and converted to a proportional voltage output. The voltage output from the transducer is then relayed to a strip chart recorder and computer. The machine code and computer programs written for this system enable the computer to read the voltage output and to calculate the average velocity, force, work and power for each swimming stroke or for any given time period. An illustration of the graphic recording is shown in Fig. 17.14.

We have recently modified this system to use the control mechanism system from a Cybex™ ergometer. In this system the wire is attached to a cycle wheel fitted to the center shaft of the Cybex™. The advantage of this system is that it provides a more easily calibrated mechanism that is truly isokinetic.

Determining body fatness

Most sports are negatively affected by excess body weight and fat. That is to say, a lean body is quicker and generally performs better than one with large amounts of fat. In some cases, one's fitness is judged by fatness—lower body fat indicates a higher level of physical fitness. This is not the case among swimmers, since fat provides buoyancy, thereby reducing the energy required to stay on the surface of the water. Of course, extreme excesses of fat will alter the body's contour and increase drag. The ideal level of body fat for the best performances has not been established. Thus, we can only examine the body composition of élite swimmers and assume that they represent a near optimal level of body fatness.

It should be realized that about 80% of the fat in the body is stored beneath the skin (i.e., subcutaneous fat), serving as fuel for exercise and aiding in the body hormone regulation. Since there is no direct way to measure body fat, we can only rely on techniques that estimate it. Some methods are better than others, but none are perfect. Consequently, the values should not be used to compare fatness or leanness between swimmers. Rather, this information should be used to compare the swimmer to him- or herself, and to gauge the effects of training on nutritional status.

The two most widely used methods for determining body fat involve hydrostatic (underwater) weighing, and multiple skinfold measurements. Though both methods provide reliable values for estimating the percentage of body fat, the calculations are based on several assumptions which may not hold true for all swimmers.

Hydrostatic method

The body can be separated into two components: lean body mass (i.e., bone and muscle) and fatty tissue. Bone and muscle are heavier than water, whereas fat weighs 12% less than an equal volume of water. Consequently, fat floats when placed in water, and swimmers who have a great deal of body fat tend to be more buoyant. The weight of a material per unit of volume is referred to as *density*. Thus, fat is less dense than either bone or muscle. The lower the body density, the more fat it contains. Studies have been done on human cadavers to determine the fat content and compared it to body density values. As a result, we can estimate a swimmer's body fat from measurements of body weight on land and while submerged in the water. The procedures for this test are given in Appendix C. The equations for the body composition are summarized as follows:

$$\text{Density}_{(body)} = \frac{\text{Weight in air (g)}}{\left\{\dfrac{(\text{Weight in air}) - (\text{Weight in water})}{\text{Density of water (g/ml)}}\right\} - [(\text{Residual volume} + 100)].}$$

%Body fat = (495/Density) − 450
Total body fat (kg) = (%Body fat/100) ×
Body weight in air.

Where residual volume is the amount of air remaining in the lungs when the swimmer is being weighed underwater. For general screening purposes, assumed values for residual volume can be taken from Table 17.2.

Table 17.2 Estimated residual volume of the lungs

	Residual volume (ml)	
Age (years)	Females	Males
6−10	600	900
11−15	800	1100
16−20	1000	1300
21−25	1200	1500
26−30	1400	1700

Skinfold estimates

It has been reported that 50−80% of the stored fat in the body is located just beneath the skin. Thus, estimates of skinfold fat have been shown to provide a reasonably valid and reliable estimate of total body fat. The general approach to this method of estimating body fat is to measure the thickness of skinfold at various sites on the body; these measurements are subsequently inserted into an equation to estimate body density and percentage of body fat. Unfortunately, the equations that are used for predicting body density from skinfold thickness have been based on relatively few subjects and specific populations (e.g., sedentary males, females gymnasts, etc.). It should also be noted that it takes considerable practice to measure skinfolds accurately with calipers. Even among experienced technicians, differences of more than 3% can be expected with this method. Another problem associated with the skinfold method of body fat determination is that it is often not sensitive to changes in body fat during periods of training or inactivity. Nevertheless, skinfold measurements are useful for screening subjects who may be overly fat or thin and can serve as an effective, simply administered tool for monitoring body weight changes over the season.

Recommended reading

Benke, A.R. & Wilmore, J.H. (1974) *Evaluation and Regulation of Body Build and Composition*. Englewood Cliffs, New Jersey: Prentice-Hall.

Borg, G.A.V. (1982) Psychophysical bases of perceived exertion. *Med. Sci. Sports Exerc.* **14**:377−381.

Burke, E.J. & Keenan, T.J. (1984) Energy cost, heart rate, and perceived exertion during the elementary backstroke. *Phys. Sportsmed.* **12**:75−78.

Costill, D.L., Kovaleski, J., Porter, D., Kirwan, J., Fielding, R. & King, D. (1985) Energy expenditure during front crawl swimming: predicting success in middle-distance events. *Int. J. Sports Med.* **6**:266−270.

Costill, D.L., Rayfield, F., Kirwan, J. & Thomas, R. (1986) A computer based system for the measurement of force and power during front crawl swimming. *J. Swim. Res.* **2**:16−19.

Costill, D.L., Sharp, R. & Troup, J. (1980) Muscle strength: contributions to sprint swimming. *Swim. World* **21**:29−34.

Craig, A.B. & Pendergast, D.R. (1979) Relationships of stroke rate, distance per stroke, and velocity in competitive swimming. *Med. Sci. Sports* **11**:278–283.

Mader, A., Heck, H. & Hollmann, W. (1976) Evaluation of lactic acid anaerobic energy contribution by determination of post-exercise lactic acid concentration of ear capillary blood in middle distance runners and swimmers. In Landing, F. & Orban, W, (eds) *Exercise Physiology*. Florida: Symposia Specialists, pp. 187–199.

Medbø, J.I., Mohn, A-C., Tabata, I., Bahr, R., Vagge, O. & Sejersted, O.M. (1988) Anarobic capacity determined by maximal accumulated O_2 deficit. *J. Appl. Physiol.*

64:50–60.

Robertson, R.J. (1982) Central signals of perceived exertion during dynamic exercise. *Med. Sci. Sports Exerc.* **14**:390–396.

Sharp, R.L., Vitelli, C.A., Costill, D.L. & Thomas, R. (1984) Comparison between blood lactate and heart rate profiles during a season of competitive swim training. *J. Swim. Res.* **1**:17–20.

Troup, J.P. & Daniels, J.T. (1986) Swimming economy: an introductory review. *J. Swim. Res.* **2**:5–9.

Chapter 18

Biomechanical evaluation

The use of films and video has increased our knowledge of swimming mechanics. Although early studies showed that freestyle swimmers were bending their arms under water, coaches of the day were teaching swimmers to keep their arms straight during the pull. The landmark study by Brown and Counsilman (1971) demonstrated that swimmers were stroking in diagonal directions, which contradicted the idea of pushing the arm and hand directly backward. Work by Plagenhoff (1971) and Barthels and Adrian (1971, 1974) confirmed these observations.

We are now entering a new phase where film and video are being used to diagnose the mechanics of swimmers. The forward velocities of swimmers' centers of gravity (Maglischo et al., 1987; Mason et al., 1989; Huijing et al., 1988) and hips have, variously, been used for this purpose. Unusual decelerations during a single stroke cycle and failure to accelerate adequately usually signal stroke defects. Measurements of the center of gravity provide the most accurate diagnostic tool. Hip velocities are sometimes inaccurate, particularly in the butterfly and breaststroke, because they can misrepresent the velocity of swimmers' centers of mass during certain phases of the stroke cycle. Movements of swimmer's hips fail to take into account changes in the positions of other body parts. Nevertheless, they are reasonably accurate for diagnostic purposes. The accelerations and decelerations of swimmers' forward velocities are generally similar to those of their centers of gravity during certain phases of each stroke cycle. They will sometimes be different in magnitude and slightly out of phase, however (Brown and Counsilman, 1971). The advantage in measuring hip movements lies in the fact that velocities can be calculated faster. Therefore, they speed the dissemination of information to swimmers. This method requires locating the position of only one body part on each frame of film or tape. Center-of-gravity calculations, on the other hand, necessitate measuring the location of 19–21 body parts on each frame. So, hip velocities provide a fast but somewhat inaccurate diagnostic tool while center-of-gravity measurements are more accurate but also more time-consuming.

Recent development of a device called a *velocity meter* has enabled coaches to benefit from the combination of television and computer technology (Costill et al., 1987). This device was described in Chapter 17. Briefly, it consists of a harness and line that swimmers attach to their neck or hips. When they swim down the pool the line is pulled over the wheel of a generator. A velocity meter is shown as part of Fig. 18.1.

Measurements of the tension on the line are communicated to a computer where analog signals from the generator are converted to digital signals that represent the swimmer's velocity. In the meantime, the swimmer is being videotaped underwater with a periscope-like device. The video signal is relayed to the computer where it is mixed with the digital signal from the generator to form a combined image on the video monitor. That is, video images of the swimmer emerge overlayed with a graph of the swimmer's velocity. Video cameras tape at 30 frames per second and swimmers generally need 1 s or more to complete a stroke cycle. Thus, stepping through the videotape one frame at a time provides coaches with 30 or more pictures per stroke cycle of changes in a swimmer's velocity.

An important feature of this device is that the information can be made available immediately after the athlete completes the swim. A disadvantage is that the velocity meter measures only the linear velocity of swimmers, so the accuracy of the results is influenced somewhat by their vertical movements. Once again, the differences between these and center-of-gravity measurements are minor and trained coaches will be able to account for them in the diagnostic process.

Other attempts to measure the propulsive efficiency of swimmers have included the use of transducers that measure changes in pressure on swimmers' limbs. The swimmers wear these pressure transducers on their hands, arms or feet while they swim across the pool. The signal is relayed to a computer where pressure measurements are analyzed and stored. Swimmers

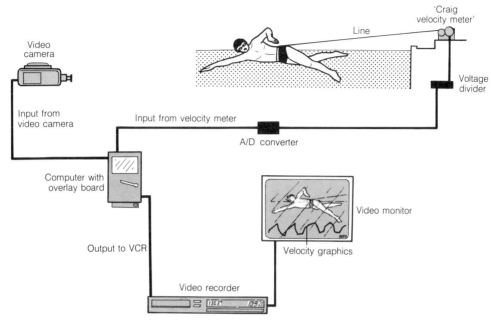

Fig. 18.1 The video-velocity meter. Courtesy of the Ball State University Human Performance Laboratory.

are also videotaped so these measurements can be coupled with the movements of their limbs to see where and how much propulsive force is being produced.

Some very sophisticated devices have been developed, though most have some serious limitations. Pressure transducers, for example, are sensitive to both movements and the depth of the water. Consequently, the simple act of stroking the hand down can register as an increase in propulsive force because the pressure of water increases as it gets deeper. This source of error must, therefore, be accounted for in the analysis. There is also no guarantee that the pressure differences registered indicate propulsive force. Transducers simply measure changes in pressure. Certain pressure differences may represent force that has been applied in the wrong direction or with an incorrect angle of attack. Therefore, some measure of forward velocity is probably also needed with this method to judge which pressure differences are propulsive.

By far the most ambitious attempt to measure the propulsive force of swimmers has been undertaken by Schleihauf (1979, 1984). He developed a method

for estimating propulsive force from measures of hand and arm velocities, directions and angles of attack. These parameters must be calculated three-dimensionally. Consequently, the measurements must be taken from matching frames of film or videotape that were recorded simultaneously from two different perspectives. One procedure for recording three-dimensional motion is illustrated in Fig. 18.2. This method yields stroke patterns from two different perspectives that, when combined, depict the directions in which the swimmer's limbs are traveling. It also results in graphs of swimmers' propulsive force and total force. One such graph was provided in Fig. 6.15.

We have gained a wealth of information from Schleihauf's work during the last two decades, including a better understanding of stroke patterns. We are also more knowledgeable about the propulsive and nonpropulsive phases of the various competitive strokes. Future developments may allow modeling of swimmers' strokes to determine if they could achieve more propulsion during certain phases of the stroke with different combinations of limb directions, angles of attack and velocities.

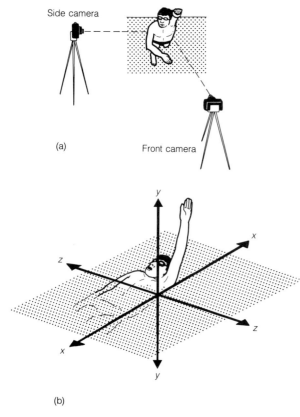

(a)

(b)

Fig. 18.2 One procedure for recording swimmers' movements for three-dimensional analysis. (a) Three-dimensional cinematography. The cameras are placed at 90° angles to one another. The swimmer is filmed from the front and side simultaneously. (b) Three axes of motion. Swimmers' forward−backward movements are filmed on the *x* axis. The up−down movements are recorded on the *y* axis and the in-and-out movements are on the *z* axis.

Although the information gained has been valuable, it should be noted that this method yields only an estimate of propulsion. The accuracy of that estimate will be only as good as the accuracy of the measurements taken from the film or tape. The difficulty in getting precise measurements lies in the fact that they are taken from tiny images of the hands, arms, feet and legs appearing in these frames. To make matters worse, these images are often partially obscured by turbulence or other parts of swimmers' bodies. Schleihauf has continued to improve upon the accuracy of his technique by using taping from both sides with three or more cameras. This is done so that each body part can be located on at least two tapes at all times. Another innovation has been the marking of body parts with lights that can be more easily located on tape.

A final method for measuring swimming propulsion is called the MAD (measuring active drag) system (Toussaint *et al.*, 1983). It consists of a series of pads mounted under water. Pressure on the pads is measured by force transducers whose signals are stored and analyzed by computer.

A series of these pads is spaced over the length of a pool so they correspond to a swimmer's stroke length. Swimmers propel their bodies forward by grasping the handle in front and pulling and pushing their bodies past it. The hand should make contact with another pad immediately they release the one behind so there is no delay between applications of propulsive force.

With the MAD system, all of the force swimmers produce is used to propel the body forward and none is lost to the water. This is because they are pushing against the solid pads. Consequently, their mean propulsive force should equal the mean opposing drag force. Propulsive forces are calculated from the forces registered on the transducers and then averaged.

Measurements of active drag, mechanical and propelling efficiency have been recorded in various studies (Hollander *et al.*, 1988; Huijing *et al.*, 1988; Toussaint *et al.*, 1988). In general, drag increases were proportional to the square of velocity increases. Measurements of $\dot{V}O_2$ have been used in conjunction with the MAD system to measure mechanical efficiency. In this case, the oxygen cost for free swimming at a given velocity was compared to the cost for swimming at the same velocity on the MAD system. Uses for this device are still being developed.

Recommended reading

Barthels, K.M. & Adrian, M.J. (1971) Variability in the dolphin kick under four conditions. In Lewillie, L. & Clarys, J.P. (eds) *First International Symposium on Biomechanics in Swimming, Waterpolo and Diving Proceedings*. Brussels: Université Libre de Bruxelles Laboratoire de l'Effort, pp. 105−118.

Barthels, K. & Adrian, M.H. (1974) Three dimensional spatial hand patterns of skilled butterfly swimmers. In Clarys, J.P & Lewillie, L. (eds) *Swimming II*. Baltimore, Maryland: University Park Press, pp. 154−160.

Brown, R.M. & Counsilman, J.E. (1971) The role of lift in

propelling swimmers. In Cooper, J.M. (ed.) *Biomechanics*. Chicago: Athletic Institute, pp. 179–188.

Costill, D.L., Lee, G. & D'Acquisto, L. (1987) Video-computer assisted analysis of swimming technique. *J. Swim. Res.* **3**: 5–9.

Hollander, A.P., de Groot, G., van Ingen Schenau, G.J., Kahman, R. & Toussaint, H.M. (1988) Contribution of the legs to propulsion in front crawl swimming. In Ungerechts, B.E., Wilke, K. & Reischle, K. (eds) *Swimming Science V*. Champaign, Illinois: Human Kinetics, pp. 39–44.

Huijing, P.A., Toussaint, H.M., Mackay, R. *et al.* (1988) Active drag related to body dimensions. In Ungerechts, B.E., Wilke, K. & Resichle, K. (eds) *Swimming Science V*. Champaign, Illinois: Human Kinetics, pp. 31–38.

Maglischo, C.W., Maglischo, E.W. & Santos, T.R. (1987) The relationship between the forward velocity of the center of gravity and the hip in the four competitive strokes. *J. Swim. Res.* **3**:11–17.

Mason, B.R., Patton, S.G. & Newton, A.P. (1989) Propulsion in breaststroke swimming. In Morrison, W.E. (ed.) *Proceedings of the VII International Symposium on Biomechanics in Sports*. Melbourne, Australia: Footscray Institute of Technology, pp. 257–267.

Persyn, U., De Maeyer, J. & Vervaecke, H. (1975) Investigation of hydrodynamic determinants of competitive swimming strokes. In Lewillie, L. & Clarys, J.P. (eds) *Swimming II*. Baltimore, Maryland: University Park Press, pp. 214–222.

Persyn, U., Van Tilborgh, L., Daly, D. *et al.* (1988) Computerized evaluation and advice in swimming. In Ungerechts, B.E., Wilke, K. & Reischle, K. (eds) *Swimming Science V*. Champaign, Illinois: Human Kinetics, pp. 341–349.

Plagenhoff, S. (1971) *Patterns of Human Motion*. Englewood Cliffs, New Jersey: Prentice-Hall.

Reischle, K. (1979) A kinematic investigation of movement patterns in swimming with photo-optical methods. In Terauds, J. & Bedingfield, E.W. (eds) *Swimming III*. Baltimore, Maryland: University Park Press, pp. 97–104.

Schleihauf, R.E. Jr (1979) A hydrodynamic analysis of swimming propulsion. In Terauds, J. & Bedingfield, E.W. (eds) *Swimming III*. Baltimore, Maryland: University Park Press, pp. 70–109.

Schleihauf, R.E. (1984) Biomechanics of swimming propulsion. In Welsh, T.F. (ed.) *1983 ASCA World Clinic Yearbook*. Fort Lauderdale, Florida: American Swimming Coaches Association, pp. 19–24.

Toussaint, H.M. (1988) *Mechanics and Energetics of Swimming*. Amsterdam: Toussaint, H.M.

Toussaint, H.M., Hollander., A.P., de Groot, G. *et al.* (1988) Measurement of efficiency in swimming man. In Ungerechts, B.E., Wilke, K. & Reischle, K. *Swimming Science V*. Champaign, Illinois: Human Kinetics, pp. 45–52.

Toussaint, H.M., van der Helm, F.C.T., Elzerman, J.R., Hollander, A.P., de Groot, G. & van Ingen Schneau, G.J. (1983) A power balance applied to swimming. In Hollander, A.P., Huijing, P.A. & de Groot, G. (eds) *Biomechanics and Medicine in Swimming*. Champaign, Illinois: Human Kinetics, pp. 165–172.

Chapter 19

Medical aspects of swimming

3 Relative rest.
4 Stretching.
5 Muscle exercise.

Cold therapy

Application of ice cups, packs, or gels will help decrease inflammation and should be done throughout the course of treatment of a strain or sprain. It is reasonable to apply ice to an injured part for 15—20 min, 4—5 times a day during the period of acute injury. After the first several days, this may be decreased to include those times immediately following activities. Application of heat is not usually as effective in treating an injury, except when used in contrast to cold therapy. Contrast therapy usually includes a short period (5—7 min) of cold, followed by 5—7 min of heat, and ending with 5—7 min of cold.

NSAIDs

These are a group of medications, of which the most common is aspirin, which tend to decrease inflammation anywhere in the body. All come in pill or capsule form. Some require a prescription in some countries, while others (e.g., aspirin) do not.

Examples are ibuprofen, naproxen, phenylbutazone etc. None are included on the International Olympic Committee's Banned Substance List. All have in common the side-effects of stomach upset and irritation in some patients. Some medications are effective in some athletes, while others are effective for others, therefore it is not uncommon for the treating physician to try several different NSAIDs to see which is most effective.

Relative rest

An injured part always benefits from rest. Unfortunately, many take this to mean complete rest from, for instance, swimming workout. In most cases, the physician, coach, trainer, and athlete should cooperate to determine a training program which will allow the swimmer to remain in physical condition, while not over-stressing the injured part. For example, when an injury occurs to the lower extremity, a pull-buoy may be employed to relieve stress on the legs, while still exercising the upper extremities. Similarly,

Introduction

Medical problems in competitive swimmers are, fortunately, relatively uncommon. As opposed to contact sports, such as boxing and wrestling, where traumatic injuries prevail, most complaints related to swimming result either from prolonged immersion in chemically treated water, or from constant, repetitive use of the extremities which leads to overuse injuries. This chapter will examine some of the more common injuries associated with competitive swimming.

Musculoskeletal problems

Sprains and strains

By definition, a *sprain* refers to an injury to a *ligament* (a structure which holds one bone to another), while a *strain* refers to an injury to a *tendon* (a structure which connects a muscle to a bone). Both are common in any sport which requires repeated use of the extremities, and swimming is no exception. Both result in inflammation of the involved part, and treatment is always directed, in part, at decreasing inflammation.

Examples are strains of the triceps muscle tendon at the elbow (which is responsible for forceful extension of the elbow during the underwater pull), and strains of the lower back muscles, particularly during breaststroke and butterfly. Sprains of the ligaments and capsule of the front of the ankle are also common because of the repeated flapping motion of the ankles in swimming.

Treatment of all these conditions follows several simple, well known patterns, which are easily carried out by the athlete.
1 Cold therapy.
2 Nonsteroidal anti-inflammatory drugs (NSAIDs).

kicking and dry-land cycle ergometry might be used for exercise to relieve stress to an injured upper extremity.

Stretching

When a ligament or tendon is suddenly pulled beyond its capacity, injury may occur. Muscles are elastic structures and can normally accommodate the full range of motion of the joints they control. Following strenuous activities and periods of inactivity, however, muscles will become less elastic and will accommodate less range of motion of their involved joints; this leads to the common feeling of stiffness. Stretching exercises prior to an activity will lengthen the muscles to be used, thereby relieving some of the stress which would otherwise fall on the attached tendons. Stretching after athletic activities allows the muscles to warm down (continued blood supply to the muscle helps remove the chemical byproducts of exercise) and helps prevent subsequent muscle spasm and stiffness.

Ballistic or bounce stretching is to be avoided in lieu of static (stretch-and-hold) stretching. While "buddy" stretching (stretching with a partner) is very popular, the athlete and coach must be careful to avoid inadvertent overstretching and injury.

Muscle exercise

Muscle imbalance plays an important role in the causation of many injuries. Identification and strengthening of weak groups of muscles can often decrease the incidence of sprains and strains of the ligaments and tendons. Quantification of muscle strength can be done either manually (resistance muscle-testing by a partner) or with one of several machines (Cybex™, Bio Dec™, etc.) commonly available through sports gyms, physical therapists, athletic trainers, etc.

Certain muscle groups are known to be weaker than others. For example, the external rotator muscles of the shoulder joint (the rotator cuff muscles) are usually much weaker than the internal rotator muscles; many feel this is a factor in causing swimmer's shoulder pain.

Shoulder pain in swimmers

Swimming is primarily an upper-extremity sport. Shoulder pain is the most common complaint of the musculoskeletal system among swimmers, with an incidence of up to 60% of élite competitors.

Anatomy

The shoulder joint is formed by two bones: the *glenoid* (or socket), which is part of the scapula (or shoulder blade), and the *humeral head*, which is the ball-shaped upper end of the arm bone (Fig. 19.1). Overlying the humeral head and providing both the point of attachment for the large deltoidius muscle and one-half of the small acromioclavicular joint is the acromion. The acromion and the coracoacromial ligament form a roof overlying the rotator cuff muscle insertion into the humeral head; the rotator cuff muscles are a group of four muscles, all of which originate from the scapula and help rotate the humeral head in the glenoid socket as the arm is moved to the overhead position.

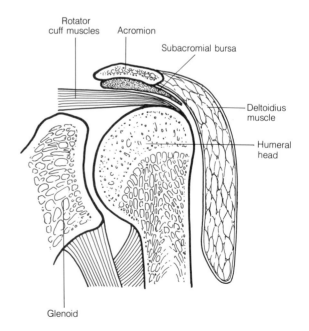

Fig. 19.1 Anatomy of the shoulder: cross-section showing the relationship of the bony and soft-tissue structures.

Between the rotator cuff muscles and the acromion is a *bursa*, or membranous sac, which usually lubricates the movement of the rotator cuff muscles under the acromion. If shoulder motion is excessive, this bursa may become inflamed (red and swollen).

The socket of the shoulder joint is small relative to the larger humeral head, allowing the shoulder joint a wide range of motion. During normal crawl swimming, the shoulder is repeatedly brought to the overhead (abducted) position, followed by a forceful adduction motion, which brings the arm back to the side. In fact, shoulder motion in the freestyle, backstroke, and butterfly strokes is mechanically very similar, so that shoulder pain occurring in any of these three strokes usually originates from the same source.

Sources of shoulder pain

It is well known that the average competitive swimmer may take as many as 750 000 strokes per arm per year over a career of some 8−12 years. Repeated impingement of the humeral head, and the rotator cuff muscles, into the overlying acromion results in inflammation of this area with subsequent pain, characteristically located diffusely about the acromion, and usually occurring just after the recovery phase of front crawl swimming.

Swimmer's shoulder is medically known as impingement syndrome (impingement of the humeral head and rotator cuff on the overlying acromion), but is often called bursitis, cuffitis, or rotator cuff syndrome. It tends to occur more often on the breathing side, is aggravated by the use of hand-paddles, and often does not affect swimmers until they are in the sixth to eighth years of their careers.

A second, newly recognized source of shoulder pain in competitive swimmers is related to instability of the shoulder joint itself. Because the shoulder joint is the most mobile of the major joints, it is also the most inherently unstable. Partial dislocation of the glenohumeral joint during each swimming stroke can lead to tears of the cartilaginous rim (the labrum) of the socket of the joint as well as inflammation of the tendon of the biceps muscle, which courses through the shoulder joint itself. Many physicians believe that it is this underlying instability which allows the humeral head to ram into the overlying acromion,

resulting in the impingement syndrome described above.

Categories of shoulder pain

For descriptive purposes, shoulder pain in swimmers may be divided into four categories.
Stage I: Pain only after heavy workouts.
Stage II: Pain during and after workouts.
Stage III: Pain which interferes with performance.
Stage IV: Pain preventing competitive swimming.

Treatment

Seven approaches to shoulder pain in competitive swimmers can be identified:
1 decreasing inflammation;
2 modalities;
3 muscle strengthening;
4 changes in technique and training;
5 mechanical measures;
6 stretching;
7 surgery.
Effective treatment of shoulder pain requires the interaction of the swimmer, the coach, an athletic trainer or physical therapist, and a physician. The physician evaluates and categorizes the problem, as well as directs the overall plan of treatment; the athletic trainer or physical therapist is responsible for application of many of the modalities used in treatment; finally, the coach and athlete are responsible for tailoring the work−rest ratio of the involved shoulder, so that the athlete can maintain the best physical condition while minimizing further pain and injury about the shoulder.

Decreasing inflammation. The response of the shoulder joint to the repeated abrasion of the humeral head on the acromion is swelling and redness of the rotator cuff muscle tendons. Measures to decrease this inflammation are effective in relieving pain, as well as decreasing swelling and allowing more relative space between the rotator cuff and the acromion.

These measures include *ice-packing* (for 15−20 min) to the shoulder on a regular basis, especially following workouts, oral *NSAIDs*, such as aspirin, ibuprofen, naproxen, etc., and *corticosteroid injections* which help directly decrease the inflammation of the subacromial bursa. Corticosteroid injections should be given judiciously, since too many injections (more than 3−4 over several months) may have deleterious, rather than beneficial, effects.

Modalities. The physical therapist or athletic trainer has available several modalities which are helpful in relieving the pain of swimmer's shoulder caused by impingement syndrome. Chief among these are the *electrogalvanic stimulation* (EGS) unit, which applies an electric current across the painful area, dispersing inflammatory cells; the *ultrasound* unit, which uses ultrasonic waves to deliver heat to the deep tissues (this can sometimes be painful, since heat will occasionally increase inflammation), and the *transcutaneous nerve stimulator* (TNS), which again uses an electrical current, but in such a way as to block the transmission of pain sensation to the brain.

Muscle strengthening. If the rotator muscles are weak, they will not be able effectively to guide the humeral head in the glenoid socket, and the overlying deltoidius muscle will pull the humeral head up into the acromion, creating an impingement syndrome. Therefore, exercises which strengthen the rotator cuff muscles are an important part of the long-term treatment plan for shoulder pain.

The swimmer performs these exercises by bending forward at the waist and lifting a hand-held weight out to the side with the elbow extended, in a "fly-away" manner (Fig. 19.2). Four sets of 15 lifts are done with the arm at 45, 90 and 135° relative to the long axis of the body, thereby strengthening the posterior, middle, and anterior rotator cuff muscles. Weight is increased according to the strength and needs of the athlete. These exercises should be continued on a regular basis throughout the entire career of the competitive swimmer to prevent shoulder pain.

Changes in technique and training. Shoulder pain is known to occur in those swimmers who have poor body roll in freestyle and backstroke, and poor body lift in butterfly. Since most swimmers use a good deal of freestyle or backstroke for their training, *increasing body roll* is usually of some help in preventing shoulder pain; both-side breathing accentuates body roll and is to be encouraged in the prevention of shoulder pain.

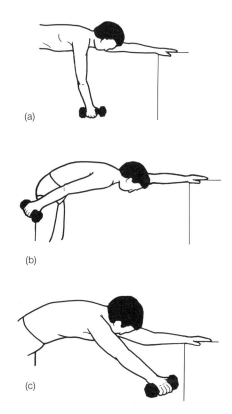

(a)

(b)

(c)

Fig. 19.2 "Fly-away" exercises for the rotator cuff muscles. (a) Bend forward and support body with uninvolved arm. Do 15 lifts directly out to the side with the elbow straight, carrying a light weight (0.5−1 kg; 1−2 lbs); repeat this 4 times. (b) Repeat the exercises (4 sets of 15 lifts) with the arm 45° behind the original position, and again (c) with the arm 45° in front of the original position.

Depending on the severity of shoulder pain, some *rest* is beneficial to the shoulder when it hurts. This might include decreasing workout distance or intensity, including a greater proportion of kicking (with the arms at the side instead of with a board and, perhaps, using fins), or including more dry-land exercises into the daily workout regimen.

It is clear that *avoiding the use of hand-paddles* is important in avoiding shoulder pain. One should also avoid rapid changes in workout mileage or intensity. Ironically, the taper period, near the end of the season, often results in more shoulder pain, secondary to the increased amount of sprint, high-intensity swims that often occurs at this time.

Mechanical measures. Use of an upper-arm band is often of help in controlling swimmer's shoulder pain. The arm band (Fig. 19.3) is a simple neoprene band which straps about the upper arm and is thought to work by decreasing the excursion of the deltoidius and biceps muscles about the shoulder.

Stretching. Preparation of the muscle–tendon unit for exercise should always include stretching. Without stretching, inflammation tends to occur at the muscle–tendon and/or the tendon–bone junction, which, in the case of the rotator cuff muscles, results in impingement syndrome.

Surgery. Surgical intervention is always a last resort, to be used when all other measures have been ineffective in controlling shoulder pain or instability. When this occurs, the usual goal of surgery is to increase the space between the acromion and the rotator cuff muscles and to remove the inflamed bursal tissues of the shoulder or to repair the lax capsular tissues of the shoulder which allow instability.

Recent developments in arthroscopy make this surgery much less of an ordeal than in the past; it can be done as an outpatient procedure and the time out of the water can be minimized. Visualization of the shoulder joint can greatly help to differentiate between impingement syndrome and instability of the shoulder.

Knee pain

Pain about the knee is known to occur in approximately 25% of competitive swimmers. There are two common causes of knee symptoms: those related to the *patella* (knee cap), and those related to the *medial structures* of the knee.

Anatomy

The knee joint is formed by the femur (thigh bone), the tibia (shin bone), and the overlying patella. The femur and tibia are held together by four ligaments named the medial collateral, the lateral collateral, and the anterior and posterior cruciate ligaments (Fig. 19.4). These ligaments allow flexion and extension of the knee, as well as a certain amount of twisting of the tibia on the femur.

The femur and the tibia are separated by two cartilages (medial and lateral menisci). The menisci serve as pads between the two bones and as guides to the normal motion of the knee.

The patella not only transmits the force of the thigh (quadriceps) muscles to the patellar ligament (and

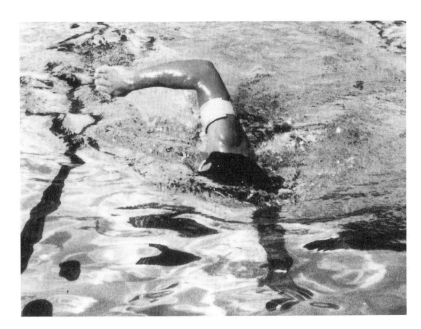

Fig. 19.3 A swimmer in the water with an upper-arm band in place.

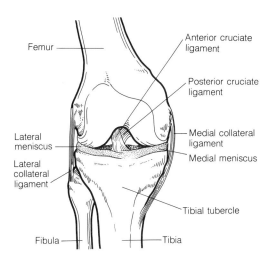

Fig. 19.4 Anatomy of the knee: normal bony and soft-tissue structures about the knee from the front. The muscles are not included.

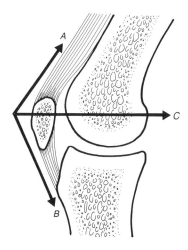

Fig. 19.5 Biomechanical diagram of the knee showing patellar compression forces. As the thigh muscle contracts, it creates force *A*, which produces the equal and opposite force *B*. These two forces produce force *C*, which is a compressive force between the knee cap and the underlying thigh bone.

thence to the tibia) during active extension of the knee, it also delivers a compressive force to the underlying femur (Fig. 19.5). This compressive force is directly related to the angle of flexion of the knee and the load applied across the joint by the quadriceps muscle; descending stairs creates a compressive force equivalent to $2-3 \times$ body weight between the patella and femur.

Sources of pain about the knee

The most common type of pain about the knee in swimming is related to patellar compression pain and is commonly known as patellofemoral pain or *chondromalacia*.

Repeated flexion and extension of the knee in all four strokes (and especially in breaststroke) can result in pain characteristically located about the kneecap; it is aggravated by walking up and down stairs, squatting, kneeling, prolonged sitting and, of course, kicking in swimming (as well as pushing off the wall and the overuse of fins). Occasionally, there will be mild swelling after activities. There is usually no pain medially, laterally or posteriorly; while there may be symptoms of catching, there is rarely locking (complete inability to move) of the knee. Noise

(grinding, grating, etc.) is not unknown, but is not directly related to any damage about the knee.

Occasionally, the patella becomes unstable and dislocates either partially or completely, producing pain about the knee cap as well as symptoms of buckling and giving way (Fig. 19.6). This can be a truly disabling problem, particularly for a breaststroke swimmer, because the valgus configuration of the knee (Fig. 19.7) with each kick predisposes the patella to dislocate. Pushing the knee cap laterally will cause the swimmer a sensation of instability (a positive *apprehension test*).

The second, better known type of knee pain in competitive swimmers is related to the medial collateral ligament and breaststroke (swimmer's or *breaststroker's knee*). An effective breaststroke kick requires a valgus, or knock-kneed, position of the knee. This repeatedly stretches the medial collateral ligament, resulting in pain. Actual rupture of the medial collateral ligament rarely, if ever, occurs, but it is common to have enough pain about this ligament that breaststroke kicking (and swimming) must be discontinued.

When pain is located at the medial joint line, the treating physician must consider the possibility of a torn medial meniscus. This is uncommon unless an

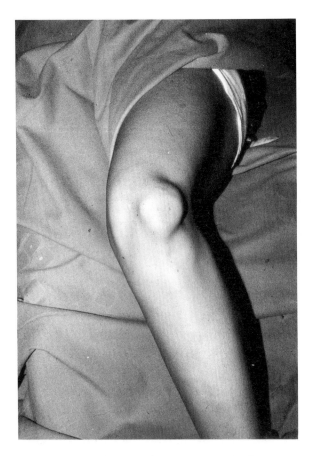

Fig. 19.6 Dislocated patella. Knee joint from the front demonstrating a knee cap which is unstable laterally.

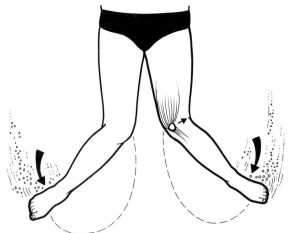

Fig. 19.7 Valgus forces during breaststroke kicking. The normal breaststroke kick emphasizes a valgus, or knock-kneed, configuration of the knee joint with each kick.

injury has been sustained while participating in another activity. A fold (plica) in the membranous lining of the knee joint may also cause pain at the medial joint line of the knee; however, again, this is less common and should only be entertained as a secondary diagnosis.

Treatment of knee pain

Knee pain in competitive swimming is usually related to the intensity of workout and is, therefore, self-limited. Relative rest is always a part of the treatment for both of the above conditions. In general, avoiding hard starts and turns, as well as doing a lot of pulling (with a pull-buoy) during training, will spare the knee the overuse which produces the discomfort. Land

exercises to strengthen the quadriceps muscles while avoiding flexion (straight-leg raising and short-arc extension exercises) are helpful for patellofemoral complaints, while all exercises which avoid valgus stress of the knee will help breaststroker's knee.

NSAIDs are sometimes helpful, as is regular ice-packing. A knee brace (Fig. 19.8) fashioned from neoprene, with a hole surrounding the knee cap, will help control excessive motion of the patella and, therefore, decrease pain. These braces can often be worn during workouts.

Surgical intervention for knee pain in swimmers is rarely indicated; it is often unsuccessful in allowing the swimmer to return to kicking with decreased pain. The exception to this is the athlete with an unstable patella or a torn meniscus. In these cases, there is usually no choice other than surgically to stabilize the kneecap or remove (or repair) the torn meniscus.

Swimmer's ear

Ear disease is common among the general population, especially in the younger age groups. Swimmers spend a great deal of time in the water and are, therefore, more susceptible to these problems than the normal population.

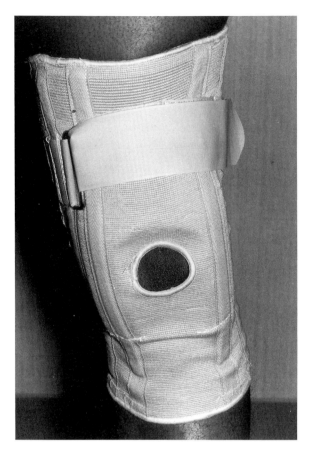

Fig. 19.8 Neoprene patellar stabilizing brace. Such a brace can help prevent excessive movement of the patella.

Anatomy

The ear is made up of the outer, middle, and inner ear (Fig. 19.9). The outer (or external) ear consists primarily of the external ear canal. Separating the outer from the middle ear compartments lies the tympanic membrane (eardrum). Small bones (ossicles) connect the inner aspect of the eardrum to the middle ear and transmit sound to nerves in the inner ear which facilitate hearing. Sense of balance is also controlled by structures in the inner ear.

Otitis externa

The most common ear problem among competitive swimmers is acute and chronic otitis externa. This condition is so prevalent that it is commonly called *swimmer's ear*.

The external ear is normally lubricated with cerumen (wax), which traps foreign materials and prevents fungal and bacterial infection. Constant irrigation of the external ear with pool water causes a loss of this normal wax, leading to drying and cracking of the skin of the canal and to repeated infections. The most common infecting organisms are *Pseudomonas, Staphylococcus, Escherichia coli*, and *Enterobacter aerogenes*. All infections of the external ear canal cause pain and swelling about the outer ear; untreated, such an infection can spread to the middle ear (across the eardrum) and lead to loss of hearing.

Since bacteria thrive in a basic environment, all ear drops are acidic in nature; they will often contain an antibiotic. Coloymycin or Cortisporin otic drops are examples of preparations available for treatment of otitis externa. The drops should be applied at least 4 times per day for the first few days; if the external ear canal is swollen closed, a wick may be inserted, both to hold the canal open, and to allow the drops to penetrate into the canal.

After the acute symptoms have subsided, it is best to continue with over-the-counter ear drops (made up of alcohol and a very mild acid such as vinegar) on a 2−3 times per week basis, especially during the swimming season when the constant exposure to water places the ear canal at risk.

Otitis media

As the name implies, otitis media refers to an infection of the middle ear. The eustachian tube, which normally allows communication of the middle ear with the throat, may become occluded because of inflammation and swelling. The resulting negative pressure in the middle ear causes pain and, occasionally, drainage of tissue fluid into the throat. Pain can be excruciating and the eardrum may become perforated. A fever is not uncommon with otitis media.

Chronic infection can lead to chronic hearing loss and loss of balance. Treatment is with oral (and rarely intravenous) antibiotics; antibiotic ear drops alone are not usually useful. Occasionally, and especially in young children, a surgeon might make a small hole (and place a small tube) in the eardrum to relieve the

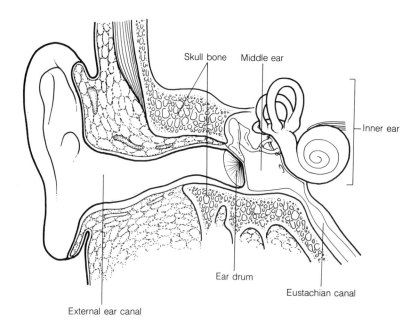

Skull bone   Middle ear

Inner ear

Ear drum

Eustachian canal

External ear canal

Fig. 19.9 Anatomy of the ear: cross-section.

pressure and the pain of a middle-ear infection. Once the tube is removed, the hole will heal. While such holes in the eardrum are in place, the patient must keep the ear dry, either by avoiding swimming or with occlusive ear plugs.

Exostoses

Long-time exposure to cold water may predispose a swimmer to a bony growth in the external ear called a bony *exostosis*. If the exostosis is sufficiently large, it will predispose the swimmer to ear infections, since water gets trapped by the excess bone in the external canal, macerating the skin of the ear. Extra attention to drying the ear (using over-the-counter ear drops) may prevent the growth of such an exostosis; however, occasionally, these bony growths require surgical removal.

Foreign bodies

Foreign bodies, such as sand, small particles, and bugs, occasionally get lodged in the external ear canal. Besides the irritation and discomfort of such a loose body, the real danger is that the swimmer will try to remove the foreign body with a cotton-swab or other such device. This will cause maceration of the skin

(predisposing to infection) or tympanic membrane (the eardrum). If the foreign body does not dislodge easily, it should not be removed with instrumentation except by a physician.

Chronic itching

Long-term itching of the ear is usually due to eczematous dermatitis, or dryness and flaking of the skin of the outer ear canal. The most usual cause is instrumentation of the outer ear in an attempt to treat either an infection or foreign body. Treatment is application of topical steroids and avoiding instrumentation of the outer ear.

Training considerations

Most common ear conditions need not keep the swimmer from training, although the early painful stages of otitis externa, and a perforation of the eardrum (either from infection or as a result of surgery) may require some time out of the water. Since constant immersion is the culprit, water can be kept out of the ears with any of several commercially available or custom-made ear plugs, usually in combination with a bathing cap. Appropriately treated, ear problems should not pose a serious threat to performance.

Eye problems in competitive swimmers

Anatomy

The human eye is a globe into which light enters, falling upon the retina at the back of the globe, which transmits signals to the brain, which are interpreted as vision (Fig. 19.10). Light is focused on the retina by the lens, which sits between the anterior and posterior chambers of the eye, and is surrounded by the iris, which is the colored part of the eye. The front of the eyeball, which allows the light to cross to the lens, is the cornea, which is surrounded by the conjunctiva. The conjunctiva is a membrane which covers the *sclera* (white) of the eye and the inside of the upper and lower eyelids.

Since swimmers spend so much time in the water, problems involving the eye are related mainly to those structures exposed to the water, specifically the cornea and the conjunctiva.

Problems with the cornea

Corneal edema

With prolonged exposure to pool water, swelling (edema) of the exposed cornea will occur, resulting in abnormal bending of light rays as they pass through the cornea and producing the halos around lights that swimmers know so well. The eye may also become sensitive to light.

Chlorine keratitis

Loss of the superficial cells of the cornea from prolonged exposure to chlorinated water will produce a sensation of something in the eye, as well as pain. This will usually resolve in 1−2 days, but will recur whenever the swimmer is exposed to chlorinated water; swim goggles, especially during practice sessions, have reduced this problem considerably.

Problems with the conjunctiva

The conjunctiva is most commonly affected by infection or, more commonly, inflammation. Conjunc-

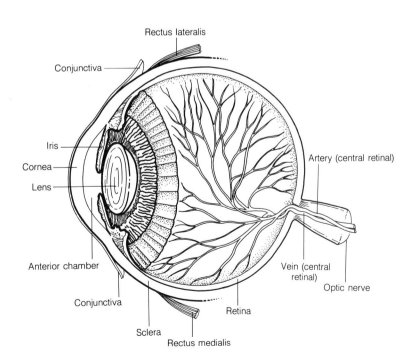

Fig. 19.10 Anatomy of the eye: cross section.

tivitis, or inflammation of the conjunctiva, causes the characteristic red-eye appearance of the orbit. The usual cause of this is chemical irritation from prolonged exposure to pool or salt water. Common treatment with ophthalmic irrigation solutions is effective in decreasing this inflammation; the use of swim goggles has decreased the incidence of conjunctivitis considerably over recent years.

Chlorination of pools has eliminated nearly all infectious diseases of the conjunctiva. Most infections of the conjunctiva can be treated with topical antibiotic solutions. Keratoconjunctivitis caused by trachoma (so-called inclusion conjunctivitis or TRIC) is treated with oral tetracycline antibiotics; this is a form of conjunctivitis seen much more commonly in third-world countries and is directly affected by water sanitation.

Viruses can also cause infections of the eye, the well known examples being the keratoconjunctivitis caused by the herpes virus (which is the leading cause of blindness in the US), and adenovirus, which can cause infection not only of the eye, but also of the throat; it is, therefore, known as pharyngoconjunctival fever. This results in a severe sore throat, muscle aches and pains, and a red eye. Cortisone preparations should not be used in the treatment of these illnesses as they may enhance permanent scarring of the cornea.

Once again, fortunately, most swimmers now use swim goggles, which will nearly eliminate the risk of inflammation or infections of the eye.

Exercise-induced bronchospasm

Asthma is a common chronic disease characterized by periodic episodes of shortness of breath. For any of several reasons (allergies, infections, drug and chemical sensitivities, and exercise), the passageways (bronchi) that carry air to the lungs become narrowed (bronchospasm), causing difficulty with breathing.

It is estimated that 60–90% of all asthmatics are susceptible to exercise-induced bronchospasm (EIB). EIB also affects about 40% of children who have hayfever or other allergies. It may be mild or moderate and can affect persons taking their prescribed medication for asthma. It can occur in adults who have been symptom-free for long periods of time, in those who have never had other respiratory illness, and in those who have grown out of other types of allergies.

The symptoms of EIB can be varied: a feeling of tightness in the chest, cough, wheezing, shortness of breath and fatigue are common. Stomach cramps can be a symptom, particularly in young children.

The typical attack does not appear during exercise, but only after exercise ends. It starts abruptly, lasts from a few minutes to 2 h, and usually stops spontaneously. Its symptoms are severe, and can often be controlled with bronchodilator medications.

Diagnosis

The diagnosis of EIB is based on a careful history of difficulty in breathing associated with exercise. Lung function tests are then done after a controlled period of exercise; a 15% drop in lung function during exercise usually indicates EIB is present; often wheezing is audible with a stethoscope.

Treatment

Swimming is one of the sports of choice for all asthmatics, since most workouts are done in a relatively warm, humid, atmosphere, and are not in proximity to other factors (pollen, air pollutants, etc.) which might cause asthma.

Proper medications will allow most athletes with EIB to perform without detriment. The most widely used is theophylline, which comes in capsule or tablet form and must be monitored by a physician.

Beta-adrenergic (β_2) agonists are also very commonly used and are usually administered with inhalers. Their effect is mainly on the lungs and onset of action is very rapid. Recently, several beta-adrenergic agonists have been removed from the International Olympic Committee List of Banned Substances since they have little or no effect on the heart or circulation:
1   bitolterol (Tornalate);
2   orciprenaline;
3   rimiterol;
4   terbutaline (Brethaire);
5   salbutamol (Albuterol, Ventolin, Proventil).

Another medication used to prevent asthma attacks is cromolyn sodium (Intal). Intal reduces the release of the chemicals that induce bronchospasm; therefore, it is most effective in preventing an attack of EIB, but has little effect on an attack which is already in progress. It is available both as a metered-dose inhaler and as an inhaled powder and should be used regularly before exercise activities.

If an asthma attack is particularly severe, one of a family of corticosteroid medications may be necessary. Once again, these medications are acceptable by the International Olympic Committee for the treatment of asthma (and EIB); however notice must be given by the athlete and treating physician. It is important to note that certain medications used to treat attacks of asthma, such as compounds containing epinephrine, ephedrine, pseudoephedrine, metaproterenol, and isoproterenol, are banned from use by athletes because of their cardiovascular effects.

Summary

Competitive swimming is one of the most popular of Olympic sports. Competition is keen among all countries of the world. Injury or illness, when it occurs, is relatively uncommon. This chapter has been intended to familiarize the reader with the more common medical problems which affect the competitive swimmer as well as to outline some of the more common treatment modalities available to swimmers and their coaches.

Recommended reading

Ciullo, J.V. (ed.) (1986) *Clinics in Sports Medicine: Swimming*, vol. 5. Philadelphia: W.B. Saunders.

McMaster, W.C. (1986) Anterior glenoid labrum damage: a painful lesion in swimmers. *Am. J. Sports Med.* **14**: 383–387.

Richardson, A.B., Jobe, F.W. & Collins, H.R. (1980) The shoulder in competitive swimming. *Am. J. Sports Med.* **8**: 159–163.

Richardson, A.B. (1986) The biomechanics of swimming: the shoulder and knee. In Ciullo, J.V. (ed.) *Clinics in Sports Medicine: Swimming*, vol. 5. Philadelphia: W.B. Saunders, pp. 103–114.

Richardson, A.B. (1987) Orthopedic aspects of competitive swimming. In *Clinics in Sports Medicine: Arthroscopy*, vol. 6. Philadelphia: W.B. Saunders, pp. 639–645.

Schleihauf, R.E. (1979) A hydrodynamic analysis of swimming propulsion. In Terauds, J. & Bedingfield, E.W. (eds) *Swimming III*. Baltimore, Maryland: University Park Press, pp. 39–44.

Troup, J. & Reese, R. (1983) *A Scientific Approach to the Sport of Swimming*. Gainesville, Florida: Scientific Sports Inc.

Appendices

Appendix A

Blood lactate analysis

Lactic acid is the end-product of glycolysis and accumulates in muscle and blood when aerobic and other metabolic pathways are unable to keep up with the removal of pyruvate. In exercise physiology, it has long been used as an indicator of anaerobic metabolism and, consequently, of the relative intensity of an exercise bout. In more recent years it has been measured during a variety of protocols of progressively increasing exercise loads to identify that exercise intensity where lactate levels abruptly increase over resting levels. This *lactate threshold* is taken as a stress point in one's submaximal aerobic exercise capacity, and is used to indicate an exercise intensity around which to design a training program and to follow improvements.

Lactic acid is measured enzymatically according to the following reaction:

$$\text{Lactic acid} + \text{NAD} \xrightarrow{\text{LDH}} \text{pyruvic acid} + \text{NADH}$$

$$\text{Pyruvate} + \text{hydrazine} \longrightarrow \text{pyruvate hydrazone,}$$

where NAD is nicotinamide adenine dinucleotide, LDH is lactate dehydrogenase, and NADH is the reduced form of nicotinamide adenine dinucleotide.

The NADH is read on a spectrophotometer at 340 nm or on a fluorometer using those filters suitable for reading NADH. The measure of the NADH produced is the measure of lactic acid. The kinetics of the reaction, however, are very unfavorable since the Michaelis constants are large and the equilibrium lies on the side of pyruvate reduction. For these reasons it is necessary to force the reaction to its end-point by using a large excess of LDH and NAD, a high pH, and hydrazine to bind out pyruvate to keep the reaction going. Even so, the reaction is slow and takes a relatively long incubation.

Nevertheless, the procedure is easy and straight-forward. Commercial kits are available for the spectrophotometer (Sigma 826-UV), and several recipes can be found in the literature. The following kitchen method is inspired by some of these.

Mix a reagent cocktail from the following stocks. Stocks are kept refrigerated, except for NAD, which is kept frozen. Begin by mixing the buffer in a volume of water close to the desired volume (Table A.1).

The pH of this reagent should be kept above 9.2. The ideal pH for the reaction would be 9.7−10. A 1 mmol·l^{-1} glycine/hydrazine stock can be mixed together as one reagent to allow for only one pipetting. Hydrazine hydrate (Sigma H-0883) is a convenient form of hydrazine to use for mixing. NAD is less expensive if bought in bulk (Sigma N-7004) than if bought in preweighed vials. The LDH should be from bovine heart (Sigma L-2625 is suitable) and can be diluted to a working stock concentration of 300−400 u·ml^{-1}. More concentrated stocks can be used, but

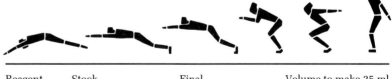

Table A.1 Preparation of reagents for lactate analyses

Reagent	Stock	Final	Volume to make 25 ml
Glycine	1 mol·l^{-1}	0.32 mol·l^{-1}	8 ml
Hydrazine hydrate	20 mol·l^{-1} (100%)	0.32 mol·l^{-1}	0.4 ml
NAD	100 mmol·l^{-1}	2.4 mmol·l^{-1}	0.6 ml
LDH	400 u·ml^{-1}	15 u·ml^{-1}	1 ml

pipet volumes will have to be adjusted accordingly. A lactate standard (Sigma 826-10) can be run with the samples as a control, but it is not needed for the calculations if the absorptivity of NADH is used. Care must be taken that the lactate in the sample does not overpower the capacity of the reagent cocktail. The ratio of NAD to lactate should not fall below 20:1. This means that with the present cocktail, a blood sample which is 18 mmol·l^{-1} in lactic acid can be measured without falling below that ratio, provided the blood was prepared in a threefold dilution with perchloric acid, of which 0.02 ml (20 µl) was used in 1 ml of cocktail (see the procedure below). If lactate concentrations higher than that are expected, the sample volume can easily be reduced to 0.01 ml (10 µl). The procedure is as follows.

1   Prepare a perchloric acid (PCA) extract of whole blood or serum. This can be done conveniently in a two- or threefold dilution. Have on hand a 0.6– 0.8 mol·l^{-1} PCA (5.2–7 ml 70% PCA per 100 ml H$_2$O) which is kept cold, preferably on ice. A threefold dilution can be prepared by pipetting 0.5 ml of blood into 1 ml of cold PCA. Cap the tube and shake it until it all turns chocolate brown. Centrifuge hard for about 10 min and decant the supernatant into a clean tube. This can be stored in the refrigerator or frozen for later analysis. Before analysis, the tube should be centrifuged briefly again to produce a clear extract.

2   Pipet 1 ml of reagent cocktail into 12 × 75 mm or 10 × 75 mm culture tubes. Run duplicates, at least for standards and blanks.

3   Pipet 0.02 ml (20 µl), or some reasonably convenient volume, of sample, standard, or PCA for the blanks into the reagent cocktail. Vortex.

4   Incubate at 37°C for 20–30 min or at room temperature for about 1 h.

5   Set the spectrophotometer to 340 nm and zero on the blank. Read a second blank to check for any possible contamination and zero on the lower of the two.

6   Read and record the absorbance of the samples (and standards).

7   Calculate the results using either the absorptivity of NADH or the standard. (The Sigma standard is 4.44 mmol·l^{-1}.)

Example
Absorbance of sample = 0.314

Millimolar extinction coefficient of NADH = 6.22
PCA dilution of blood = 3
Dilution of sample (20 µl) in the reagent (1 ml) = 51
(0.314/6.22) × 3 × 51 = 7.72 mmol·l^{-1}
The molecular weight of lactic acid is 90
(mmol·l^{-1}/10) × 90 = mg·dl^{-1}
(7.72/10) × 90 = 69.5 mg/dl.

In this assay it is very important to keep in mind that lactate is abundant on your fingers. It is very easy to contaminate the culture tubes as you are pipetting the samples. This usually manifests itself by an unstable blank that keeps drifting up as it is zeroed on the spectrophotometer. What happens is that the lactate contamination on the rim of the culture tube is washed into the cuvette as the blank or sample is poured in. An automatic sampling system on the spectrophotometer goes a long way toward avoiding this.

Fingertip or earlobe blood can be collected in 20– 30 µl capillary tubes and deproteinized in 100 µl PCA in 400 µl microcentrifuge tubes. The heparinized 30 µl capillary tubes and pipettor made by Boehringer Mannheim for their Reflotron instrument are quite handy here (catalogue numbers 832375 and 832359, respectively). The capillary tubes have a plug in them to stop the blood at exactly 30 µl, and the pipettor pushes all the blood cleanly into the PCA tubes. Other sizes of microcentrifuge tubes and other pipet volumes can, of course, be used.

Procedure for the fluorometer

Blood lactate can easily be done on the fluorometer as well as on the spectrophotometer. But since lactate concentrations in blood are so high, it seems convenient to work on the spectrophotometer, especially if your spectrophotometer is equipped with an automatic sampler. The advantage of the fluorometric method is that the tubes used for the analysis would not have to be decanted into a cuvette to be read. The disadvantage is that the PCA extract of blood needs to be diluted and neutralized in another preparation step, and smaller pipet volumes (5–10 µl) ought to be used for high blood concentrations. Other disadvantages of the fluorometer are a sometimes troublesome blank fluorescence and the need to read, record and calculate more numbers.

Table A.2 Reagents for the fluorometric analyses of lactate

Reagent	Stock	Final	Volume to make 25 ml
Glycine	1 mol·l^{-1}	100 mmol·l^{-1}	2.5 ml
Hydrazine	20 mol·l^{-1}	100 mmol·l^{-1}	0.125 ml
NAD	0.1 mol·l^{-1}	0.2 mmol·l^{-1}	0.05 ml (50 µl)
LDH	5000 u·ml^{-1}	8 u·ml^{-1}	See below

Mix the following reagent cocktail in the usual way. (Table A.2). If a 1 mol·l^{-1} glycine/hydrazine stock is mixed as in the spectrophotometer procedure, only one pipetting is necessary. The pH of the cocktail should be adjusted to 9.6–9.8. A more concentrated LDH stock allows one to use smaller volumes and thus to introduce less ammonium sulfate into the reagent. The procedure is as follows.

1 Prepare a PCA extract of blood or serum as before. On the day of the assay, neutralize an aliquot of this with some convenient volume of potassium hydroxide (KOH). For example, a second threefold dilution of the PCA extract can be done by adding two parts of a 0.4 N KOH to every part of PCA extract. In 10 × 75 mm culture tubes, place 0.25 ml PCA extract and 0.5 ml 0.4 N KOH. This will produce a light potassium perchlorate precipitate, which should be settled with a quick centrifugation.

2 Mix the reagent without the LDH and pipet 1 ml of this into 10 × 75 mm borosilicate glass culture tubes. Run standards and blanks at least in duplicate.

3 Pipet 5–20 µl of neutralized extract or standard, and water for blanks, into the appropriate tubes. The lactate standard should be $0.5–1 \text{ mmol·l}^{-1}$. Alternatively, 1–2 µl of the Sigma lactate standard (4.44 mmol·l^{-1}) can be used, plus a volume of water to equal the volume of samples, but remember that you did this when it comes time to do the calculations.

4 Read and record the initial fluorescence of all tubes.

5 Prepare an LDH mix that will allow you to aliquot ~8 u into each tube. To do this in 25-µl aliquots with the stock concentration of LDH given above, add ~30 µl of the 5000 u·ml^{-1} stock to 0.5 ml of reagent cocktail (or buffer). Then pipet 25 µl of this into all the tubes. Vortex.

6 Let the reaction proceed to its end-point — about 20–30 minutes.

7 Read and record the final fluorescence of all tubes.

8 Calculate the change in fluorescence of the samples and standards, and the change in fluorescence of the blanks. Subtract the change in fluorescence of the blanks from the change in fluorescence of the samples and standards. Then calculate the lactate values in the usual way.

$$dF_{\text{samp}}/dF_{\text{std}} \times \text{mmol·l}^{-1} \text{ conc}_{\text{std}} \times \text{dilutions of sample} = \text{mmol·l}^{-1} \text{ conc}_{\text{blood}}.$$

Example
Initial fluorescence of sample = 7
Initial fluorescence of standard = 6
Initial fluorescence of blank = 6
Final fluorescence of sample = 60
Final fluorescence of standard = 80
Final fluorescence of blank = 13
Concentration of the standard = 0.5 mmol·l^{-1}
Sample, standard, and blank volume = 0.02 ml (20 µl)
Reagent volume = 1 ml
Dilutions of the blood: threefold in PCA, threefold in KOH

$46/67 \times 0.5 \text{ mmol·l}^{-1} \times 3 \times 3 = 3.09 \text{ mmol·l}^{-1}.$

Normal values

Resting blood levels of lactic acid are normally very low, about $0.3-1.3$ mmol·l^{-1}. As exercise intensity increases, lactic acid begins to accumulate in the blood. For a totally aerobic run of $5-10$ miles, it may be about 2 mmol·l^{-1}. After a progressive test for $\dot{V}_{O_2 \max}$, it may rise to about $7-15$ mmol·l^{-1}. After an intense interval workout that "stacks" lactate, it may be as high as $25-30$ mmol·l^{-1}.

Appendix B

Calculation of oxygen uptake

Since the volume of all gases is directly affected by variations in temperature (T) and barometric pressure (PB), it is necessary to convert all expired gas volumes to the same (0°C) temperature, barometric pressure (760 mmHg) and to eliminate the water content (dry). The calculations are referred to as the STPD (standard temperature and pressure, dry) correction and can be determined as follows:

$$\dot{V}_{E\,(STPD)} - \dot{V}_{E\,(observed)} \times [273/(T_G + 273)] \times P_B - P_{H_2O}$$

where T_G = temperature of gas and P_{H_2O} can be obtained from the equation in Fig. B.1.

$$P_{H_2O} = 6.195 + 0.059\,T_G + (0.024\,T_G^2) + (7.836 \times 10^{-5}\,T_G^3).$$

In the measurement of total body oxygen uptake ($\dot{V}_{O_2}$) only expired air is collected and analyzed. However, $\dot{V}_{O_2}$ is determined from the difference between the volume of oxygen entering ($\dot{V}_{I_{O_2}}$) and leaving ($\dot{V}_{E_{O_2}}$) the lung. For that reason we must calculate the volume of air ($\dot{V}_I$) and oxygen ($\dot{V}_{I_{O_2}}$) being inspired. If a correction is made for the nitrogen concentration in the expired air, then we can calculate ($\dot{V}_I$) as follows:

$$\dot{V}_I = \dot{V}_E \times (\%N_2 \text{ in expired air})/79.04.$$
$$\dot{V}_E - \text{volume of expired (STPD) per unit of time}$$
(usually per min).

Since oxygen and carbon dioxide are only fractions of the total gas inspired and expired, we must sample the expired gas and analyze it for both O_2 and CO_2. Inspired air is assumed to contain 0.03% CO_2 and 20.93% O_2. After determining the O_2 and CO_2 concentrations in the expired air it is possible to calculate the volume of O_2 and CO_2 entering and leaving the lungs:

$$\dot{V}_{I_{O_2}} = \dot{V}_{I(STPD)} \times 0.2093$$
$$\dot{V}_{E_{O_2}} = \dot{V}_{E(STPD)} \times F_{E_{CO_2}}.$$

Therefore, the volume of oxygen consumed ($\dot{V}_{O_2}$) by the body can be determined as follows:

$$\dot{V}_{O_2} = \dot{V}_{I_{O_2}} - \dot{V}_{E_{O_2}}$$

and the volume of carbon dioxide can be determined by:

$$\dot{V}_{CO_2} = \dot{V}_{E_{CO_2}} - \dot{V}_{I\,CO_2}.$$

Body size

Normally a large person requires more energy and oxygen than a small person to do a given task such as swimming or running. For that reason we often correct $\dot{V}_{O_2}$ for differences in body weight as follows:

$$\dot{V}_{O_2}\,(ml \cdot kg^{-1} \times min) = \dot{V}_{O_2}/\text{body weight (kg)}$$

or for swimmers it is more appropriate to calculate the $\dot{V}_{O_2}$ per unit of body weight measured in the water:

$$\dot{V}_{O_2}\,(ml \cdot kg^{-1} \text{ weight in water} \times min) = \dot{V}_{O_2}/\text{underwater weight (kg)}.$$

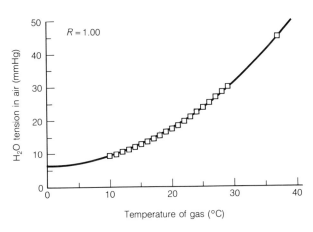

Fig. B.1 Water vapor tension at various air temperatures.

Appendix C

Procedures for hydrostatic weighing

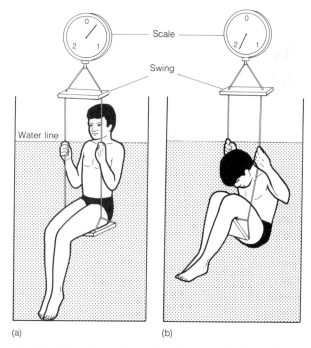

Fig. C.1 (a) Position before subject is weighed. (b) Position while subject is weighed.

1   The subject should urinate and expel, as much as possible, any gas or feces in the bowels.

2   The subject should shower thoroughly, using soap, and should be especially thorough in hairy areas of the body. It is not necessary to soap the head, but it must be thoroughly soaked. Be sure swimming apparel is thoroughly soaked, inside and out.

3   After showering, the subject should not dry off and should report immediately to the weighing area.

4   Attach a weight (2–3 kg), if necessary, around the subject's waist to insure that the subject will sink properly when weighed.

5   The weighing of the individual underwater is easily accomplished by having the individual sit on a chair or bar supported by a scale in an enclosed body of water. The seat should be located just below the buttocks. Be sure air bubbles are removed from the hair, body, and from inside the swimming suit.

6   The subject should practice the underwater weighing procedure as he or she sits by forcefully expelling as much air as possible from the lungs.

7   During the weighing process, the subject should repeat the procedure in step 6. However, while forcibly expelling all the air, the subject must submerge him or herself while sitting on the chair,

and remain stationary until as much air has been expelled as possible. There will be considerable fluctuation in the scale readings when the subject is blowing out the air, and these will become stable within a relatively narrow range when all the air is expelled. The subject should be instructed to remain underwater and stationary for at least 10–15 s following complete expiration (Fig. C.1).

8   Repeat the weighing procedure at least 8–10 times. Selection of the best underwater weight should be based on one of three criteria: (i) the highest obtained weight if it was observed more than twice;

Table C.1 Density of water at varied temperatures

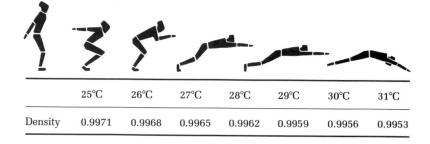

	25°C	26°C	27°C	28°C	29°C	30°C	31°C
Density	0.9971	0.9968	0.9965	0.9962	0.9959	0.9956	0.9953

(ii) the second highest weight if it was observed more than once and if the first criterion was not attained; and (iii) the third highest weight if neither the first nor the second criterion was attained. This method of selection is used to reduce the possibility of underestimating the actual underwater weight of the subject who attained the highest values during the first 5–7 trials.

9 After the last weighing, determine the tare weight (weight of the chair underwater). Subtract the weight from the subject's underwater weight to find the true underwater weight. Have the subject dry him or herself thoroughly and weigh on land to the nearest 50 g. Fill in the following form.

Subject's name: .... Gender .... Age ....

Dry weight (kg) .... Underwater weight (kg) ....

Temperature of water ....°C

Density of water (DH_2O) .... (see **Table C.1**)

Vital capacity (BTPS) .... liters

Residual lung volume (RLV) .... liters

Estimated gastrointestinal gas 0.100. liters (constant)

Index